About the Author

Helen Wiseman graduated in Biochemistry from King's College London and there obtained a PhD on the mechanisms of action of tamoxifen. Subsequent appointments have enabled Dr Wiseman to continue her research on tamoxifen, with current efforts focusing on its cardioprotective action. She has published extensively in this field. Dr Wiseman is a Lecturer in the Department of Nutrition and Dietetics at King's College London and Secretary of the London Branch of the Institute of Biology.

29.95

Tamoxifen

Molecular Basis of Use in Cancer Treatment and Prevention

Tamoxifen

Molecular Basis of Use in Cancer Treatment and Prevention

Helen Wiseman
Department of Nutrition and Dietetics
School of Life, Basic Medical and Health Sciences
Kings College London, UK

JOHN WILEY & SONS
Chichester · New York · Brisbane · Toronto · Singapore

Telephone: National Chichester (0243) 779777
International +44 243 779777

Other Wiley Editorial Offices

John Wiley & Sons, Inc., 605 Third Avenue,
New York, NY 10158-0012, USA

Jacaranda Wiley Ltd, 33 Park Road, Milton,
Queensland 4064, Australia

John Wiley & Sons (Canada) Ltd, 22 Worcester Road,
Rexdale, Ontario M9W 1L1, Canada

John Wiley & Sons (SEA) Pte Ltd, 37 Jalan Pemimpin #05-04,
Block B, Union Industrial Building, Singapore 2057

Library of Congress Cataloging-in-Publication Data

Wiseman, Helen.
Tamoxifen, molecular basis of use in cancer treatment and prevention / Helen Wiseman.
p. cm.
Includes bibliographical references and index.
ISBN 0 471 94316 9
1. Tamoxifen. 2. Breast—Cancer—Chemotherapy. 3. Breast—Cancer—Chemoprevention. 4. Cancer—Chemotherapy. I. Title.
[DNLM: 1. Tamoxifen. 2. Breast Neoplasms—drug therapy. 3. Neoplasms–prevention & control. 4. Candida—drug effects. QV 269 W814t 1994]
RC280.B8W497 1994
616.99′449061—dc20
DNLM/DLC
for Library of Congress 94-18163
CIP

British Library Cataloguing in Publication Data

A catalogue record for this book is available from the British Library

ISBN 0 471 94316 9

Typeset in 10/12 pt Palatino by
Mathematical Composition Setters Ltd, Salisbury, Wiltshire.
Printed and bound in Great Britain by Biddles Ltd, Guildford, Surrey.

Contents

Preface

Currently there is considerable interest in the potential use of tamoxifen not only to treat breast cancer but also to prevent it. This prospective role as a major chemopreventative agent has attracted controversy relating to the possibility of long term side-effects of tamoxifen therapy; in addition, the likely beneficial side-effects of tamoxifen therapy, such as protection against cardiovascular disease and osteoporosis, are also considered in this book. It is emerging that tamoxifen may be useful in the treatment of a number of other cancers in addition to breast cancer. These present and future uses of tamoxifen, including its potential as an anti-*Candida* and antiviral agent, make the understanding of its actions at a molecular level very important, and the author is particularly interested in the contribution to this of the reported membrane-mediated mechanisms of action of tamoxifen. This exciting area of research is likely to be vital also to the development of new derivatives of tamoxifen aimed at overcoming the problem of the development of eventual resistance to tamoxifen.

I would like to thank the following people for their support and encouragement of my research on tamoxifen, initiated in the School of Life, Basic Medical and Health Sciences, King's College London: Professor Henry Arnstein, Dr Michael Cannon, Professor Peter Quinn, Professor Harold Baum, Dr Catherine Rice-Evans (UMDS, Guy's), Professor David Wilkie (UCL) and Professor Barry Halliwell. Special thanks are due also to Verity Waite, Publishing Editor in Medicine and to Lesley Winchester, Senior Production Editor in Life Sciences at John Wiley & Sons, Chichester.

Helen Wiseman
London
July 1994

1

Importance of Understanding the Anticancer Action of Tamoxifen at a Molecular Level

INTRODUCTION

It is recognised that drugs have the ability to elicit multiple responses at therapeutic doses: some of these are referred to as unwanted side-effects if they cause discomfort or harm to the patient! Drugs are chosen, and developed to reach particular body tissues and associated target sites by selected routes of administration. Nevertheless, the chemical insight required to predict their interaction with the body's biochemical complexity is often incomplete—despite extensive experimental and computer-aided modelling studies. Drug receptors are now recognised to be particular proteins with a high affinity for the appropriate drug. Some of these receptors are located in the membrane (and additionally may be enzymes in some cases). In addition, genotoxic drugs, or their metabolites, are likely to interact with nuclear (or mitochondrial) DNA.

TAMOXIFEN: A DRUG WITH MULTIPLE PHARMACOLOGICAL ACTIONS

Tamoxifen is a non-steroidal triphenylethylene that is nevertheless likely to be capable of adopting a structural conformation that resembles the steroid nucleus. Despite the frequent diagrammatic depiction of tamoxifen in other molecular conformations, the molecular basis of the clearly recognised antioestrogen (and partial oestrogen agonist) action of tamoxifen is likely to be through this resemblance to steroids such as 17β-oestradiol. Indeed, a tamoxifen metabolite, 4-hydroxytamoxifen, which often displays a greater biological activity than tamoxifen itself, more closely resembles 17β-oestradiol owing to the presence of a hydroxyl group at an analogous location in the ring in 4-hydroxytamoxifen that corresponds to the steroid ring A. However, tamoxifen also displays an equally notable resemblance to the important membrane-located sterol cholesterol in human cell membranes (see Figure 1.1). Cholesterol and tamoxifen (and derivatives) have been shown to protect membranes, and membrane-model systems such as liposomes, against free radical-mediated lipid peroxidation (see Chapter 8). Observation of this protective action of tamoxifen and its derivatives (and also of 17β-oestradiol) can be

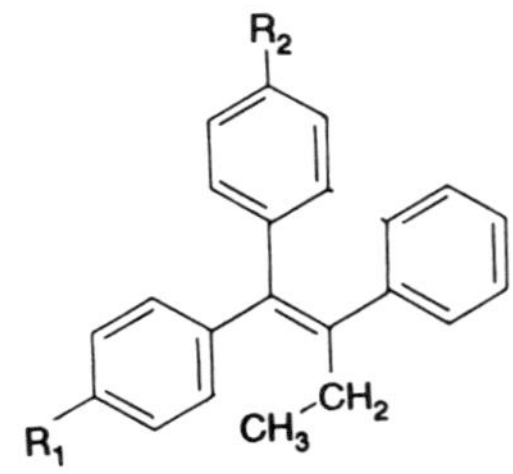

Tamoxifen R_1 = H, R_2 = $OCH_2CH_2N(CH_3)_2$
4-Hydroxytamoxifen R_1 = OH, R_2 = $OCH_2CH_2N(CH_3)_2$

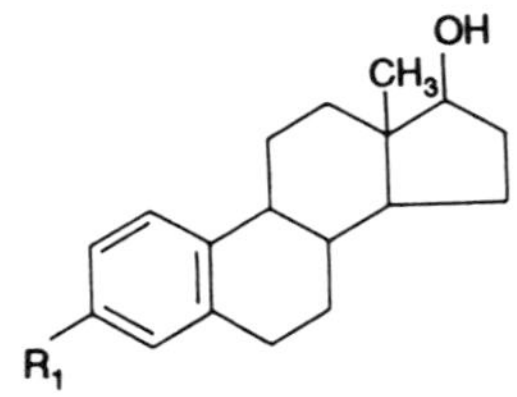

17β-Oestradiol R_1 = OH

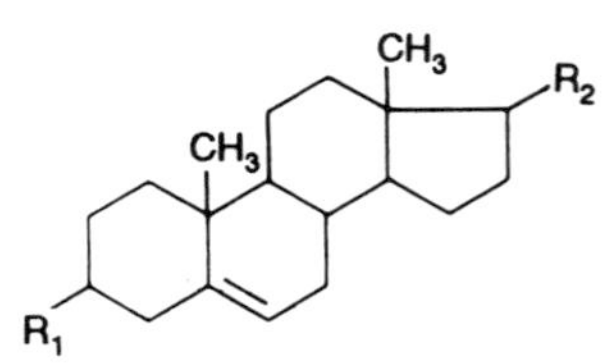

Cholesterol R_1 = OH, R_2 = $CH(CH_3)(CH_2)_3CH(CH_3)_2$

Figure 1.1. Structural similarity of tamoxifen to 17β-oestradiol and cholesterol

attributed to molecular modulation of the membrane environment by the interaction of sterols (and molecules with the ability to mimic them) with the particular fatty acid side-chains present in membrane phospholipids. Post-menopausal oestrogen receptor-negative breast cancer patients can also benefit from adjuvant tamoxifen therapy, and some of the oestrogen receptor-independent responses of cancer cells to tamoxifen may therefore be attributed to such interactions of tamoxifen with cellular membranes. This concept could lead to the development of new designer forms of tamoxifen and related drugs that may be of improved efficacy in the treatment and prevention of breast cancer. Furthermore, the ability of tamoxifen and its derivatives to protect human low-density lipoproteins (LDL) against oxidative damage may contribute to its cardioprotective action and this is discussed in Chapter 8.

OUTLINE OF CHAPTER CONTENTS: FOCUS ON TAMOXIFEN—A MULTIPLE TARGET-SITE DRUG

Chapter 2—An introduction to the chemistry and pharmacology of tamoxifen

This chapter deals briefly with the chemistry and pharmacology of tamoxifen. This includes a brief history of its unusual route to acceptance and use as a treatment for breast cancer via a research programme aimed at the antioestrogen oral contraceptive market. Tamoxifen is the *trans* isomer; the irradiation of solutions of tamoxifen with ultraviolet light results in the formation of the *cis* isomer, and also substituted phenanthrenes formed by cyclisation reactions. These reactions provide some indication of the ability of this molecule to adopt steroid-like conformations (see above and Chapter 8).

Chapter 3—Metabolism and toxicology of tamoxifen: an overview

This chapter deals with the metabolism and toxicity of tamoxifen and considers the relationship between these in rat liver, where toxicity is manifest as liver cancer. Tamoxifen undergoes metabolism in the liver, where biotransformation is mainly by particular members of the cytochromes P-450 superfamily of enzymes; this leads to the formation of metabolites including the more potent molecule 4-hydroxytamoxifen and also *N*-desmethyltamoxifen. This metabolism of tamoxifen has led to the study of the efficacy of 4-hydroxytamoxifen in a number of model systems, including the MCF-7 human breast cancer cell line discussed in Chapter 5. A feature of tamoxifen is its general very low acute toxicity (oral LD_{50} is around 3 g/kg in mice and 2.5 g/kg in rats). Although concern has been expressed that tamoxifen can cause liver cancer in rats as a result of its metabolism, currently there is no convincing evidence for this in humans. Indeed, tamoxifen is generally well tolerated in breast cancer patients (see also Chapter 4).

Chapter 4—An overview of the clinical use of tamoxifen in the treatment and prevention of breast cancer

This chapter presents an overview of the therapeutic use of tamoxifen in the treatment of breast cancer. Consideration is also given to dietary indications in the development of breast cancer, in addition to the obligatory discussion of hormonal and gene factors. Tamoxifen is also starting to be used with some success in the treatment of a number of other cancers, including malignant gliomas, malignant melanoma and hepatocellular carcinoma. Some side-effects of tamoxifen therapy are indicated in this chapter. A major issue exists in the desirability of the use of tamoxifen as a chemopreventive agent in apparently healthy women but who have a higher than normal risk of developing breast cancer because of a family history of this disease. The evidence suggests that chemoprevention with tamoxifen in such cases is likely to be justified and in the future this basis for selection of women for chemoprevention may be extended when information on individual genetic disposition becomes available through gene-location studies of human chromosomes. Any long-term risks would, as always, have to be weighed against the perceived likely benefit to the individual. In addition, administration of tamoxifen may confer additional benefits to treated individuals, in lowering the risk of development of other diseases such as cardiovascular disease and osteoporosis. Nevertheless, some concern has been expressed concerning the long-term safety of tamoxifen, given prophylactically, in relation to perceived risks of development of endometrial cancer and retinopathy.

Chapter 5—Oestrogen receptor-mediated mechanisms of anticancer action of tamoxifen

This chapter presents a discussion of the important oestrogen receptor-dependent mechanisms of the anticancer action of tamoxifen, especially in human breast cancer cells. This refers to the action of tamoxifen on cancer cell growth, including the consideration of cell cycle parameters. An account is given also of molecular studies on the structure of the oestrogen receptor and its interaction with tamoxifen and its derivatives. In this connection the ability of tamoxifen to affect cancer cell gene transcription and translation (protein synthesis) is outlined. In addition, studies on the action of tamoxifen in animal models of hormone-dependent cancer are reviewed.

Chapter 6—Modulation by tamoxifen of oncogenes and growth factors and the problem of tamoxifen resistance in breast cancer

In this chapter the modulating action of tamoxifen on oncogenes (and proto-oncogenes) is reviewed, along with its action on cellular growth factors in the modulation of cancer cell growth. Cell-signalling events are of particular interest, especially where transmembrane events may regulate cancer cell growth. Cytokine-mediated effects in breast cancer cells are of particular interest, and these are discussed in relation to the effects of tamoxifen and oestrogens and other compounds on breast cancer cells. The development of resistance to tamoxifen in populations of breast cancer cell is discussed in relation to tumour progression from hormone sensitivity to insensitivity. Some of this progression involves loss of active receptors, while the involvement of abnormal receptors cannot be ruled out.

Chapter 7—Inhibitory action of tamoxifen on enzymes involved in the synthesis of oestrogens and in signal transduction: importance to anticancer action?

This chapter deals with the interesting topic of the ability of tamoxifen to bind to some well-known enzymes, including those involved in oestrogen synthesis, and thereby inhibit their action. This subject is an important part of mainstream biochemistry where action is due to binding, often at high affinity, which results in a hindering of substrate access or to conformational changes in the enzymes that are incompatible with the catalytic conversion of the substrate. Inhibition of calcium-dependent enzymes are reviewed here, including inhibition of protein kinase C. This enzyme has been shown to be important in the phosphorylation system responsible for the transduction of membrane signals, cellular regulation and tumour promotion. In addition, an evaluation is made of the antioestrogen binding site (AEBS), which has been studied using synthetic ligands. A review is presented of the important subject of the inhibition by tamoxifen of cytochrome P-450-dependent enzymes involved in the pathway of cholesterol biosynthesis.

Chapter 8—Antioxidant action of tamoxifen in membranes and lipoprotein particles: role in the anticancer, anti-multidrug resistance and cardioprotective actions of tamoxifen

This chapter emphasises the importance of the assessment of the membrane antioxidant ability of tamoxifen and related compounds in the understanding of their anticancer and cardioprotective action. Membrane structure and lipid peroxidation are outlined, followed by a discussion of free radical mediated lipid peroxidation in membranes. Measurement of lipid peroxidation is discussed, and its inhibition by tamoxifen and related compounds is explained in terms of the molecular modulation of membrane fluidity. Emphasis is placed on the mimicry of the structural antioxidant action of cholesterol in membranes by tamoxifen and related compounds that leads to the ability of these substances to inhibit lipid peroxidation in membranes. Details are given of the use of computer-aided molecular-modelling studies and the calculation of a parameter that quantitates the efficacy of structural antioxidants relative to cholesterol, termed the cholesterol coefficient (Cc). This stabilisation of membranes against lipid peroxidation through decreased membrane fluidity has important implications for the ability of tamoxifen to inhibit the growth of cancer cells. In this connection the membrane antioxidant of tamoxifen is discussed in relation to the involvement of second messenger systems in the growth of cancer cells. Furthermore, prevention of the formation of the free radical intermediates and products of lipid peroxidation, especially in the nuclear membrane, is likely to contribute to the anticarcinogenic action of tamoxifen. Protection of human low density lipoproteins (LDL) by tamoxifen is likely to contribute to the beneficial cardiovascular effects of tamoxifen treatment. The ability of tamoxifen, and also antifungal azoles, to reverse multidrug resistance is also discussed.

Chapter 9—Inhibitory action of tamoxifen in a yeast tumour model and the potential anti-*Candida* and antiviral use of tamoxifen

This chapter examines the ability of tamoxifen to inhibit growth in a yeast tumour model: emphasis is given to the possibility that tamoxifen and related compounds could be useful anti-*Candida* agents for therapeutic purposes. Infection with the pathogenic yeast *Candida albicans* is of increasing clinical importance, especially in relation to immunocompromised patients including patients with AIDS. In addition to its clinical potential as an anti-*Candida* agent, tamoxifen may have potential as an antiviral agent and this possibility is discussed. The growth of yeast is inhibited by several anticancer drugs, including tamoxifen and its derivatives. Indeed tamoxifen appears to be more effective than the azole antifungal drug ketoconazole, which also has a membrane antioxidant ability. Some drugs target particular subcellular sites such as the mitochondrion and induce the *petite* mutation: tamoxifen does not appear to act in this way. It is of interest that an oestrogen-binding protein has been detected in yeast, although it does not appear to interact with tamoxifen. Other potential target sites for tamoxifen in yeast are discussed, including protein kinase C and cytochromes P-450. The features of the biosynthesis of DNA, RNA and of protein are presented; however, these do not appear to be the primary target for the inhibition of yeast growth, nor indeed for the inhibition of the growth of the SK-OV-3 human tumour cell line by tamoxifen. The pro-oxidant and antioxidant activities of anticancer drugs in the yeast tumour model is discussed from a mechanistic viewpoint, which is especially interesting now that a specific antioxidant protein has been isolated and characterised from yeast. There are clear advantages in using the yeast tumour model for the study of growth inhibition by drugs including tamoxifen and its derivatives. These include the ease with which yeast can be grown and genetically manipulated, and the rapid attainment of results. Manipulation of yeast genetics is readily achieved, including the use of recombinant DNA transformants that contain human genes. Progress is being made rapidly in the complete sequencing of the yeast genome, in addition to the studies in the human genome project. In addition, basic information on yeast itself can be obtained, which includes here the enhancement by tamoxifen of the membrane antioxidant action of ergosterol (the main membrane sterol in yeast) when the yeast lipid fraction is extracted and incorporated into liposomes: a tamoxifen enhancement coefficient has been calculated that quantifies this ability.

Chapter 10—Tamoxifen: brief outline of future possibilities in disease control in relation to drug design strategies

The concluding chapter of this book presents a brief outline of the present status of tamoxifen, and the future possibilities for the use of tamoxifen and designer derivatives in human therapy. These relate mainly to the treatment of breast cancer and other cancers; nevertheless, the proposed chemopreventive use of tamoxifen may well confer other health advantages including cardiovascular benefits.

TAMOXIFEN AS A STRUCTURAL MIMIC OF CHOLESTEROL IN CELL MEMBRANES

Advances in the understanding at the molecular level of the various modes of action of tamoxifen (see Figure 1.2) and related drugs should facilitate their therapeutic application. Some of these advances are discussed here, often in terms of molecular interactions in cells and model systems. Particular attention is drawn to the identification of the cholesterol-mimicking ability of tamoxifen and related compounds in cell membranes (see Chapter 8). This is indicated by protection by tamoxifen and related compounds from the lipid peroxidation caused by free radical attack on membranes. Modulation of cell membrane fluidity may be

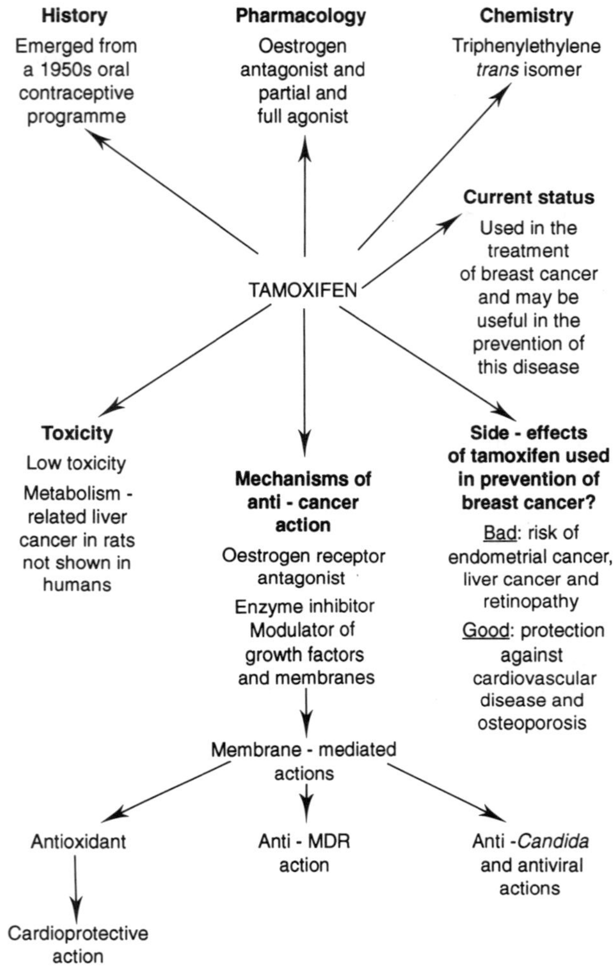

Figure 1.2. An overview of tamoxifen

primarily responsible both for this protective action of tamoxifen and for its ability to inhibit the growth of cancer cells. This inhibition of cell growth may arise from changes in cell membrane-associated signalling processes directed to the cell nucleus by the second messenger molecular cascades that modulate gene expression.

2

An Introduction to the Chemistry and Pharmacology of Tamoxifen

A BRIEF HISTORY

Tamoxifen (1-(*p*-dimethylaminoethoxyphenyl)-1,2-*trans*-diethyl-but-1-ene) (marketed by ICI as the monocitrate salt, under the proprietary name Nolvadex) emerged from a late 1950s research programme aimed at developing an antioestrogen oral contraceptive. Currently, interest in the use of triphenylethylenes (of which tamoxifen is the best-known example) as oral contraceptives has largely been replaced by interest in their use in both the treatment and prevention of breast cancer. Early work showed that stilbene and triphenylethylene displayed weak oestrogenic properties in the mouse. Further studies of structure–activity relationships led to the synthesis of diethylstilboestrol a potent non-steroidal oestrogen mimic (Dodds *et al.*, 1938a, 1938b). However it was not until 1958 that MER-25 (ethamoxytriphetol) (1-*p*-(2-diethylaminoethoxyphenyl)-1-phenyl-2-*p*-methoxyphenyl-ethanol), the first non-steroidal compound to show good oestrogen antagonist activity (in both intact and spayed female rats), was discovered. MER-25 was found to have antifertility activity in rats, which stimulated interest in the possible uses of antioestrogens as contraceptives. Clinical trials with MER-25 were discontinued because of its low potency and its toxicity (reviewed in Furr and Jordan, 1984 and Richardson, 1988).

A basic ether derivative of triphenylchloroethylene, MRL-41 (also known as clomiphene or chloramiphene, 1-[*p*-β-diethylaminoethoxyphenyl]-1,2 diphenyl–2-chloroethylene), also showed antioestrogenic properties and inhibited implantation but unfortunately induced ovulation and so was discarded as an antifertility agent. Clomiphene can be used in the induction of ovulation in some anovulatory patients. Triphenylmethylethylene was found to be slightly beneficial in the treatment of some breast cancers, but was also a potent oestrogen in laboratory animals (Richardson, 1988).

This compound, consequently was replaced by its basic ether derivative ICI 42 043, which inhibited implantation of the fertilised ovum in rats at doses lower than that at which it displayed oestrogenic activity, (Richardson, 1988). This finding resulted in compounds of this chemical series being developed as contraceptives and ICI 45,960 was selected for further study. ICI 45 960 was then superseded by its analogue, tamoxifen (ICI 46 474) (Richardson, 1988).

SYNTHESIS AND PHYSICAL AND CHEMICAL CHARACTERISTICS

Tamoxifen and its *cis* isomer are synthesised from the appropriately substituted desoxybenzoin. This involves the preparation of the alkanol by standard methods and then the olefinic link is generated in an acid-catalysed elimination reaction. This process yields an approximately 1 : 1 mixture of the *trans* and *cis* forms, which can then be separated by fractional crystallisation: tamoxifen, the *trans* isomer, has two unsubstituted phenyl groups in the *trans* configuration and ICI 47 699 is the corresponding *cis* isomer. Nolvadex contains less than 1% of the *cis* isomer. The configuration of tamoxifen and *cis*-tamoxifen was originally determined by a combination of dipole moment measurements and nuclear magnetic resonance (NMR) spectroscopy and it has now been confirmed by X-ray crystallography (Richardson, 1988). Chemical characteristics of tamoxifen (free base M_r 371.5 or monocitrate salt M_r 563.6) include that it is a fine, white and odourless crystalline powder, which is only slightly soluble in water but highly soluble in ethanol, methanol, acetone and toluene (in addition to other organic solvents).

Tamoxifen is sensitive to ultraviolet (UV) light, especially when it is in solution. The UV photolysis products are the *cis* isomer, and the substituted phenanthrenes formed by cyclisation of both isomers. The substituted phenanthrenes formed are produced by dehydrogenation of cyclised intermediates subsequent to the partial isomerisation of tamoxifen (Wilson and Reunitz, 1993).

Tamoxifen in powder form is stable for at least five years, provided that it is protected from moisture and light: it is substantially pure, and contains less than 1% of the *cis* isomer.

BASIC PHARMACOLOGY

Tamoxifen has complex pharmacological properties and can behave either as a pure oestrogen agonist, a partial agonist or as an antagonist, depending on the species studied, the target organ examined and the endpoint measured (see Figure 2.1). The activity of tamoxifen has been investigated in a number of different species and target tissues (reviewed in Furr and Jordan, 1984). It has been found that tamoxifen was a partial oestrogen agonist in the uterus (uterine weight test) in the rat and oestrogenic (uterine weight test and vaginal smear test) in the mouse. Further studies, however, have shown that although tamoxifen is oestrogenic in short-term tests (Jordan *et al.*, 1990), in long-term therapy tamoxifen has been reported to suppress mouse mammary tumorigenesis (Jordan *et al.*, 1991).

Action in different species

A brief summary is given of the basic pharmacological action of tamoxifen in a number of different species (reviewed in Furr and Jordan, 1984).

The pharmacology of tamoxifen in the rat is dependent upon the target tissue being examined and the biochemical endpoint being measured: thus only the overall effects of tamoxifen are discussed. Administration of tamoxifen to ovariectomised rats leads to vaginal cornification, although tamoxifen will also inhibit the vaginal cornification induced by oestradiol. The results of uterine weight tests in both immature and ovariectomised rats indicate that tamoxifen is also a partial agonist in the uterus. Indeed, a comparative study of the actions of tamoxifen and oestrogen has been reported in the ovariectomised rat (Kalu *et al.*, 1991). Oestrogens and antioestrogens have been demonstrated to affect the food intake and body weight of rats (Gray *et al.*, 1993), and tamoxifen has been shown to mimic the effects of oestrogens on food intake, body weight and body

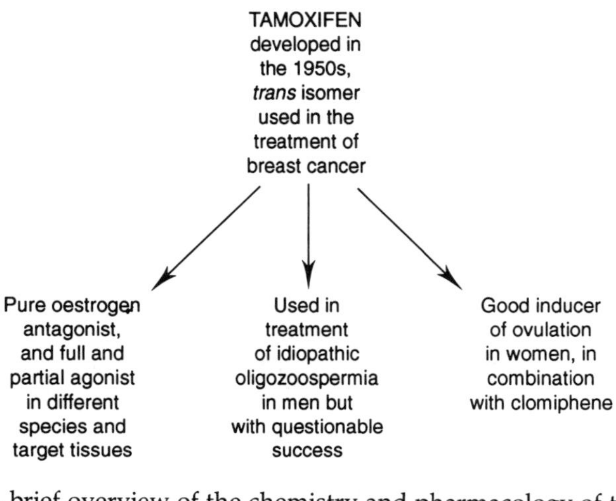

Figure 2.1. A brief overview of the chemistry and pharmacology of tamoxifen and its use in fertility treatment

composition in rats (Wade and Helle, 1993) and tamoxifen and oestrogen both protect the rat muscle against physiological damage (Koot *et al.*, 1991).

The pharmacological effects of tamoxifen in the rabbit, like those in the rat, are dependent on the endpoint of the assay, measured. Tamoxifen at high doses (1–5 mg/rabbit) was found to be sufficiently oestrogenic to prime the uterus to respond to progesterone and also antagonised the luteotrophic effect of oestrogen, reduced circulating progesterone and terminated pregnancy.

In hens, tamoxifen at levels of 0.005% or 0.05% in the diet reduced plasma calcium concentrations, which probably reflects an antioestrogenic effect of the drug on the synthesis of calcium-binding proteins in the liver. This effect is in contrast to the activity of oestrogens in the hen. In the chick, tamoxifen and 4-hydroxytamoxifen were pure antagonists of oestrogen-stimulated growth of the oviduct. Also it has been shown in the hen that tamoxifen increased basal luteinising hormone (LH) levels, increased the sensitivity of the pituitary gland to luteinising hormone releasing hormone (LHRH) and decreased the LH response to progesterone. These findings are all consistent with tamoxifen acting as an antioestrogen.

In the pig-tailed monkey (*Macaca nemestrina*) tamoxifen suppressed ovulation and the usual increase in plasma progesterone during the luteal phase. The action of tamoxifen can be explained on the basis of interference with the action or biosynthesis of oestrogen and suggests that tamoxifen is a pure antioestrogen in the pig-tailed monkey.

Tamoxifen is oestrogenic in the mouse, but only under strictly defined conditions. In mature ovariectomised mice, tamoxifen given orally was oestrogenic in the vaginal smear test. Tamoxifen was also oestrogenic in the ovariectomised mouse in the three-day uterine weight test.

Action in oestrogen target tissues

The agonist and antagonist actions of tamoxifen, demonstrated by the differences in response of the uterus of different animal species, can also be seen when the actions of tamoxifen in particular target tissues of the species are compared (reviewed in Furr and Jordan, 1984).

In the uteri of immature and of ovariectomised rats, although tamoxifen increases wet weight and DNA content it acts as only a partial oestrogen agonist. Marked differences between the effects of oestrogens and anti-oestrogens (such as tamoxifen) on cell division in the uterus have been found. For example oestradiol increased the mitotic activity of luminal epithelial cells (of the uterine endometrium), whereas tamoxifen and 4-hydroxytamoxifen were much less effective. Progesterone receptor synthesis increased in response to both tamoxifen and 4-hydroxytamoxifen treatment in uteri of both immature and ovariectomised rats. The concentration of progesterone receptors was similar after treatment with both tamoxifen and 4-hydroxytamoxifen to that obtained with oestradiol. However, the total uterine content of progesterone receptors was less after administration of tamoxifen and 4-hydroxytamoxifen compared with oestradiol. The uterus is known to respond to oestrogens by stimulation of cell proliferation. For example, in the classical uterotrophic assay in immature rodents, oestrogens have been found to cause fluid retention and cell proliferation, and indeed tamoxifen has species-specific oestrogen-like effects. However, 4-hydroxytamoxifen and other 4-hydroxylated triphenylethylenes generally show fewer oestrogenic properties than unhydroxylated ones, while ICI 164 384 (a steroidal pure oestrogen antagonist) has no oestrogenic activity in this model (Kangas, 1992). In addition, the tamoxifen analogue 4-iodotamoxifen had a similar partial agonist activity to tamoxifen in the immature rat and mouse uterotrophic assays and this was greater than that observed with pyrrolidino-4-iodotamoxifen (Chander *et al.*, 1991). Furthermore, pyrrolidino-4-iodotamoxifen caused a dose-dependent inhibition of oestrogen-induced vaginal cornification, whereas tamoxifen and 4-iodotamoxifen did not. It is of interest that the agonist and antagonist effects of tamoxifen have also been studied in the female mouse brain (McKenna *et al.*, 1992).

The oestrogen-stimulated release of prolactin by the pituitary gland of ovariectomised rats was partially inhibited by tamoxifen treatment. Additionally, tamoxifen inhibited the cyclic release of prolactin at the pro-oestrus phase. Although these effects suggest antioestrogenic activity for tamoxifen, it did not inhibit the oestrogen-induced secretion of prolactin. Furthermore, tamoxifen caused an increase in pituitary oestrogen receptors, an oestrogenic effect which could indicate that tamoxifen has no anti-oestrogenic effect at the level of the pituitary. Moreover, tamoxifen, unlike oestrogen, did not stimulate prolactin release; and oestradiol-stimulated prolactin synthesis by immature rat pituitary cells can be inhibited by either tamoxifen or 4-hydroxytamoxifen. Following ovariectomy in mature female rats the LH and follicle-stimulating hormone (FSH) levels increased progressively. Short-term (five days) therapy of ovariectomised rats with tamoxifen (250 μg per rat daily) did not reduce LH levels in the serum, whereas long-term therapy (200 μg per rat daily for up to four weeks) resulted in a consistent decrease in LH value. In comparison, FSH secretion appears to be less responsive to antioestrogens in the ovariectomised rat.

The liver and also other tissues such as breast and bone respond to oestrogens by regulation of specific protein synthesis. The regulation of gene expression is a complex process and oestrogens may turn oestrogen-responsive genes on or off. Furthermore, some of the proteins produced can act as growth factors, while the function of others is still unknown. In the liver of both rats and monkeys a well-defined oestrogen receptor system has been found, through which both oestrogens and anti-oestrogens may exert some of their effects. The effect of tamoxifen was similar in the liver of both rats and monkeys.

During tamoxifen treatment changes in several liver proteins have been observed in patients with breast cancer that are likely to be oestrogen modulated, e.g. serum sex steroid hormone binding globulin (SHBG), plasma antithrombin III and other non-specialised plasma proteins. The plasma protein profile of these patients has been found to resemble that of patients undergoing administration of oestrogen; for example, the plasma antithrombin III was slightly decreased and SHBG was elevated. These effects are discussed further in Chapter 4. The effects of antioestrogens such as tamoxifen in the mammalian liver are therefore mostly oestrogenic in nature. These findings are in contrast to the observed effects on the liver of the rooster, where specific oestrogen-stimulated protein synthesis (of apolipoprotein B) was inhibited by administration of tamoxifen and no agonist action was observed.

Pharmacological activity of tamoxifen metabolites

A brief outline is given below of the basic pharmacological activity of the tamoxifen metabolites 4-hydroxytamoxifen, *N*-desmethyltamoxifen and also the oestrogenic metabolite, metabolite E (reviewed in Furr and Jordan, 1984), which are formed in the liver by the action of particular cytochromes P-450 (see Chapter 3). The metabolism of tamoxifen is dealt with in further detail in Chapter 3.

4-Hydroxytamoxifen binds to the oestrogen receptor with much greater affinity than tamoxifen: indeed the affinity of 4-hydroxytamoxifen was at least as great as that of oestradiol. 4-Hydroxytamoxifen showed a very slow dissociation rate from the oestrogen receptor, in common with oestradiol and in contrast to tamoxifen, and will also translocate the oestrogen receptor to the nucleus. 4-Hydroxytamoxifen was approximately 100-fold more potent than tamoxifen in inhibiting the growth of the oestrogen receptor-positive human breast cancer cell line, MCF-7, and this correlates well with its higher relative binding affinity for the oestrogen receptor. It can act as a pure antioestrogen, inhibiting the secretion of the oestrogen-induced 46 kDa protein by MCF-7 cells. The duration of action of 4-hydroxytamoxifen was much shorter than tamoxifen *in vivo* because of the greater ability of this metabolite to be conjugated and excreted. This shorter half-life of 4-hydroxytamoxifen was probably also responsible for its lower potency than tamoxifen, following chronic dosing in the dimethylbenz(*a*)anthracene (DMBA)-induced rat mammary tumour model (this model is discussed further in Chapter 5). 4-Hydroxytamoxifen was similar to tamoxifen in that it showed partial agonist action and stimulated uterine weight increases in immature rats, and progesterone receptor synthesis. It was, however, a full agonist in the ovariectomised mouse, and was equipotent with tamoxifen in inhibiting implantation when administered on day 4 of pregnancy in rats. It is of interest that 4-hydroxytamoxifen, as found for oestradiol, can induce peroxidase activity in the oestrogen-primed immature rat uterus—an effect which can be antagonised by tamoxifen.

N-Desmethyltamoxifen has a low relative binding affinity for the oestrogen receptor, similar to that of tamoxifen, in rat uterus and human mammary cancer tissue. It has similar biological properties to tamoxifen in that it will antagonise the oestrogen-induced increase in the uterine weight in immature rats, although it was found to be less potent than tamoxifen. *N*-Desmethyltamoxifen was also a partial agonist and did not suppress completely the oestrogen-induced increase in uterine weight. Additionally, *N*-desmethyltamoxifen prevented implantation in rats if given on day 4 of pregnancy; and it suppressed the growth of the DMBA-induced rat mammary tumour *in vivo* and in MCF-7 cells *in vitro*.

Removal of the basic sidechain from tamoxifen results in the formation of metabolite E, which is a full oestrogen agonist and will cause a full agonist response on the immature rat uterus, both on uterine weight and histology, and will induce progesterone receptor synthesis. In addition, metabolite E has a lower affinity than tamoxifen for the oestrogen receptor in the rat and lamb uterus.

Action on fertility and pregnancy

Tamoxifen was found to terminate pregnancy when administered orally to rats during the first few days after mating. The time of maximum effectiveness of tamoxifen is at days 3 and 4 and this coincides with the time of a surge in plasma oestradiol that is thought to be vital for implantation. Tamoxifen can inhibit oestrogen-dependent implantation and this effect can be reversed by oestrone administration. Low doses of tamoxifen (0.1 mg/kg), administered on day 19 or 20 of pregnancy delayed parturition, whereas high doses (0.5 mg/kg) accelerated parturition. Although the mechanism of action of tamoxifen in accelerating parturition is unknown, the delay in parturition may involve an inhibition of prostaglandin biosynthesis because the administration of natural or synthetic prostaglandins was found to reverse the effects of tamoxifen. There is evidence that prostaglandin biosynthesis is mediated by oestrogen in the rat and guinea-pig uterus. The inhibitory effects of tamoxifen on prostaglandin biosynthesis have been demonstrated in uterine homogenates from guinea-pigs *in vitro* and in pseudopregnant rats *in vivo*: tamoxifen may interact directly with the enzyme prostaglandin synthetase. In addition the effects of tamoxifen on uterine prostaglandin production and luteal function in non-pregnant guinea-pigs have been studied (Poyser, 1993). It is of interest also that tamoxifen increases plasma oestrogen-binding equivalents and has an oestradiol agonist effect on histologically normal pre-menopausal and post-menopausal endometrium. Studies have been reported on the effect of tamoxifen on the endometrium (Uziely *et al.*, 1993) in the mid-luteal phase (Swahn *et al.*, 1993).

A method of ovulatory induction in women has been reported that involves the use of combination therapy with tamoxifen and clomiphene, administered as citrate salts (Suginami *et al.*, 1993). A randomised cross-over study with clomiphene citrate alone and clomiphene citrate–tamoxifen citrate combination therapies was carried out for 20 normo-prolactinaemic anovulatory women. The rates for the clomiphene citrate–tamoxifen citrate combination therapy of ovulatory/treated, pregnant/treated and pregnant/ovulatory cycles were 42 of 56 (75%), 3 of 47 (6.4%) and 3 of 35 (8.6%) respectively, whereas those for clomiphene citrate alone were 25 of 57 (43.9%), 1 of 48 (2.1%) and 1 of 21 (4.8%). Clomiphene citrate in combination with tamoxifen citrate was thus more effective in ovulation induction than clomiphene citrate alone and all the pregnancies were normal and single. Furthermore, none of the treatments was accompanied by any notable side-effects.

Action in males

Tamoxifen is finding a use in the adjuvant therapy of carcinoma of the human male breast (Ribeiro and Swindell, 1992; Coffman, 1993) and this is discussed further in Chapter 4.

It has been shown that tamoxifen reduces the weight of the accessory sex organs in male rats when administered daily in high doses (100 mg/kg) for short periods or in lower doses (2 and 20 mg/kg) for longer periods. The action of oestradiol and tamoxifen on the mullero-regressive activity of the chick embryonic testis has been assayed *in vivo* by organotypic grafting (Stoll *et al.*, 1993). Tamoxifen (20 mg per day for three weeks) has also been used in men to determine whether the action of testosterone on the somatotropic axis is direct, or requires the aromatisation of testosterone to oestradiol (Weissberger and Ho, 1993). In normal men, and in hypogonadal men receiving testosterone replacement, tamoxifen reduced 24 h mean serum growth hormone (GH) levels, mean GH pulse amplitude and serum insulin-like growth factor 1 (IGF-1), whereas testosterone treatment increased all of these parameters. It was concluded that testosterone plays an important part in the modulation of the male somatotrophic axis in adulthood and that this is partly dependent on the aromatisation of testosterone to oestradiol.

Tamoxifen has been used in human males in the treatment of idiopathic oligozoospermia (Krause *et al.*, 1992; Sterzik *et al.*, 1993; Kotoulas *et al*; 1994). Modulation of immunoradiometric and bioactive FSH secretion and clearance has been measured in young and elderly men during treatment with tamoxifen (Urban *et al.*, 1992). However, there does not appear to be any conclusive evidence of the usefulness of tamoxifen in the treatment of idiopathic oligozoospermia. In a controlled study of idiopathic oligozoospermia with tamoxifen versus placebo, although there was a significant increase in serum testosterone levels in the tamoxifen-treated group, the increases in FSH hormone levels and in sperm count in the tamoxifen treated group were not statistically significant. Furthermore, serum levels of LH and the percentage of motile and abnormal sperm were similar in both groups (Krause *et al.*, 1992). It is of related interest that the effect of hydrogen peroxide on polyspermic fertilisation in the sea urchin is modulated by tamoxifen (Rosenkranz *et al.*, 1991).

REFERENCES

Chander, S.K., McCague, R., Luqmai, Y., Newton, C., Dowsett, M., Jarman, M., Coombes, R.C. (1991) *Cancer Research* **51**, 5851–5858.

Coffman, B.L. (1993) *Annals of Internal Medicine* **118**, 749.

Dodds, E.C., Goldberg, L., Lawson, W., Robinson, R. (1938a) *Nature London* **141**, 247–248.

Dodds, E.C., Lawson, W., Noble, R.L. (1938b) *Lancet* **i**, 1389–1391.

Furr, B.J.A., Jordan, V.C. (1984) *Pharmacology and Therapeutics* **25**, 127–205.

Gray, J.M., Schrochk, S., Bishop, M. (1993) *American Journal of Physiology* **264**, R124–1218.

Jordan, V.C., Lababidi, M.K., Mirecki, D.M. (1990) *European Journal of Cancer* **26**, 718–721.

Jordan, V.C., Labibidi, M.K., Langanfahey, S. (1991) *Journal of the National Cancer Institute* **83**, 492–495.

Kalu, D.N., Salerno, E., Liu, C.C., Echon, R., Ray, M., Garzazapta, M., Hollis, B.W. (1991) *Bone and Mineral* **15**, 109–124.

Kangas, L. (1992) *Acta Oncologica* **31**, 143–146.

Koot, R. W., Amelink, G. J., Blankenstein, M. A., Bar, P. R. (1991) *Journal of Steroid Biochemistry and Molecular Biology* **40**, 689–696.

Kotoulas, I. G., Cardamatis, E., Michopoulos, J., Michopoulos, D., Dounis, A. (1994) *Fertility and Sterility* **6**, 911–914.

Krause, W., Holland-Moritz, H., Schramm, P. (1992) *International Journal of Andrology* **15**, 14–18.

McKenna, S.E., Simon, N.G., Cologerclifford, A. (1992) *Hormones and Behaviour* **26**, 536–344.

Posyer, N.L. (1993) *Journal of Reproduction and Fertility* **98**, 307.

Ribeiro, G., Swindell, R. (1992) *British Journal of Cancer* **65**, 252–254.

Richardson, D.N. (1988) *Drug Design and Delivery* **3**, 1–14.

Rosenkranz, M., Lim, J.S., Frenkel, K., Troll, W. (1991) *Biological Bulletin* **181**, 346.

Sterzik, K., Rosenbuch, B., Mogck, J., Heyden, M., Lichtenberger, K. (1993) *Archives of Gynecology and Obstetrics* **252**, 143–148.

Stoll, R., Ichas, F., Faucounau, N., Maraud, R. (1993) *Anatomy and Embryology* **187**, 379–384.

Suginami, H., Kitagawa, H., Nakahashi, N., Yano, K., Matsubara, K. (1993) *Fertility and Sterility* **59**, 976–979.
Swahn, L., Bygdeman, M., Seppala, M., Johannisson, E., Ceka, S. (1993) *Human Reproduction* **8**, 193–200.
Urban, R.J., Dahl, K.D., Lippert, M.L., Velhuis, J.D. (1992) *International Journal of Andrology* **13**, 579–586.
Uziely, B., Lewin, A., Brufman, G., Dorembus, D. (1993) *Breast Cancer Research and Treatment* **26**, 101–106.
Wade, G.N., Helle, H.W. (1993) *American Journal of Physiology* **264**, R1219–1223.
Weissberger, A.J., Ho, K.K. (1993) *Journal of Clinical Endocrinology and Metabolism* **76**, 1407–1412.
Wilson, S., Reunitz, P.C. (1993) *Journal of Pharmaceutical Sciences* **82**, 571–574.

3

Metabolism and Toxicology of Tamoxifen: An Overview

CYTOCHROMES P-450 INDUCTION AND ACTIONS

Cytochromes P-450 are phase I drug-metabolising enzymes and are a family of haemoproteins with spectral peaks close to 450 nm (reduced iron:carbon monoxide complex) which catalyse a wide range of mono-oxygenase reactions. These enzymes have a very important role in the oxidative metabolism of a wide range of compounds such as endogenous steroid hormones, environmental carcinogens and structurally diverse drugs of a lipophilic nature, including many antitumour drugs (Le Blanc and Waxman, 1989). Cytochromes P-450 carry out *C*-, *N*- and *S*-hydroxylations and dehalogenations, in addition to dealkylations and deaminations.

The cytochrome P-450 genes are named with the root 'CYP' and gene families are designated by numbers (subfamilies are represented by letters followed by a number for the individual gene: Gonzalez and Nebert, 1990). Several distinct classes of mammalian P-450 inducers have been characterised that activate transcription of one or more P-450 genes. These include polycyclic aromatic hydrocarbons, some benzoflavones and 2,3,7,8,tetra-chlorodibenzo-*p*-dioxin (TCDD), which all induce two genes in the CYP1 family via an aromatic hydrocarbon (Ah) receptor-mediated enhancement of transcriptional rates. Phenobarbitone (PB) and terpenoids increase the transcriptional rates of genes in the CYP2B and CYP2C subfamilies and in the CYP3 and CYP6 families. Glucocorticoids and peroxisome proliferators activate transcription of genes in the CYP3 and CYP4 families respectively, and adrenocorticotrophic hormone positively regulates the cyclic AMP-mediated expression of P-450 genes encoding enzymes involved in steroid synthesis.

In eukaryotic cells most of the cytochromes P-450 are located in the endoplasmic reticulum. The components of the cytochrome P-450 mono-oxygenase system are well established. Two main proteins are involved: cytochrome P-450 (a haemoprotein containing the protoporphyrin IX group) and cytochrome P-450 reductase (a flavoprotein containing one flavine adenine dinucleotide (FAD) and one flavine mononucleotide (FMN) group). The cytochrome P-450 component contains the substrate and oxygen binding sites, whilst the reductase transports electrons from NADPH (reduced form of nicotinamide adenine dinucleotide phosphate) to the cytochrome P-450 component. Metabolism by this cytochrome P-450-dependent mixed-function oxidase system has been reported in both laboratory animals and man and in corresponding tissues and extracts, for many antitumour drugs including tamoxifen. Extensive studies have been made on cytochromes P-450: for example, PB induction of cytochrome P-450 gene expression has been studied (Waxman and Azaroff, 1992) and the regulation of cytochrome P-450 gene expression has been investigated in human breast and colon cancer xenografts (G. Smith *et al.*, 1993b). It is also of interest that expression of the CYP1A1 gene in MCF-7 breast cancer cells is potentiated by co-treatment with TCDD and 12-*o*-tetradecanoyl phorbol-13-acetate (Moore *et al.*, 1993). Furthermore, α-naphthoflavone (αNF) and 6-methyl-1,3,8-trichlorodibenzofuran (MCDF) inhibited TCDD-induced CYP1A1 gene expression in MCF-7 cells and also decreased the accumulation of the Ah receptor complex (Merchant *et al.*, 1993). TCDD (10^{-9} M) also inhibited the 17β-oestradiol-induced proliferation of MCF-7 cells, and co-treatment with αNF (10^{-8} to 10^{-6} M) resulted in a concentration-dependent decrease in the antioestrogenic action of TCDD. Tamoxifen (10^{-7} M) also inhibited 17β-oestradiol-induced proliferation of MCF-7 cells and αNF did not affect the tamoxifen-mediated antiproliferative response.

TAMOXIFEN METABOLISM

The metabolism of tamoxifen has been investigated in both laboratory animals and female patients. It has been shown that in the rat, dog, rhesus monkey (Fromson *et al.*, 1973a) and man (Fromson *et al.*, 1973b; Lien *et al.*, 1988, 1989) that tamoxifen is well absorbed and, after oral administration, is extensively metabolised by cytochrome P-450-dependent hepatic mixed-function oxidases to form tamoxifen metabolites including 4-hydroxytamoxifen and *N*-desmethyltamoxifen (see Figure 3.1). Furthermore two acidic metabolites of tamoxifen (tamoxifen acid and 4-hydroxytamoxifen acid) have been identified in the rat (Reunitz and Nanavati, 1990). In addition, a 4-hydroxy *N*-desmethyl metabolite of tamoxifen has been reported in human bile (Lien *et al.*, 1988, 1989), indicating that tamoxifen metabolites are capable of undergoing further change. It is of interest that evidence has been found for superoxide formation during hepatic metabolism of tamoxifen (Turner *et al.*, 1991).

Further studies (Mani *et al.*, 1993a, 1993b) have shown that in rat liver microsomes incubated with tamoxifen the three major products were the polar metabolites of tamoxifen: tamoxifen *N*-oxide, *N*-desmethyltamoxifen

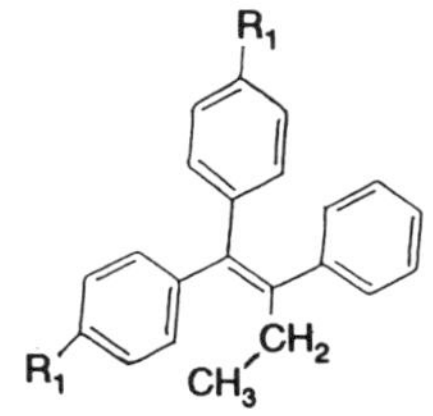

	R_1	R_2
Tamoxifen	H	$OCH_2CH_2N(CH_3)_2$
4-Hydroxytamoxifen	OH	$OCH_2CH_2N(CH_3)_2$
N-Desmethyltamoxifen	H	$OCH_2CH_2NHCH_3$

Figure 3.1. Metabolites of tamoxifen

and 4-hydroxytamoxifen (a flavin-containing monooxygenase (FMO) catalysed the formation of tamoxifen *N*-oxide). The *N*-demethylation and 4-hydroxylation reactions were inhibited by carbon monoxide and by the cytochrome P-450 inhibitor SKF-525A, suggesting the involvement of P-450 monooxygenase in these reactions. Furthermore, antibodies to NADPH:P-450 reductase also inhibited *N*-demethylation and 4-hydroxylation. It is of interest that *N*-demethylation was higher in the male rat, whereas 4-hydroxylation was higher in the female. The participation of multiple P-450s was demonstrated by enhanced *N*-demethylation in rats treated with PB, pregnanolone-16α-carbonitrile (PCN) or methylcholanthrene (MC). There is evidence that tamoxifen *N*-demethylation in the rat is catalysed by the cytochrome P-450 families 3A, 1A and 2C.

Human liver microsomes formed tamoxifen metabolites at a much lower rate than rat microsomes. Inhibitors of FMO diminished the accumulation of *N*-oxide by human liver microsomes, which suggests an involvement of FMO in this reaction. Furthermore, tamoxifen *N*-oxide can be reduced to tamoxifen in human (or rat) microsomes by NADPH and this suggests that the *N*-oxide metabolite may act as a storage form for tamoxifen *in vivo*. The formation of *N*-desmethyl and 4-hydroxy metabolites in human microsomes was decreased by the use of inhibitors, and tamoxifen *N*-demethylation in the human is catalysed only by the cytochrome P-450 family 3A. This is in agreement with an earlier study that identified the cytochrome P-450 family 3A as the enzymes involved in the *N*-demethylation of tamoxifen in human liver microsomes (Jacolot *et al.*, 1991). Furthermore, it has been found that the metabolism of tamoxifen by human liver microsomes is not mediated by cytochrome P-450 2D6 (Blankson *et al.*, 1991).

It has been suggested that tamoxifen is metabolised by rat and human liver microsomes into a reactive intermediate (txf*), which binds irreversibly to microsomal proteins in the presence of NADPH and oxygen. This binding is inhibited by carbon monoxide—inhibitors of cytochrome P-450 and antibodies to rat NADPH:P450 reductase—indicating catalysis by the cytochrome P-450 (Mani and Kupfer, 1991). Glutathione and cysteine inhibited the binding of tamoxifen but did not affect cytochrome P-450-mediated metabolism of tamoxifen to microsomal protein and, therefore, were either reacting with txf* or competing for the same binding site on microsomal protein. Inactivation of the FMO diminished this binding, suggesting that P-450 and FMO catalyse the reactions leading to the formation of txf*. However, it was also shown that *N*-desmethyltamoxifen and tamoxifen *N*-oxide, which are the principal P-450 and FMO metabolites respectively, were not on the major route of txf* formation: thus txf* was not an aldehyde derived from tamoxifen nitrone.

Metabolic activation of tamoxifen and its inhibitory action on metabolic reactions

4-Hydroxytamoxifen but not tamoxifen (both at 50 nM) inhibited the oestradiol-stimulated growth of MCF-7 cells, and rescue with oestradiol (10 μM) overcame this growth inhibition. In BG-1 (ovarian carcinoma) cells both 4-hydroxytamoxifen and tamoxifen inhibited oestradiol-stimulated growth, and this was again overcome with oestradiol, suggesting that BG-1 cells have an intrinsic ability to hydroxylate and thus metabolically activate tamoxifen by conversion to 4-hydroxytamoxifen (Pavlik *et al.*, 1991).

A study using the rat as an animal model for tamoxifen biotransformation showed that a dose of 30 mg/kg of tamoxifen resulted in an accumulation of tamoxifen and its *N*-desmethyltamoxifen and 4-hydroxytamoxifen metabolites in liver tissue. This finding suggests that the disposition of tamoxifen itself as well as that of other drugs (which may be administrated with it) may be subject to modification, affecting both the efficacy and safety of these agents (Meltzer *et al.*, 1984). Furthermore, it has been found that tamoxifen inhibits the action of the four androstenedione hydroxylase pathways (Reid and Murray, 1989). Tamoxifen, 4-hydroxytamoxifen and *N*-desmethyltamoxifen were shown by *in vitro* competitive substrate experiments to be essentially equipotent as inhibitors of mixed-function oxidases and the inhibitory effect was more pronounced towards Type I binding substrates. Spectral binding studies of substrates to cytochrome P-450 showed that tamoxifen produces a classical Type I spectrum and competitively displaces ethylmorphine and aminopyrine from their protein Type I binding site (tamoxifen species do not bind directly to the Type II iron binding site of cytochrome P-450).

Tamoxifen and its metabolites may also act as inhibitors of microsomal mixed-function oxidase systems, primarily by interaction at or near the

Type I binding site of cytochrome P-450, hence inhibiting the further metabolism of tamoxifen and other co-administered drugs. In the clinical situation, where tamoxifen is administered twice daily for long periods, it may interfere therefore with both its own metabolism and the metabolism, and likely detoxification, of other drugs. This is of great importance because tamoxifen is being evaluated clinically in combination with potent cytotoxic agents, many of which exhibit low therapeutic indices and thus potential toxicity.

Metabolism of tamoxifen itself was also found to be sensitive to the presence of other compounds and this could also be of importance clinically. Indeed, in breast cancer patients the metabolism of tamoxifen has been shown to be altered by the simultaneous administration of medroxy-progesterone acetate (see Chapter 4) (Reid *et al.*, 1992). Pre-treatment of rats with known inducers of microsomal oxidases, for example PB and 3-methylcholanthrene, resulted in not only the expected increase in metabolic activity corresponding to increased liver microsomal protein (per gram of liver) and cytochrome P-450 levels, but also caused significant changes in the levels of tamoxifen metabolites.

Excretion

It has been shown by the use of [^{14}C]tamoxifen that tamoxifen and its metabolites are mostly excreted via bile, into faeces, as glucuronides and other conjugates. Indeed very little tamoxifen was found to be eliminated as unchanged drug. In primates, including man, although urinary excretion is greater than in rodents it is still only a minor route of elimination of the drug. It has also been found that the 4-iodo derivative of tamoxifen was metabolised four times more slowly than tamoxifen by isolated rat hepatocytes and there was very little formation of glucuronide conjugates (McCague *et al.*, 1990). This is likely to be advantageous therapeutically because 4-iodotamoxifen, which has a higher affinity for the oestrogen receptor and is a better growth inhibitor of the human breast cancer cell line MCF-7 than tamoxifen, is likely to have a greater duration of action than tamoxifen in the body.

The bioconversion of tamoxifen by microorganisms has been studied, and it was found that only *Streptomyces rimosus* (ATCC 2234) was able to metabolise tamoxifen to 4-hydroxytamoxifen. The yield of 4-hydroxytamoxifen was 10% and was chemically identified by two-dimensional nuclear magnetic resonance (NMR) spectroscopy (El-Sharkawy, 1992). However, a number of microorganisms were found to be capable of biotransforming tamoxifen to tamoxifen *N*-oxide and *N*-desmethyltamoxifen (El-Sharkawy, 1992).

TISSUE DISTRIBUTION AND PHARMACOKINETICS

Following the intravenous injection of spayed female mice with [^{14}C]tamoxifen, levels of radioactivity after about 4 h were higher in liver, lung, adrenal, kidney, pancreas, uterus, salivary glands and mammary tissue than in blood. Studies have shown the similarities and differences in the metabolites, pharmacodynamics and pharmacokinetics of tamoxifen in rats and mice compared to breast cancer patients (Robinson *et al.*, 1991). The distribution of tamoxifen and its metabolites in rat and human tissues during steady-state treatment has also been reported (Lien *et al.*, 1991a). In addition, the adsorption of tamoxifen and its 2-methyl derivative has been studied in cell cultures (Chamart *et al.*, 1993).

The serum concentrations of tamoxifen, *N*-desmethyltamoxifen and 4-hydroxytamoxifen under steady-state conditions in women with breast cancer have been measured in a number of different investigations. The concentration of tamoxifen in the blood was approximately 300 ng/ml after chronic doses of 20 mg twice daily. These studies showed also that the concentration of *N*-desmethyltamoxifen was about 50% higher than that of tamoxifen (i.e., approximately 460 ng/ml at a dose of 20 mg twice daily), while that of 4-hydroxytamoxifen was very low: approximately 3 ng/ml at 10 mg twice daily and approximately 6 ng/ml at 20 mg twice daily (reviewed in Furr and Jordan, 1984). The serum levels of tamoxifen and tamoxifen metabolites have been measured also in patients on long-term tamoxifen therapy for breast cancer (Langanfahey *et al.*, 1990). In addition, the distribution of tamoxifen and its metabolites into brain tissue and brain metastases has been measured in patients with breast cancer (Lien *et al.*, 1991b). The pharmacokinetics and bioavailability of tamoxifen in healthy volunteers have been determined (Herrlinger *et al.*, 1992).

In addition, the anticancer agent aminoglutethimide has been shown to decrease the serum concentrations of tamoxifen and its metabolites (Lien *et al.*, 1990), and this has important implications for co-administration of these drugs. After daily doses of 40 mg tamoxifen, tumour biopsy samples from women contained mean concentrations of tamoxifen of 25.1 (range 5.4–117), *N*-desmethyltamoxifen of 52 (range 7.8–210) and 4-hydroxytamoxifen of 0.53 (range 0.29–113) ng/mg protein (reviewed in Furr and Jordan, 1984). These values are roughly in proportion to the concentration in plasma. Similar results were obtained when the levels of tamoxifen and tamoxifen metabolites were measured in the cytosol of breast tumour biopsy samples (Murphy *et al.*, 1987).

It has been shown by the administration of [^{14}C]tamoxifen to dogs, rats, mice, rhesus monkeys and women that tamoxifen has a long half-life (Fromson *et al.*, 1973a, 1973b). Furthermore the plasma elimination half-life of tamoxifen in healthy male volunteers was also long (208 h) and equal to that of *N*-desmethyltamoxifen (De Vos *et al.*, 1989). In addition, the serum elimination half-life of tamoxifen and its metabolites in patients with breast cancer has been measured (De Vos *et al.*, 1992). Furthermore, phase I and phase II metabolites of tamoxifen have been analysed in breast cancer patients (Poon *et al.*, 1993). It is of interest that oestrogenic tamoxifen metabolites have been identified in tamoxifen-resistant human breast cancer (Wiebe *et al.*, 1992). Tamoxifen resistance is a serious problem in the therapeutic use of this drug and this is discussed in Chapter 6.

ASSAY PROCEDURES FOR DETECTION AND MEASUREMENT

Assay methods have been developed for detecting and measuring tamoxifen, *N*-desmethyltamoxifen and 4-hydroxytamoxifen levels, using either thin-layer chromatography (TLC), high-performance liquid chromatography (HPLC) or gas chromatography/mass spectrometry (GC/MS). The compounds are estimated by ultraviolet (UV) fluorescence after conversion to phenanthrene derivatives either before or after TLC or HPLC. Alternatively, following gas–liquid chromatography, the ratio of peak heights of the molecular ion of a tamoxifen derivative and an internal standard is used to determine tamoxifen concentrations by high-resolution mass spectrometry. Two-dimensional NMR spectrospcopy has been used to identify 4-hydroxytamoxifen (El-Sharkawy, 1992). An HPLC-based analysis of tamoxifen and its major human metabolites has been reported (Bethou and Dreano, 1993). In addition, a quantitative measurement of 4-hydroxytamoxifen in human plasma and in mammary tumours has been carried out using a combined gas chromatography/negative ion chemical ionisation mass spectrometry method (Girault *et al.*, 1993).

TOXICITY, TERATOLOGY AND CARCINOGENICITY

Tamoxifen has been reported to have virtually no side-effects in female breast cancer patients (Powles *et al.*, 1989; 1990). Furthermore, very little difference in acute toxicity between tamoxifen and placebo was observed (Powles *et al.*, 1989, 1990; Jordan, 1993). However, some adverse effects of tamoxifen in rat liver have been reported although such cases in humans are very rare, and there is also some concern about its effect on the endometrium (Seoud *et al.*, 1993; Demuylder and Neven, 1993; Uziely *et al*, 1993). Furthermore, tamoxifen-induced asthma has been reported (R.P. Smith *et al.*, 1993).

Tamoxifen has a very low acute toxicity (oral LD_{50} in mice approximately 3 g/kg and in rats 2.5 g/kg); however, chronic dosing does produce changes in the reproductive organs (Richardson, 1988). Teratogenic tests showed that offspring of rats treated with tamoxifen had a deformity of the rib cage called wavy ribs or 'kinky ribs'. The period after organogenesis was found to be the critical time of pregnancy during which the drug had to be administered to cause this deformity. The deformity was caused by the restriction in growth of the uterus due to tamoxifen, hence causing mechanical constriction of normal rib growth; thus it is not a true teratogenic effect. In fact this deformity disappeared by the time the young were weaned. In humans, for the 85 women who have become pregnant while on tamoxifen no fetal abnormalities have been reported (Clark, 1993). However, tamoxifen and teratogenicity in humans remains a subject of considerable importance and indeed pregnancy while receiving tamoxifen therapy is not recommended (Vancutsem and Williams, 1993). Furthermore, careful follow-up of children born to women who received tamoxifen during pregnancy is likely to be a good precaution.

Induction of hepatocarcinoma in the rat

Tamoxifen has been reported to cause liver cancer in the rat (Dragan *et al.*, 1991; Bignall, 1993; Williams *et al.*, 1993) but not in mice, and although the mechanism of this action of tamoxifen is not clearly understood it is likely to be related to its metabolism and there is a considerable difference between metabolism in the rat and in humans. It is of associated interest that tamoxifen has been reported to cause hepatocellular damage and agranulocytosis (Ching *et al.*, 1992), and conversely tamoxifen can prevent the induction of hepatic neoplasia by zeranol, which is an oestrogenic food contaminant (Coe *et al.*, 1992).

In a one-year study, tamoxifen was able to induce hepatocarcinoma in Sprague–Dawley rats (Hirsimaki *et al.*, 1993) and similar results were found in a two-year carcinogenicity study of tamoxifen in Alderly–Park Wistar-derived rats (Greaves *et al.*, 1993). When tamoxifen and also its derivative toremifene were studied in a 52-week toxicity study (including a 13-week recovery period) liver tumours were found in four out of five rats at the highest dose level of tamoxifen (45 mg/kg per day) and these were hepatocellular carcinoma in three rats; but no tumours were found in the toremifene-treated rats dosed at 48 mg/kg per day (Hirsimaki *et al.*, 1993). This difference in the hepatocarcinogenicity and DNA adduct-forming ability between the tamoxifen derivative toremifene and tamoxifen has also been reported in female Cr1-CD(BR) rats (Hard *et al.*, 1993a, 1993b). The role of DNA adducts in mutation and cancer is well recognised (see review by Hemminki, 1993). Furthermore, in the tamoxifen-treated animals, electron microscopic analysis showed elevation of the volume densities of peroxisomes, mitochondria and residual bodies in non-neoplastic hepatocytes, and in the neoplastic hepatocytes the volume density of nuclei was slightly elevated (Hirsimaki *et al.*, 1993). This proliferation of peroxisomes and mitochondria may thus be related to tumour development in tamoxifen-treated rats.

Tamoxifen can covalently modify the DNA of rodents, and DNA adducts have been found in the livers of female Sprague–Dawley rats injected with tamoxifen and measured using ^{32}P post-labelling (Han and Liehr, 1992; Shimomura *et al.*, 1992). The genotoxic potential of tamoxifen has also been measured in this way in female Fischer F344/N rats, DBA/2 and C57B1/6 mice and human MCL-5 cells (White *et al.*, 1992). It is likely that the extensive metabolism of tamoxifen to its highly reactive epoxide metabolites is responsible for the formation of the observed DNA–tamoxifen adducts in the rat. Furthermore, the genotoxicity of tamoxifen and tamoxifen epoxide in human lymphoblastoid cells containing human cytochromes P-450 has been reported (Styles *et al.*, 1993). In addition, a mechanistic hypothesis for the formation of DNA–tamoxifen adducts following hepatic oxidative metabolism has been proposed (Potter *et al.*, 1994). An increased yield of glutathione *S*-transferase (GST-P)-positive liver pre-neoplastic foci induced by diethylnitrosamine (DENA) or ethylnitrosourea (ENU) in rats pretreated with oestradiol or tamoxifen has been reported (Servais and Galand, 1993). Furthermore, in a human cell line genetically engineered to express several human cytochromes, tamoxifen (at micromolar doses) induced micronuclei by a clastogenetic mechanism (Phillips and Venitt, 1993).

Examination of the effects of tamoxifen on cytochrome P-450 isoenzymes and associated monooxygenase activities in the livers of female Fischer rats and C57B1/6 and DBA/2 mice has shown that total microsomal cytochrome P-450 was not induced in the livers of rats given tamoxifen (45 mg/kg daily for four days) (White *et al.*, 1993). However, the metabolism of benzyloxy- and pentoxyresorufins to resorufins was increased by 30- to 60-fold and ethoxyresorufin *O*-deethylase was induced 2.5-fold. The hydroxylations of testosterone and its oxidation to androstenedione were all increased, and generally tamoxifen produced a mixed pattern of induction with a significant PB-like component. The hydroxylation pathway was not induced in either mouse strain. In rats, tamoxifen pre-treatment resulted in 2- to 3-fold increases in both CYP2B1 and 3A1 proteins. Similar patterns of induction were observed with toremifene and droloxifene (3-hydroxytamoxifen), which are considered to be non-carcinogenic in rats: these tamoxifen derivatives are cleared much faster than tamoxifen and in therapeutic trials three times as much has to be administered to achieve the same efficacy (see Chapter 10). No induction of these monooxygenase activities was observed in C57B1/6 mice and there was only a small increase in benzyloxy- and pentoxyresorufin metabolism in DBA/2 mice. It has been suggested that the induction of cytochrome P-450-dependent activities by tamoxifen may result in accelerated liver metabolism of this drug, which has important implications for its conversion to genotoxic metabolites;

and the difference in inducibility of cytochrome P-450 monooxygenase activities in mice compared to rats suggests that differences in metabolism in these two species may contribute to their different carcinogenic responses. The carcinogenicity of tamoxifen cannot, however, be readily explained on this basis because the non-carcinogenic analogues toremifene and droloxifene (3-hydroxytamoxifen) are also cytochrome P-450 isoenzyme inducers. However, metabolic activation (see above) may still be important because the very small structural differences between tamoxifen and its analogues could result in the generation of metabolites of very different genotoxic potential (droloxifene and toremifene do not produce an increase in modified DNA bases). Furthermore, promoter action on spontaneously initiated genotoxic damage to liver DNA cannot be ruled out at this stage, however.

The activation by metabolism of some compounds is important in their displayed toxicity, and indeed carcinogenicity; small differences, however, in molecular structure can determine the ability of a compound to be carcinogenic through its metabolism. It is important to establish if the effects observed for tamoxifen in rats are pertinent to man (this is discussed further in Chapter 4). It has been suggested that this could be tested in breast cancer patients taking tamoxifen using ^{32}P post-labelling for the presence of tamoxifen–DNA adducts in liver (Phillips and Venitt, 1993); however, preliminary results in a small number of liver biopsy samples from women being treated with tamoxifen showed no significant difference from the control population in terms of presence of ^{32}P post-labelling adducts and indicate that the observed carcinogenicity of tamoxifen in the rat appears not to be relevant to man.

REFERENCES

Bethou, F., Dreano, Y. (1993) *Journal of Chromatography* **616**, 117–128.

Bignall, J. (1993) *Lancet* **341**, 1086.

Blankson, E.A., Ellis, S.W., Lennard, M.S., Tucker, G.T., Rogers, K. (1991) *Biochemical Pharmacology* **42**, S209–S211.

Chamart, S., Haocq, M., Leclercq, G., Devleeschouwer, N. (1993) *International Journal of Pharmaceutics* **99**, 59–66.

Ching, C.K., Smith, P.G., Long, R.G. (1992) *Lancet*, **339**, 940.

Clark, S. (1993) *Lancet* **342**, 168.

Coe, J.E., Ishak, K.G., Ward, J.M., Ross, M.J. (1992) *Proceedings of the National Academy of Sciences USA* **89**, 1085–1095.

Demuylder, X., Neven, P. (1993) *Cancer Journal* **6**, 111–115.

De Vos, D., Mould, G., Stevenson, D. (1989) *Current Therapeutic Research* **46**, 703–708.

Devos, D., Slee, P.H.T.J., Stevenson, D., Briggs, R.J. (1992) *Cancer Chemotherapy and Pharmacology* **31**, 76–78.

Dragan, Y.P., Xu, Y.D., Pitot, H.C. (1991) *Preventative Medicine* **20**, 15–28.

El-Sharkawy, S.H. (1992) *Pharmacology Acta Helvetica* **67**, 15–19.
Fromson, J.M., Pearson, S., Bramah, S. (1973a) *Xenobiotica* **3**, 693–709.
Fromson, J.M., Pearson, S., Bramah, S. (1973b) *Xenobiotica* **3**, 711–714.
Furr, B.J.A., Jordan, V.C. (1984) *Pharmacology and Therapeutics* **25**, 127–205.
Girault, J., Istin, B., Fourtillan, J.B. (1993) *Biological Mass Spectrometry* **22**, 395–402.
Gonzalez, F.J., Nebert, D.W. (1990) *Trends in Genetics* **6**, 182–186.
Greaves, P., Groonetillete, R., Nunn, G., Iophan, J., Oston, T. (1993) *Cancer Research* **53**, 3919–3924.
Han, X.L., Liehr, J.G. (1992) *Cancer Research* **52**, 1360–1363.
Hard, G.C., Iatropoulos, M.J., Jordan, K., Radi, L., Kaltenberg, O.P., Imondi, A.R., Williams, G.M. (1993a) *Cancer Research* **53**, 4534–4541.
Hard, G.C., Williams, G.M., Iatropoulos, M.J. (1993b) *Lancet* **342**, 444–445.
Hemminki, K. (1993) *Carcinogenesis* **14**, 2007–2012.
Herrlinger, C., Braunfels, M., Fink, E., Kinzig, M., Metz, R., Sorgel, F., Vergin, H. (1992) *International Journal of Clinical Pharmacology Therapeutics and Toxicology* **30**, 1487–1488.
Hirsimaki, P., Hirsimaki, Y., Nieminen, L., Payne, B.J. (1993) *Archives of Toxicology* **67**, 49–54.
Jacolot, F., Simon, I., Dreano, Y., Beaune, P., Riche, C., Berthou, F. (1991) *Biochemical Pharmacology* **41**, 1911–1919.
Jordan, V.C. (1993) *British Medical Journal* **307**, 1371–1378.
Langanfahey, S.M., Tormey, D.C., Jordon, V.C. (1990) *European Journal of Cancer* **26**, 883–887.
Le Blanc, G.A., Waxman, D.J. (1989) *Drug Metabolism Reviews* **20**, 395–439.
Lien, E.A, Solheim, E.K., Kvinnsland, S., Ueland, P.M. (1988) *Cancer Research* **48**, 2304–2308.
Lien, E.A., Solheim, E., Lea, O.A., Lundgren, S., Kvinnsland, S., Ueland, P.M. (1989) *Cancer Research* **49**, 2175–2183.
Lien, E.A., Anker, G., Lonning, P.E., Solheim, E., Ueland, P.M. (1990) *Cancer Research* **50**, 5851–5857.
Lien, E.A., Solheim, E., Ueland, P.M. (1991a) *Cancer Research* **51**, 4837–4844.
Lien, E.A., Wester, K., Lonning, P.E., Solheim, E., Ueland, P.M. (1991b) *British Journal of Cancer* **63**, 641–645.
Mani, C., Kuppfer, D. (1991) *Cancer Research* **51**, 6052–6058.
Mani, C., Gelboin, H.V., Park, S.S., Pearce, R., Parkinson, A., Kuppfer, D. (1993a) *Drug Metabolism and Disposition* **21**, 645–655.
Mani, C., Hodgson, E., Kuppfer, D (1993b) *Drug Metabolism and Disposition* **21**, 657–661.
McCague, R., Parr, I.B., Haynes, B.P. (1990) *Biochemical Pharmacology* **40**, 2277–2283.
Meltzer N.M., Stang, P., Sternson, L.A. (1984) *Biochemical Pharmacology* **33**, 115–123.
Merchant, M., Krishnan, V., Safe, S. (1993) *Toxicology and Applied Pharmacology* **120**, 179–185.
Moore, M., Narasimhan, T.R., Steinberg, M.A., Wang, X., Safe, S. (1993) *Archives of Biochemistry and Biophysics* **305**, 483–488.
Murphy, C., Fotsis, T., Pantzar, P., Adlercreutz, H., Martin, F. (1987) *Journal of Steroid Biochemistry* **28**, 609–618.
Pavlik, E.J., Nelson, K., van Nagell, J.R., Jr, Gallion, H.S., Donaldson, E.S., DePriest, P., Meares, K., van Nagell, J.R. (1991) *Gynecology and Obstetrics* **42**, 245–249.
Phillips, D.H., Venitt, S. (1993) *Lancet* **341**, 1486.

Poon, G.K., Chui, Y.C., McCague, R., Lonning, P.E., Feng, R., Rowlands, M.G., Jarman, M. (1993) *Drug Metabolism and Disposition* **21**, 1119–1124.
Powles, T.J., Hardy, J.R., Ashley, S.E., Farrington, G.M., Cosgrove, D., Davey, J.B., Dowsett, M., McKinna J.A., Nash A.G., Sinnett, H.D., Tillyer, C.R., Treleaven, J.G. (1989) *British Journal of Cancer* **60**, 126–131.
Potter, G.A., McCague, R., Jarman, M. (1994) *Carcinogenesis* **15**, 439–442.
Powles, T.J., Tillyer, C.R., Jones, A.L. (1990) *European Journal of Cancer* **26**, 680–683.
Reid, A.D., Horobin, J.M., Newman, E.L., Preece, P.E. (1992) *Breast Cancer Research and Treatment* **22**, 153–156.
Reidy, G.F., Murray, M. (1989) *Biochemical Pharmacology* **38**, 195–199.
Reunitz, P.C., Nanavati, N.T. (1990) *Drug Metabolism and Disposition* **18**, 645–648.
Richardson, D.N. (1988) *Drug Design and Delivery* **3**, 1–14.
Robinson, S.P., Langanfahey, S.M., Johnson, D.A., Jordan, V.C. (1991) *Drug Metabolism and Disposition* **19**, 36–43.
Seoud, M.A.F., Johnson, J., Weald, J.C. (1993) *Obstetrics and Gynecology* **82**, 165–169.
Servais, P., Galand, P. (1993) *International Journal of Cancer* **54**, 996–1001.
Shimomura, M., Higashi, S., Mizumoto, R. (1992) *Japanese Journal of Cancer Research* **83**, 438–444.
Smith, G., Harrison, D.J., East, N., Rae, F., Wolf, H., Wolf, C.R. (1993) *British Journal of Cancer* **68**, 57–63.
Smith, R.P., Dewar, J.A., Winter, J.H. (1993) *Lancet* **341**, 772.
Styles, J.A., Davies, A., Lim, C.K., De Matteis, F., Stanley, L.A., White, I.N.H., Yuan, Z.X., Smith, L.L. (1993) *Carcinogenesis* **15**, 5–10.
Turner, M.J., Fields, C.E., Everman, D.B. (1991) *Biochemical Pharmacology* **41**, 1701–1705.
Uziely, B., Lewin, A., Brufman, G., Dorembus, D. (1993) *Breast Cancer Research and Treatment* **26**, 101–106.
Vancutsem, P., Williams, G.M. (1993) *Lancet* **342**, 873–874.
Waxman, D.J., Azaroff, L. (1992) *Biochemical Journal* **281**, 577–592.
White, I.N.H., Dematteis, F., Davies, A., Smith, L.L, Crofton-Sleigh, C., Venitt, S., Hewer, A., Philips, D.H. (1992) *Carcinogenesis* **13**, 2197–2204.
White, I.N.H., Davies, A., Smith, L.L, Dawson, S., Dematteis, F. (1993) *Biochemical Pharmacology* **45**, 21–30.
Wiebe, V.J., Osborne, C.K., McGuire, W.L., Degregario, M.W. (1992) *Journal of Clinical Oncology* **10**, 990–994.
Williams, G.M., Iatropoulos, M.J., Djordjevic, M.V., Kaltenberg, O.P. (1993) *Carcinogenesis* **14**, 315–318.

4

An Overview of the Clinical Use of Tamoxifen in the Treatment and Prevention of Breast Cancer

BREAST CANCER: A BRIEF OVERVIEW

Breast cancer is the most common single cause of death in women aged 35–54 years, and in the UK alone there are approximately 24 000 new cases of breast cancer each year and 15 000 deaths. A family history of breast cancer on the maternal side is considered to be an important risk factor: risk of developing the disease is two-fold if one first-degree relative has the disease, and this rises to a four-fold risk with two first-degree relatives affected. If the relative had bilateral breast cancer the risk is further increased to about five-fold. Other risk factors include nulliparity or late age at first childbirth and also an early menarche (with onset of ovulatory cycles) and a late menopause. These factors are all associated with ovarian function and with prolonged exposure to the known mitogen, oestrogen, which is important in the promotion phase of breast cancer (see below). Early pregnancy (and possibly breast feeding) may confer protection by resulting in differentiation of the breast cells such that they are no longer sensitive to the mitogenic effects of oestrogen. However, studies on the levels of circulating oestrogen have not yielded a conclusive correlation, probably because of cyclical variability in pre-menopausal women and the very low levels found in post-menopausal women. It is of interest that most plasma oestrogen is bound to sex hormone binding globulin (SHBG); and levels of SHBG are inversely correlated with breast cancer, suggesting that it is the free oestradiol (biologically active) levels that are important and may be a more useful marker of risk than the total level of protein-bound hormone.

Dietary indications in the development of breast cancer

It is thought that 40% of circulating oestrogens are of dietary origin; thus diet is also a factor to consider. Dairy produce is a major source of oestrogens as a result of oestrogen synthesis by gastrointestinal bacteria from cholesterol and bile acids. The level of free oestradiol can be decreased by switching from an average diet (fat providing 40% of calories) to a low-fat diet (20% of calories) and this may be related to elevated SHBG levels (for a brief review of dietary fat and breast cancer see Whittemore and Henderson, 1993 and Freedman *et al.*, 1993). It is of interest that the combined effects of tamoxifen adjuvant therapy (see below) and a low-fat diet on serum binding proteins and oestradiol bioavailability have been studied in post-menopausal women with breast cancer (Rose *et al.*, 1992, 1993). In animal experiments both ovarian-dependent and -independent mammary tumour growth is promoted by a high-fat diet (probably related to fatty acid composition and not total fat content), suggesting that mammary growth stimulation by fatty acids is independent of synthesis of oestrogen in the ovary. In addition, dietary restriction reduces the incidence of *N*-nitroso-*N*-methylurea (NMU)-induced mammary tumours (see Chapter 5) in rats (Chevalier *et al.*, 1993). In one human study post-menopausal women with malignant breast cancer showed increased levels of plasma lipids, total cholesterol, low-density lipoprotein (LDL) cholesterol, very-low-density lipoprotein (VLDL) cholesterol, phospholipids, triacylglycerols and free fatty acids, and decreased levels of high-density lipoprotein (HDL) cholesterol, compared to control subjects (Kumar *et al.*, 1991). These profiles were measured before surgery, which is known to cause changes. Other studies have shown a poorer response to treatment in women with a high fat intake during diagnosis. However, these changes may be as a consequence of altered lipid metabolism arising from the disease or of the risk factors associated with the disease.

Together with prophylactic treatment with tamoxifen, considerable interest has focused on a restricted fat diet as a means of preventing breast cancer; however, this would have to be started early in life (as shown by the major dietary changes observed in migrant studies), and the likelihood of sufficient compliance to have a major effect on this risk factor (high-fat diet) may be unlikely in most cases (Cuzick, 1992). A new study proposed by the US National Institutes of Health (NIH) is aiming to ascertain whether low-fat diets will prevent breast cancer in 160 000 post-menopausal women (Culliton, 1993).

Dietary factors, however, may be important in prolonged survival from breast cancer (Rohan *et al.*, 1993). A better dietary intervention than restricted dietary fat intake alone may be the additional intake of oils that contain particular fatty acids, such as the ω-3 fatty acids found in fish oils, as these have been found to inhibit the growth of breast cancer cell lines *in vitro* and to reduce the production of 16α-hydroxysterone, which may be a promoter of breast cancer. Furthermore, γ-linolenic acid is known to be toxic to human breast cancer cells in culture (Cantrill *et al.*, 1993).

Protection against oxidative damage: use of antioxidants

It is likely that an unfavourable intake of fat can contribute to an increased risk of heart disease in an individual. Particularly important in this respect is the consideration of supplementation with dietary antioxidants such as vitamins C, E and β-carotene to prevent the oxidative damage by free radicals to membrane lipids and lipoproteins that is important in the development of heart disease (and oxidative damage to DNA, which increases the risk of cancer); this is discussed further in Chapter 8. In this connection a prospective study of the intake of vitamins C, E and A and the risk of breast cancer has been reported (Hunter *et al.*, 1993). Furthermore, the effect of the breast cancer treatments themselves on plasma antioxidant levels should be taken into consideration in relation to dietary supplementation with antioxidant vitamins. In one study of 71 women with breast cancer and 95 women with benign breast disease, it was found that in those patients not given post-surgical adjuvant drug therapy levels of α-carotene, lycophene and α- and γ-tocopherol did not change over time (Potischman *et al.*, 1992). On the contrary, those given chemotherapy showed increased levels of retinol and α- and γ-tocopherol, and those on antioestrogen therapy showed increased levels of α-tocopherol. Overall, although the concentrations of carotenoids (lycophene, α-carotene and β-carotene) did not change in breast cancer patients, increased levels of β-carotene were found in patients not receiving drug treatment, and decreased levels in patients receiving antioestrogen treatment.

Development of breast cancer: hormonal and genetic factors

Benign breast disease and in particular atypical epithelial hyperplasia and lobular hyperplasia have been associated with an increased risk of breast cancer. These risk factors are of importance in relation to assessing the likely risk of an individual and thus whether inclusion in the preventive trials with tamoxifen can be recommended. Breast cancers most probably arise in the epithelial cells of the terminal ductal lobular unit. Optimal proliferation of these cells in normal epithelium occurs during the luteal (progestagenic) phase of the menstrual cycle. Oestrogens and progestins (synthetic derivatives of progesterone) are important for both the genesis of human breast cancer and growth of these tumours, once formed (see review by King, 1993). Progestins are likely to be the predominant mitogen for normal breast epithelium, and oestrogens assume this role in neoplastic epithelium. The main evidence that oestrogens are the major adverse factor in the development of human breast cancer is based on the ability of oestrogens to generate mammary tumours in rodents, epidemiological evidence of increased risk with increased exposure to oestrogens, the mitogenic effects of oestrogens on human breast cancer cell lines and the usefulness of antioestrogens such as tamoxifen in treating established breast cancer (King, 1991); the role of the oestrogen receptor is discussed in detail in Chapter 5. The ability of oestrogens to greatly stimulate the proliferation of established breast cancer cells is in contrast to the effects seen *in vivo* with normal epithelial cells and indicates either an increased or changed sensitivity to oestrogen. Increased levels of the oestrogen receptor in neoplastic epithelium may sensitise these cells to oestrogen, which then becomes the main steroidal mitogen. However, although high doses of progestins induce regression of some breast cancers they only weakly inhibit the proliferation of human breast cancer cell lines, and it is not yet clear whether physiological levels of progestins decrease the rate of growth of breast cancer cells (King, 1991, 1993). It is of interest in this connection that a novel molecular graphics study of steroid interactions with a protein, which has relevance to the understanding of the mechanism of steroid recognition, using the anti-progesterone antibody DB3 has been reported (Arevalo *et al.*, 1993).

Considerable effort has been put into studying the genetics of breast cancer (Devillee and Cornelisse, 1990) and into assessing the clinical importance of screening for inherited breast cancer with DNA markers (Lalle *et al.*, 1993; Powles and Baum, 1993). A breast and ovarian cancer susceptibility gene (BRCA1) has been mapped to chromosome 17q12–q21. The majority of families with breast and ovarian cancer seem to be linked to the BRCA1 locus, whereas only 45% of families with site-specific breast cancer are linked to this locus. DNA markers may therefore be of use in identifying pre-clinical cancer in women at very high risk of breast and ovarian cancer in selected families. Human breast tumours have been identified also with translocations involving 12q13–q15 as the sole cytogenetic abnormality (Rohen *et al.*, 1993) and it is of related interest that gene deletion has been proposed as a new target for cancer chemotherapy (Frei, 1993). Neurofibromatosis type 2 (NF2) is a monogenic dominantly inherited disease predisposing carriers to develop nervous system tumours, and the NF2 gene from chromosome 22 has been identified (Rouleau *et al.*, 1993). However, chromosome 22 losses have been reported in tumours outside the nervous system, including those of the breast, and it will be interesting to see if NF2 has any involvement in breast cancer (Kinzler and Vogelstein, 1993).

The biological and endocrinological factors in the development of breast cancer risk from menopausable oestrogen replacement therapy has been discussed (Zumoff, 1993). In addition, life events have been studied in relation to breast cancer prognosis (Barraclough *et al.*, 1993). It was found in 204 patients with operable breast cancer that severe life events were not associated with increased risk of relapse within 42 months of diagnosis, and these negative results persisted in the longer term (more than five years). This is in contrast to earlier studies (Ramirez *et al.*, 1989, 1992) in which the relapsed patients showed more severe life events than the controls.

THERAPY: SOME INVESTIGATIONS AND FINDINGS

Adjuvant therapy

Tamoxifen has been used in the treatment of breast cancer for over 20 years and is probably the most prescribed anticancer drug in the world (see Figure 4.1). It is an orally effective, synthetic, non-steroidal oestrogen antagonist, and also a partial agonist (see Chapter 2) The benefits of tamoxifen were first observed in women with metastatic breast cancer, with approximately 30–60% of patients with metastatic breast cancer responding to tamoxifen treatment. In primary breast cancer the use of tamoxifen as adjuvant therapy prolongs the disease-free survival period and can increase the overall survival period (see below and review by Plowman, 1993). Tamoxifen can produce regressions also in woman with fibrocystic changes including pre-cancerous ones. Although tamoxifen was originally introduced for the treatment of advanced disease in post-menopausal women, it is now also available for the palliative treatment of pre-menopausal women with oestrogen receptor-positive breast cancer. In pre-menopausal women, oophorectomy or radiation-induced menopause is currently the more usual antioestrogenic procedure; this results in remission in approximately 30% of patients.

Tamoxifen is frequently prescribed as an adjuvant to surgery in the treatment of breast cancer. The efficacy of adjuvant therapy in pre-menopausal

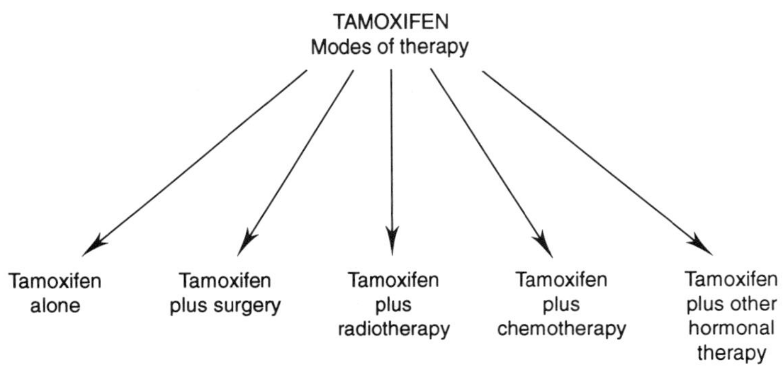

Figure 4.1. Modes of therapy with tamoxifen

women has been assessed (Smith and Hillner, 1993). Furthermore, the efficacy of adjuvant tamoxifen in early breast cancer is considered to be partly independent of oestrogen receptor status (Benson and Baum, 1993). Tamoxifen increases disease-free survival and overall survival rates when given as an adjuvant systemic type of therapy in women with early breast cancer. In one study the effect of adjuvant tamoxifen versus placebo was investigated in elderly women with node-positive breast cancer, and in this study the women were followed-up in the long term and eventual causes of death recorded (Cummings *et al.*, 1993). The effect of adjuvant tamoxifen has been studied in the Cancer Research Campaign (CRC) adjuvant breast trial (Riley *et al.*, 1992) and a study of adjuvant treatment with tamoxifen of lymph node-negative breast cancer in post-menopausal women has also been reported (Kurz *et al.*, 1992). The occurrence of primary tumours in breast cancer patients in a randomised trial of adjuvant tamoxifen therapy has been studied (Rutqvist, 1991). Furthermore, adjuvant endocrine therapy (ovarian ablation and tamoxifen) in addition to cytotoxic polychemotherapy can prevent the recurrence of breast cancer and prolong overall survival (Rutqvist, 1991): in clinical trials in post-menopausal women with node-negative breast cancer, between two and five years of adjuvant tamoxifen therapy provides a survival advantage. The positive effect of tamoxifen as part of adjuvant chemo-endocrine therapy for breast cancer has also been reported (Uchino *et al.*, 1994).

Although tamoxifen has been used as sole therapy for breast cancer in the elderly patient (Foudraine *et al.*, 1992) it has been suggested that treating such patients with tamoxifen alone is no longer justified (Dixon, 1992). Treatment with tamoxifen and optimal surgery versus tamoxifen alone has been studied in a CRC trial with elderly women with breast cancer (Bates *et al.*, 1991). Furthermore, the effectiveness of mastectomy versus tamoxifen as initial therapy for operable breast cancer in elderly patients has been assessed in a five-year follow-up period and a retrospective study has been made of surgical resection plus tamoxifen in the treatment of breast cancer in elderly patients (Martelli *et al.*, 1993).

The usefulness of tamoxifen in axillary node-negative breast cancer has been studied in terms of multisystem benefits and risks (Love, 1992a). In addition, a study has been reported of 62 cases of mammary carcinoma treated with tamoxifen (30 mg per day for six months with a follow-up period of a further six months) as adjuvant and monotherapy, in which after four weeks of treatment a significant improvement in well-being and tumour status was established for a total of 48 of the cases and treatment was reported to be well tolerated (Polubiec *et al.*, 1991). However, side-effects of adjuvant tamoxifen (Leake, 1991) and symptoms associated with tamoxifen treatment in post-menopausal women (Love *et al.*, 1991a) have also been reported (see below). It is of interest that 20 mg of tamoxifen taken once daily has been reported to be bioequivalent to 10 mg twice daily, with no difference in relative risk (Buzdar *et al.*, 1994).

Tamoxifen in combination with chemotherapy

The interaction of tamoxifen with chemotherapy has been studied. It appears that chemotherapy reduces the effect of tamoxifen in patients less than 50 years old and this may be because a greater proportion of younger women have oestrogen receptor-negative tumours. Tamoxifen has several oestrogen receptor independent effects (see Chapters 6–9) and it is possible that these may be inhibited by chemotherapy (A'Hern *et al.*, 1991). It is clear that adjuvant tamoxifen and chemotherapy generally prolongs life and increases disease-free survival of women with breast cancer. A randomised adjuvant trial is in progress to evaluate the addition of tamoxifen to chemotherapy in patients with primary breast cancer, and the results at five years have been reported (Toi *et al.*, 1992). A trial of chemotherapy versus tamoxifen, versus chemotherapy plus tamoxifen in node-positive, oestrogen receptor-positive breast cancer patients is in progress, and a report has been made at seven years (Boccardo *et al.*, 1992). In addition the results of two randomised trials of adjuvant systemic therapy are available. These tested chemotherapy alone, with doxorubicin (adriamycin)–cyclophosphamide (AC) versus doxorubicin–cyclophosphamide–tamoxifen (30 mg per day for two years) or chemotherapy with CMF (cyclophosphamide–methotrexate–fluorouracil) versus tamoxifen. These trials were in 747 women with histologically proven node-positive breast cancer (Kaufmann *et al.*, 1993). It was found in low-risk patients (i.e., relatively good prognosis) that CMF and tamoxifen were equally effective, although in women 49 years old or under CMF was superior to tamoxifen, whereas in those 50 years old or over the opposite was found. In high-risk patients (i.e., relatively poor prognosis) a combination of AC plus tamoxifen was no better than AC, although in women 50 years old or over the addition of tamoxifen to AC resulted in a significantly higher disease-free survival and a better overall survival compared to those women who received AC alone. These somewhat complicated findings suggest that further trials are necessary to determine the role of combined simultaneous or sequential chemoendocrine adjuvant treatment, compared to each single therapy alone.

In pre-menopausal women with early-stage breast cancer, chemotherapy added substantial clinical benefit, whereas tamoxifen alone was most effective in oestrogen receptor-positive patients (Smith and Hillner, 1993). Combined therapy is effective for all women but again is most beneficial in oestrogen receptor-positive patients, although the possible beneficial side-effects of tamoxifen in reducing cardiovascular and osteoporosis mortality (see below) may suggest that combined treatment is desirable for all pre-menopausal women with breast cancer (Smith and Hillner, 1993). It has also been found, in a study of 105 patients with operable breast cancer, that prior adjuvant chemotherapy negatively influenced response to tamoxifen at relapse such that the overall survival of treated and control patients was identical (de Takats *et al.*, 1993).

Tamoxifen in combination with other endocrine therapy

The effect of endocrine therapy with medroxyprogesterone acetate, 4-hydroxyandrostenedione or tamoxifen on plasma concentrations of insulin-like growth factor (see Chapter 6) has been investigated in women with advanced breast cancer (Reed *et al.*, 1992). Medroxyprogesterone acetate (500 mg per day) and aminoglutethimide (55 mg twice daily) have also been used and compared in 257 post-menopausal breast cancer patients who had become resistant to tamoxifen (Garcia-Giralt *et al.*, 1993). Overall it was found that the median time to progression was significantly longer with aminoglutethimide (an inhibitor of aromatase, an enzyme involved in oestrogen synthesis) therapy. Phase III trials comparing aminoglutethimide to tamoxifen in women with metastatic breast cancer have also been reported (Gale *et al.*, 1994). In one study the timing of surgery during the menstrual cycle was investigated in relation to the survival of pre-menopausal women with operable breast cancer (Badwe *et al.*, 1991). Furthermore, the cyclical use of tamoxifen and high-dose medroxyprogesterone acetate in advanced oestrogen receptor-positive breast cancer has been reported (Gundersen, 1991). In addition, steroid hormone agonists, as well as antagonists, have been studied in relation to the treatment of breast cancer (Dreicer and Wilding, 1992). In one study patients who had failed to respond to prior hormonal therapy with tamoxifen and a progestational agent, and patients who had responded to prior hormonal therapy, were treated with fluoxymesterone as a third-line of endocrine therapy for advanced breast cancer (Schifeling *et al.*, 1992). Here it was concluded that third line hormonal therapy with fluoxymesterone can only be recommended as a temporising measure in patients with indolent disease who have responded to prior hormonal therapy. Randomised clinical trials of tamoxifen in combination with progestins for metastatic disease are also in progress (Parazzini *et al.*, 1993).

Tamoxifen in combination with retinoids

Retinoids are synthetic analogues or derivatives of vitamin A (and isomers) and have been shown to inhibit malignant transformation in cells, including breast cancer cells *in vitro* that have already undergone a degree of de-differentiation to the malignant phenotype. Retinoids are thought to increase the activity of growth factors such as the negative growth factor, transforming growth factor β (see Chapter 6). The chemopreventive effect of one retinoid, fenretinide, against carcinogen-induced rodent mammary cancer is well established. The usefulness of tamoxifen in combination with retinoids in breast cancer chemoprevention has been assessed (Costa *et al.*, 1993). Furthermore, the combination of tamoxifen plus fenretinide is more effective than tamoxifen or fenretinide alone in preventing rat mammary cancer. However, less is known about its direct antitumour ability or indeed its toxicity in humans when used in combination with tamoxifen. It has been reported that in a phase I/II trial in women with oestrogen receptor-positive or progesterone receptor-positive breast cancer, previously untreated for metastatic breast cancer and subsequently treated with tamoxifen (20 mg per day) plus fenretinide (100, 200, 300 or 400 mg per day), there were no adverse effects on renal, hepatic, haematological or lipid values; it can be concluded that tamoxifen administered with fenretinide appears to be non-toxic (Cobleigh *et al.*, 1993). Retinoids also have potential for use in the prevention of breast cancer, which is discussed in relation to tamoxifen (see below). It is of related interest that a phase II evaluation has been made of interferon added to tamoxifen (see Chapter 6) in the treatment of metastatic breast cancer (Macheledt *et al.*, 1991).

Tamoxifen as a clinical anti-multidrug resistance agent

It is of interest that high-dose oral tamoxifen is being tested as a potential multidrug resistance reversal agent in combination with vinblastine in phase I clinical trials (Trump *et al.*, 1992). Tamoxifen-treated stage IV breast cancer patients show a reduced occurrence of *mdr-1* amplification compared to patients treated with other endocrine therapies (Lonn *et al.*, 1993). The gene *mdr-1* codes for the P-170 glycoprotein drug-efflux pump responsible for the multidrug resistance effect in tumour cells. The cellular basis for this action of tamoxifen is discussed in Chapter 8. However, other studies have suggested a possible link between the expression of P-glycoprotein and clinical resistance to tamoxifen (Keen *et al.*, 1994) and the cellular basis of this problem is discussed in Chapter 6.

Treatment of male breast cancer

Trials on the use of adjuvant tamoxifen therapy for male breast cancer (MBC) (see Chapter 2) have shown that significant improvement in disease-free survival can be achieved with few side-effects. In one study started in 1976, male patients with stage II and operable stage III breast cancer were given adjuvant tamoxifen for one year (increasing to two years in 1988), where the primary treatment consisted of radical mastectomy or simple mastectomy with radiotherapy; disease-free survival at five years was 56% in tamoxifen treated patients compared to 28% in non-tamoxifen treated patients (Ribeiro and Swindell, 1992).

USE IN TREATMENT OF CANCERS OTHER THAN BREAST CANCER (Figure 4.2)

Pancreatic adenocarcinoma

Pancreatic adenocarcinoma tissue contains oestrogen binding sites, and some studies have suggested that tamoxifen increases the survival of patients with this form of cancer. In one clinical trial 80 patients (50 women and 30 men) with biopsy-documented irresectable or incompletely resected ductal pancreatic adenocarcinoma were treated with tamoxifen (20 mg twice daily). It was found that tamoxifen-treated patients with irresectable or incompletely resected ductal pancreatic carcinoma had a prolonged survival benefit and that this benefit was most obvious in women over 60 years old (Wong and Chan, 1993). However, in another randomised placebo-controlled clinical trial of tamoxifen (20 mg twice daily) in 44 patients with biopsy-proven irresectable pancreatic carcinoma, no significant difference in the duration of survival of patients treated with tamoxifen or placebo was found (Taylor *et al.*, 1993; Morris, 1993). Furthermore, tamoxifen or cyproterone acetate (an antiandrogen) in combination with the luteinising hormone releasing hormone (LHRH) agonist buserelin in nine patients with irresectable pancreatic adenocarcinoma was found to be ineffective (Swarovsky *et al.*, 1993). Further large-scale studies are clearly required to accurately assess the usefulness of tamoxifen in the treatment of irresectable pancreatic carcinoma.

Malignant gliomas

The antitumour effects of tamoxifen have been studied on neuroblastoma cells *in vitro* and *in vivo* (Busse *et al.*, 1991). High dose tamoxifen has been used in the treatment of intracranial malignant gliomas (Vertosick *et al.*, 1992) and recurrent high grade gliomas (Baltuch *et al.*, 1993), and it has been reported that clinical stabilisation and tumour regression can be achieved (Baltuch *et al.*, 1993). Furthermore, a clinical and radiographic response to high-dose tamoxifen treatment has been reported in a minority of patients with recurrent malignant gliomas (Couldwell *et al.*, 1993). The protein kinase C signal transduction system is known to be important in regulating the growth rate of malignant gliomas *in vitro*, and indeed tamoxifen has been shown to inhibit the activity of protein kinase C *in vitro* at micromolar concentrations (see Chapter 7). Tamoxifen administered at doses calculated to give tissue concentrations in the micromolar range was used to treat 11 patients with malignant gliomas (anaplastic astrocytoma or glioblastoma multiforme) who had not responded to treatment with external beam radiation therapy (Couldwell *et al.*, 1993). Here treatment resulted in tumour reduction observed on radiographic images with clinical

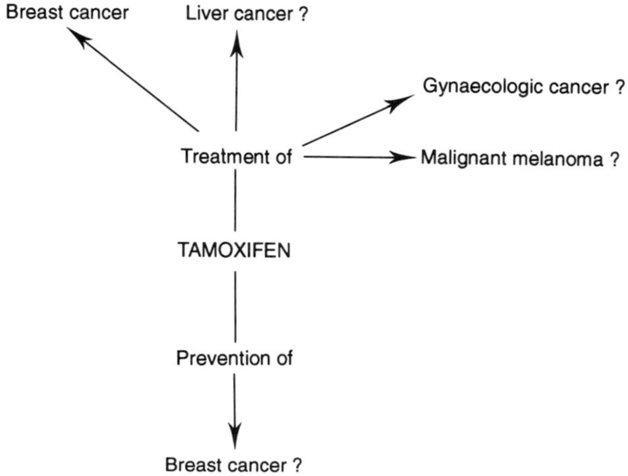

Figure 4.2. Use of tamoxifen in treatment of various cancers

improvement in three patients and halting of tumour progression clinically and radiographically occurred in one other patient.

Hepatocellular carcinoma

Tamoxifen has been reported to be of benefit in the treatment of hepatocellular carcinoma, and controlled trials have been carried out with tamoxifen in patients with unresectable hepatocellular carcinoma (Farinati *et al.*, 1990, 1992). In the earlier study, 38 consecutive cirrhotics (males and females) with unresectable hepatocellular carcinoma were allocated to either 30 mg per day tamoxifen or no treatment. Survival was significantly prolonged in tamoxifen-treated patients, with 22% survival at 12 months compared to only 5% in the untreated group (Farinati *et al.*, 1990). In 53% of tamoxifen-treated patients the levels of α-fetoprotein decreased (a decrease is a favourable prognostic index), and in this subgroup survival was further prolonged. No differences were observed between males and females, or between alcoholic and non-alcoholic cirrhosis. In the later study 32 cirrhotic patients received either 30 mg per day tamoxifen or no treatment (as above) and again survival of the tamoxifen-treated patients was significantly prolonged, with 35% survival at 12 months compared to none in the control group (Farinati *et al.*, 1992). Again no differences were observed between males and females, or between alcoholic and non-alcoholic cirrhosis, and in 40% of patients the levels of α-fetoprotein declined. From these studies it would appear that tamoxifen is effective in the palliative treatment of hepatocellular carcinoma and that an initial decline in α-fetoprotein levels may be a favourable prognostic indicator. It is of associated interest that tamoxifen has been reported to be a promising treatment for chronic hepatic impairment (Kulcsar and Kulcsar-Gergely, 1991).

Renal cell carcinoma

High-dose tamoxifen has been used in progressive, advanced renal cell carcinoma (Stahl *et al.*, 1991) and exerts antitumour effects in a small cohort of cases (Papac and Keohane, 1993). However, combined androgen (testosterone) and Provera, followed by high-dose tamoxifen therapy for metastatic renal cell carcinoma, was found to offer very little therapeutic advantage (Papac and Keohane, 1993). In this study 20 patients, most of whom had failed to respond to androgen and Provera, received tamoxifen 100 mg (twice daily) but only 10% experienced tumour response with tamoxifen. In another study of 62 patients with advanced metastatic renal cell carcinoma treated with high-dose tamoxifen (100 mg twice daily) systemic toxicity was significant (5% showed fatigue and 20% showed moderate anaemia, alopecia and malaise). Antineoplastic efficacy of tamoxifen at this dosage in this cohort of patients was marginal and consistent with the known lack of therapeutic efficacy of endocrine therapy in advanced renal cell carcinoma (Schomburg *et al.*, 1993).

Malignant melanoma

Tamoxifen is used in combination with chemotherapy in the treatment of malignant melanoma (McKeage *et al.*, 1993). High-dose cisplatin has been used with dacarbazine and tamoxifen in the treatment of metastatic melanoma (Buzaid *et al.*, 1991). In addition, metastatic melanoma has been treated with only dacarbazine plus tamoxifen (Coccini *et al.*, 1992). Sequential small phase II trials have shown that tamoxifen is an important component in these combinations (Buzaid and Murren, 1992). Furthermore, the combination of tamoxifen with cisplatin, dacarbazine and carmustine appears to be one of the most effective therapeutic regimes, with an overall response rate approaching 50%, and in some patients responses have been durable and have been found to exceed three years (Buzaid and Murren, 1992). It is of interest that cisplatin and its analogues are used in the treatment of advanced breast cancer (Smith and Talbot, 1992). Furthermore, the tamoxifen derivative toremifene has a cytostatic effect in human melanoma cell lines, and topical toremifene administration in animal models achieves high local concentrations with minimal systemic distribution and, therefore, may be a useful approach for cutaneous melanoma (Maenpaa *et al.*, 1993). The usefulness of tamoxifen in the treatment of patients with metastatic melanoma has been discussed (McClay and McClay, 1994).

Gynaecological malignancies

Tamoxifen can inhibit the growth of human endometrial cells in culture and of endometrial carcinomas in nude mice (see Chapter 5). It is of interest that although medroxyprogesterone acetate can be used in the curative and adjuvant treatment of advanced or early gynaecological cancers, treatment was more successful when medrocyprogesterone acetate was used in combination with tamoxifen (Vanderstappen and Bonte, 1992). Furthermore, in a prospective and randomised study of 540 primary endometrial cancer patients, oxyprogesterone caproate administered pre-operatively and after surgical and combined therapy from 6 to 36 months increased survival rates compared to patients who did not receive hormone treatment. In addition, combination of oxyprogesterone and tamoxifen administered additionally to surgery and combined therapy increased the survival rate at five-year follow-up by 19% (Vishnevsky *et al.*, 1993). These results suggest that adjuvant hormone therapy may have to be administered to endometrial carcinoma patients with an unfavourable disease prognosis for three years or more to obtain an increase in remission. The responsiveness of patients with advanced ovarian carcinoma to tamoxifen has been assessed in a gynaecological oncology group study of second-line therapy in 105 patients (Hatch *et al.*, 1991).

Retroperitoneal fibrosis

Retroperitoneal fibrosis is a benign condition that can have a malignant course because of obstruction and encasement of retroperitoneal structures such as the urinary system. Tamoxifen may be of benefit in the treatment of retroperitoneal fibrosis and also desmoid tumours (Loffeld and Vanweel, 1993; Benson and Baum, 1993). The shared pathology and similarities of retroperitoneal fibrosis and desmoid tumours are worth mentioning; both are tumour-like conditions with enhanced activity of mesenchymal elements (e.g., increased collagen disposition and fibroblast proliferation) and although up to a third of desmoid tumours may contain oestrogen receptors, the measured response rate of tamoxifen (and toremifene) does not correlate with oestrogen receptor status.

SIDE-EFFECTS OF THERAPY

In numerous studies and trials, tamoxifen has been shown to have only limited side-effects. The major symptomatic effects from tamoxifen treatment are vasomotor symptoms hot flushes, sweaty palms or racing heart), gynaecological symptoms (vaginal discharge, bleeding or vaginal/external genitalia irritation), depression and nausea (Love *et al.*, 1991a, 1992b).

Although, in adjuvant studies the patient drop-out rate is only around 4% because of these symptoms, a much greater loss of compliance might be expected in healthy women taking tamoxifen prophylactically (see below). In one study of 75 patients with advanced breast cancer the side-effects of tamoxifen therapy encountered in 10 patients were vaginal discharge, bleeding and hot flushes (Mohapatro *et al.*, 1992). However, hypercalcaemia, tumour flare, and hepatic, renal, cardiac, pulmonary and neurological toxicities were not encountered. When tamoxifen was used in combination with chemotherapy with cyclophosphamide, methotrexate, 5-fluorouracil and prednisone, the combined chemohormonal therapy was mostly well tolerated and any toxicities were temporary and reversible. A toxic interaction has been reported between mitomycin C and tamoxifen, leading to the occurrence of the haemolytic uraemic syndrome (Montes *et al.*, 1993). The clinical recognition and management of depression in node-negative breast cancer patients treated with tamoxifen is clearly important (Cathcart *et al.*, 1993).

As tamoxifen is currently recommended for post-menopausal breast cancer patients receiving definitive radiation therapy after limited surgery, it is of concern that carcinogenic outcome (i.e., incidence of new primary cancers) has been reported for the combined effects of adjuvant tamoxifen treatment and radiotherapy for early breast cancer (Andersson *et al.*, 1991, 1992). This is in contrast to a study of rats with small mammary tumours induced by NMU (see Chapter 5) and treated with tamoxifen, radiation or a combination of these (Kantorowitz *et al.*, 1993). It was found that high-dose radiation alone reduced the size of existing tumours, but also significantly increased the number of tumours that were detected. Tamoxifen alone also caused a reduction in tumour volume but had no effect on final incidence or number of mammary tumours, and combined treatment resulted in both the reduction in the volume of existing tumours and the suppression of the increased occurrence of additional tumours observed with radiation therapy alone. This is likely to be due to tamoxifen-induced cell cycle changes (see Chapter 5) which make the cells more susceptible to radiation inhibition. It has been suggested that in the context of fractionated, high dose radiation treatment of established breast cancers, tamoxifen may reduce subsequent tumour development and may therefore provide a useful simultaneous conjoint adjuvant therapy to post-operative radiation treatment. Further studies are thus required to assess the value of combined tamoxifen and radiation therapy in humans. It should be noted, however, that when exposed to radiation it cannot simply be assumed that all the tamoxifen molecules remain unchanged, particularly as UV radiation has been shown to convert tamoxifen into phenanthrene derivatives (see Chapter 3). A case of tamoxifen-induced radiation recall, which is an inflammatory reaction at a previously irradiated site normally associated with the administration of cytotoxic drugs and is thought to be a delayed form of radiosensitisation, has also been reported (Parry, 1992).

PREVENTION OF BREAST CANCER

Current issues in breast cancer chemoprevention with tamoxifen, in healthy women at risk of breast cancer, have been extensively discussed (Nayfield *et al.*, 1991; Baum *et al.*, 1991a, 1991b; Jordan, 1992a, 1992b; Powles, 1992; Bernstein *et al.*, 1992a; Jordan, 1993a, 1993b; Chlebowski *et al.*, 1993; Vanchien, 1993; Costa, 1993; Clark, 1993; Paterson and Geggie, 1993a; Bush and Helzlsouer, 1993; Leis, 1993; Cuzick *et al.*, 1993) (see Figure 4.3). The ability of tamoxifen to decrease the rates of second primary (or contralateral) breast cancers supports the prediction that tamoxifen can effectively suppress pre-clinical breast cancer (in four trials it decreased the rate by approximately half). Indeed, cancer in the contralateral breast has been proposed as a most appropriate marker for assessing tamoxifen as a preventive agent (Fisher and Redmond, 1991).

Consideration of the long-term effects of tamoxifen is of particular interest. The benefits of prophylactic tamoxifen therapy, including potential protection against coronary heart disease and osteoporosis, in addition to decreasing the risk of breast cancer should outweigh any risk of deleterious side-effects, although this high benefit/risk ratio remains to be demonstrated in large-scale trials.

Breast cancer prevention trials

A double-blind placebo-controlled feasibility trial has been carried out at the Royal Marsden Hospital, London, with 200 women to study the logistical and ethical problems of using tamoxifen in high-risk women to prevent breast cancer (Powles *et al.*, 1990; Jones and Powles, 1992). In a preventive trial involving a large number of healthy women the ethical problems are quite different from those in a chemotherapy trial of patients who already have a disease. This is because although only a small number of women are likely to gain clearly demonstrated protective benefit in these preventive trials, all the women are exposed to the possibility of a long-term unknown chronic toxicity, including the theoretical possibility of hepatocellular carcinoma (see below and Chapter 3). In this trial participation was based on fully informed consent, and eligible healthy volunteers (examination and mammography were used to exclude breast cancer patients) were offered regular follow-up and screening and could withdraw at will. The volunteers were randomised to receive tamoxifen (20 mg per day) or placebo for two years. Overall, little difference in the acute toxicity between the tamoxifen and placebo groups was found, with

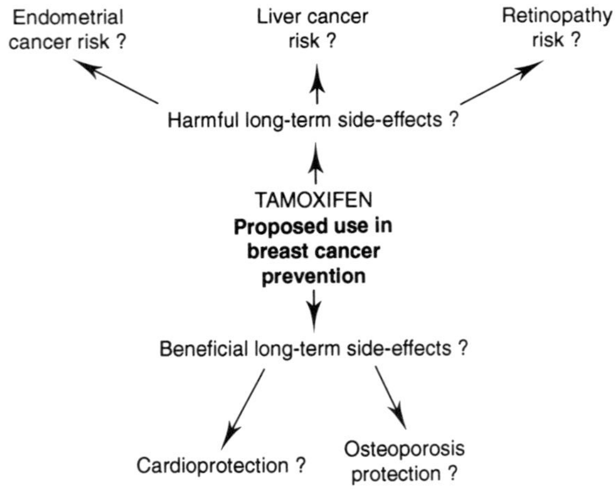

Figure 4.3. Possible side-effects of tamoxifen

the possible exception that hot flushes were more prevalent in tamoxifen-treated women, and there were no significant differences in nausea, headaches, weight gain, depression or menstrual changes between the two groups. In addition, compliance after one year was greater than 80% in both groups and this is clearly a reflection of the relatively low toxicity of tamoxifen. The changes in lipid profiles (see below) were similar to those observed in women receiving oral contraceptives or oestrogen replacement therapy. This feasibility study has been extended to a pilot trial for up to 1000 women taking tamoxifen or placebo for up to five years (Jones and Powles, 1992), and the promising data so far achieved from the feasibility and pilot trials have led to the suggestion of a large UK prevention trial involving about 10 000 women: from this it would be hoped to detect a 25% prevention rate. Indeed in November 1993 national trials began at the Christie Hospital in Manchester (and other centres will also join this trial) with 15 000 healthy women aged 45 and over with a family history of breast cancer.

A large-scale breast cancer prevention trial, which will involve 16 000 high-risk women in the United States (The National Surgical Adjuvant Breast and Bowel Project), was launched in 1992 and so far 5000 women have been recruited (it is hoped to give half the women tamoxifen—20 mg daily for a minimum of five years—and half placebo) (Facundus *et al.*, 1993). Preventive trials with tamoxifen are being planned in many other countries: in Italy, a trial has started with 20 000 volunteers (Veronesi *et al.*, 1992; Jordan, 1993b).

GENERAL BENEFICIAL EFFECTS OF TREATMENT AND PROPHYLAXIS

There are many indications of possible beneficial effects of tamoxifen therapy, especially in relation to the incidence of coronary heart disease and of osteoporosis in women.

Cardiovascular considerations

Although hormonally related cancers are the most common causes of death in women aged 40–60 years old, after the age of 60 myocardial infarction becomes the leading cause of death and far exceeds all other causes in later years. It is likely to be of great importance, therefore, that tamoxifen has significant effects on the risk factors for coronary heart disease (CHD) and stroke. Retrospective studies on the two randomised arms of the Scottish adjuvant tamoxifen trial have shown that tamoxifen treatment significantly reduced the incidence of fatal myocardial infarction (McDonald and Stewart, 1991), and it appears that tamoxifen therapy for at least five years as an adjuvant to breast cancer has a cardioprotective oestrogen-like action in post-menopausal women.

Adjuvant tamoxifen treatment in a group of 123 consecutively and newly diagnosed women with stage I and II breast cancer resulted in a significant decrease in serum cholesterol levels compared with a control group of 81 consecutively diagnosed women with stage I and II breast cancer who were not taking a hormonal treatment or supplement (Schapira *et al.*, 1990). Decreases in serum cholesterol of more than 10 mg/dl were recorded in 72.9% of tamoxifen-treated patients compared to 35.1% of controls and of more than 40 mg/dl in 39.9% of tamoxifen-treated patients compared to 12.6% of controls; age and initial serum cholesterol level were found to be important factors in producing a decrease in serum cholesterol.

Tamoxifen treatment was found to lower total cholesterol levels by 26 mg/dl (from 216 mg/dl at baseline to 190 mg/dl after three months of treatment) and lower LDL cholesterol levels by 20% (from 138 mg/dl at baseline to 110 mg/dl at follow-up) in the Wisconsin Tamoxifen Study, which was a randomised placebo-controlled, double-blind toxicity trial in disease-free women (Love *et al.*, 1990, 1991b; Love, 1992b). These changes were maintained throughout two years of tamoxifen therapy although minor increases in triglycerides were recorded, and the long-term effects of tamoxifen on blood lipid levels in breast cancer patients have been studied (Dewar *et al.*, 1992). In addition, decreases in HDL cholesterol were observed, but no clear picture of the effect of tamoxifen on HDL cholesterol has been reported. Women with greater baseline cholesterol levels had greater decreases with tamoxifen treatment. It is of interest that plasma glucose levels, weight and diastolic and systolic blood pressure levels did not change. A reduction in cholesterol levels (15% compared to pre-treatment values) was also reported from the Royal Marsden Hospital preventive feasibility trial, which was again in disease-free women (Powles *et al.*, 1990; Jones and Powles, 1992). It is of interest also that tamoxifen has been reported to decrease total cholesterol levels after only two weeks of treatment (Love *et al.*, 1993). These changes all suggest a favourable effect on CHD risk with tamoxifen treatment. Furthermore, the antioxidant action of tamoxifen, particularly its ability to protect human low density lypoproteins (LDL) against the oxidative damage implicated in atherogenesis (see Chapter 8) is another likely benefit of tamoxifen therapy for breast cancer (Wiseman, 1994; Wiseman *et al.*, 1994).

A study of 140 post-menopausal women with surgically resected breast cancer who were disease free and participating in a study of tamoxifen toxicity (see the Wisconsin Tamoxifen Study, above) showed decreased fibrinogen levels at six months in tamoxifen-treated subjects by 52 mg/dl (from a baseline of 320 mg/dl to 268 mg/dl), and this may be associated with a decreased risk of arterial thrombosis (Love *et al.*, 1992b; Love, 1992b). Tamoxifen, however, caused a small decrease in antithrombin III levels at six months (antithrombin III levels were elevated at baseline), although no subject exhibited a clinically significant decrease in antithrombin III level and this is unlikely, therefore, to explain the small thrombophlebitis-promoting effect of tamoxifen. Similarly, although tamoxifen has been reported to cause small decreases in antithrombin III in post-menopausal women receiving long-term adjuvant therapy, associated thromboembolism was rare (Henderson *et al.*, 1993). In the Royal Marsden Hospital pilot trial (Powles *et al.*, 1990) no adverse effect on coagulation (fibrinogen/antithrombin III ratio) was detected. Although the oestrogen agonist action of tamoxifen could be responsible for the increased risk of arterial and venous thrombosis observed in breast cancer patients, studies have shown no increased incidence of thromboembolism in tamoxifen treated patients compared to placebo (Jones and Powles, 1992) and haemostatic changes and thromboembolic risk during tamoxifen (single-agent) therapy have also been examined in normal women (Jones *et al.*, 1992). The increased thromboembolic risk in breast cancer patients and its occurrence as a complication of tamoxifen therapy at a rate of one per 800 treatment years may in fact be related to the disease status and to concomitant assignment to chemotherapy.

Cardiac and thromboembolic morbidity has also been studied in post-menopausal women with early-stage breast cancer in the Stockholm randomised trial of adjuvant tamoxifen (40 mg daily for two or five years) versus no adjuvant endocrine therapy (Rutqvist and Mattsson, 1993). Short-term tamoxifen therapy was found significantly to reduce the incidence of hospital admissions due to cardiac disease. Furthermore, there was again a statistically significant reduction with the longer tamoxifen therapy period of five years. However, there was very little difference between the tamoxifen and control groups in the incidence of admissions due to thromboembolic disease. In addition, tamoxifen has been shown to reduce vasomotor symptoms over a period of time (Love and Feyzi, 1993). The effects of combined tamoxifen and medroxyprogesterone treatment (see above) for advanced breast cancer on the coagulation/fibrinolytic systems have also been considered (Fukutomi *et al.*, 1993).

Osteoporosis

In Western countries, in women over the age of 55 major bone fractures, particularly of the spine and hip resulting from osteoporosis, are responsible for as much hospitalisation as breast cancer. Studies including nuclear activation analysis and absorptiometry indicate that even though tamoxifen is usually considered to be an antioestrogen in relation to the treatment and prevention of breast cancer, it does not induce osteoporosis, thus suggesting it is acting here as an oestrogen agonist (Kalef-Ezra *et al.*, 1992). Similarly, the effects of tamoxifen on bone mineral density (Love *et al.*, 1992a; Neal *et al.*, 1993) and the effect of long-term tamoxifen treatment on bone turnover (Wright *et al.*, 1993) in women with breast cancer have been reported. The Wisconsin Tamoxifen Study found a statistically significant preservation of bone density in the lumbar spine, and a trend towards preservation of bone density was found in the radius (Love, 1992b; Love *et al.*, 1992a). Using photon absorptiometry, it was shown that in women given tamoxifen the mean bone mineral content of the lumbar spine increased by 0.61% per year compared to a decrease of 1% per year in the control group, whereas radial bone mineral density decreased to the same extent in both groups (Love *et al.*, 1992a). Tamoxifen treatment also resulted in a significant decrease in serum osteoclacin and alkaline phosphatase concentrations, but did not effect the level of serum parathyroid hormone or of 1,25-dihydroxyvitamin D. Tamoxifen has been shown to reduce bone turnover and prevent lumbar spine and proximal femoral bone loss in early post-menopausal women (Ward *et al.*, 1993). Furthermore, tamoxifen protects against steroid-induced bone loss in women (Fentiman *et al.*, 1992). Preventive treatment with tamoxifen could in the course of time be expected to lead to a 25% decrease in fracture rates in a manner similar to oestrogen (Love, 1992b).

Similarly, in laboratory animals tamoxifen decreases the rate of readsorption of trabecular bone, resulting in the preservation of bone density. Thus the bone density and mineral content of the femora were significantly decreased in ovariectomised mice compared to control animals, whereas tamoxifen-treated animals did not show a decrease in bone density, or in calcium and phosphate content of the femora (Broulik, 1991). In addition, uterine weight in tamoxifen-treated ovariectomised mice was the same as in intact controls, and these actions of tamoxifen show it is acting as an oestrogen agonist in this species. In the rat, tamoxifen prevents the oestrogen-deficiency bone loss that is caused by the LHRH agonist buserelin (Gollding *et al.*, 1992). Tamoxifen and oestrogen both affect serum osteoclacin levels in ovariectomised rats (Williams *et al.*, 1991).

Osteoarthritis

It is of associated interest that tamoxifen can inhibit the oestradiol-induced early changes in osteoarthritis (Tsai and Liu, 1992), and in contrast to its beneficial oestrogen agonist action against CHD and osteoporosis, this is fortuitously an oestrogen antagonist action. Furthermore, oestradiol has been shown to accelerate rat femoral head cartilage degradation *in vivo* and *in vitro*, as assessed by glycosaminoglycan content, and this effect is blocked by tamoxifen (Chander and Desa, 1991).

LONG-TERM SAFETY OF PROPHYLACTIC TAMOXIFEN

Endometrial cancer risk

Long-term tamoxifen therapy as a cause of the development of cancer of the endometrium in some patients is a problem that has attracted considerable attention (Wolf and Jordan, 1992; O'Connell and Arnold, 1993; Paterson and Geggie, 1993b; Rayter *et al.*, 1993; McAuliffe and Foley, 1993; Neven, 1993; Fornander *et al.*, 1993; Van Leeuwan *et al.*, 1994; Kedar *et al.*, 1994). It is of related interest, therefore, that tamoxifen can inhibit the growth of human endometrial cells in culture and of endometrial carcinomas in nude mice (see also Chapter 5). The possibility that tamoxifen can cause endometrial cancer suggests that its usefulness in the treatment of endometrial cancer (see above) and indeed in the prevention of breast cancer remains to be assessed.

It is likely to be the oestrogenic action of tamoxifen that is implicated in the development of endometrial carcinoma. Tamoxifen is known to affect the endometrium (Uziely *et al.*, 1993) and endometrial changes have been reported in post-menopausal women treated for breast cancer with tamoxifen (Seoud *et al.*, 1993; Cohen *et al.*, 1993). In addition, tamoxifen has been implicated in the formation of endometrial lesions (Neven, 1993; Neven *et al.*, 1993), and endometrial changes and lesions in post-menopausal women treated with tamoxifen have been discussed (Ugwumadu, 1993; Cohen, 1993). Endometrial abnormalities have in some cases been associated with tamoxifen therapy and a sonographic and pathogenic correlation has been made (Hulka and Hall, 1993; Goldstein, 1994). A study has been made of 17 patients with endometrial cancer that occurred during or after adjuvant tamoxifen treatment in early breast cancer (Fornander *et al.*, 1993) and tamoxifen has been reported to induce adenomyosis and adenomyomatous endometrial polyps (Ugwumadu *et al.*, 1993). Results of a case study of intestinal and pelvic endometriosis presenting as a tumour in a patient undergoing tamoxifen therapy have been reported (Hajjar *et al.*, 1993).

In one study the endometrium of 103 gynaecologically-asymptomatic post-menopausal breast cancer patients was examined (51 tamoxifen treated and 52 not tamoxifen treated) and compared with control subjects. The tamoxifen patients had a thicker endometrium and larger uterine volume (Lahti *et al.*, 1993); in addition, endometrial polyps were more frequent in the tamoxifen group. These results provide evidence for an oestrogenic long-term tamoxifen effect on the post-menopausal uterus, and this appears to be associated with an increased occurrence of polyps. Post-menopausal bleeding from unusual endometrial polyps in four women on chronic tamoxifen therapy have been reported (Corley *et al.*, 1992). In these patients the polyps demonstrated cystically dilated glands in all cases and stromal decidualisation in two of these patients. Furthermore, in one of these patients metastatic breast carcinoma was present in the polyp. In another investigation, 94 women were examined (49 on tamoxifen and 45 controls) and a greater proportion of women taking tamoxifen had endometrial cell hyperplasia compared to the controls (16% versus 9%); however, this difference was not significant and only one patient from each group had dysplastic (pre-cancerous) endometrial cells and, most importantly, no cases of invasive endometrial cancer were detected (Rayter *et al.*, 1993).

Endometrial decidual changes have also been reported in a post-menopausal woman treated with a combination of tamoxifen and megestrol acetate (Cohen *et al.*, 1992). Furthermore, tamoxifen inhibited decidual induction in pseudopregnant rats (Barkai *et al.*, 1992). Gestagens and synthetic oestrogens can cause metaplastic changes in the epithelial cells of the endometrium, and tamoxifen can act like a gestagen on the endometrium (Lang-Averous *et al.*, 1991). In this study of 31 women who were treated with tamoxifen for breast cancer, three developed endometrial endocarcinoma. It is of interest also that gestagens and tamoxifen stimulated mucinous and clear cell metaplasia, whereas squamous and tubal metaplasia are most often stimulated by oestrogens and develop in hyperplastic endometrium. In further studies seven (Malfetano, 1990) and three (Spinelli *et al.*, 1991) cases respectively of endometrial carcinoma were reported in women on tamoxifen therapy for breast carcinomas.

Gynaecological tumours in women treated for breast cancer with tamoxifen is a relatively rare problem but one that requires careful monitoring. Indeed, to date there are relatively few reports of endometrial cancer being diagnosed during adjuvant therapy with tamoxifen; however, any instances of uterine bleeding or spotting should be followed up with an endometrial biopsy.

Retinopathy risk

Tamoxifen-induced retinopathy is a rare but serious complication of tamoxifen therapy (Bentley *et al.*, 1992). In one case study a 68-year-old woman with metastatic breast carcinoma presented with tamoxifen-induced retinopathy after nine years of low-dose tamoxifen therapy (Chang *et al.*, 1992). However, when treatment with the drug was stopped partial resolution of the retinopathy occurred and improvement in visual acuity was recorded over a $2\frac{1}{2}$-year follow-up period. In another study of long-term low-dose tamoxifen therapy in 63 patients, evidence of ocular toxicity was also found (Pavlidis *et al.*, 1992). Tamoxifen was administered to these patients on a 20 mg per day basis and four patients displayed retinopathy and/or keratopathy 10, 27, 31 and 35 months respectively after the start of tamoxifen therapy. The ophthalmological findings in these patients included decreased visual acuity, bilateral macular oedema and yellow–white dots in the paramacular and foveal areas. Furthermore, corneal opacity was found in one patient. Again, upon withdrawal of tamoxifen therapy, almost all ocular abnormalities were found to be reversible, except for the corneal opacity.

Is tamoxifen generally safe?

The molecular and cellular basis of the problem of the DNA adducts reported in rat liver has been discussed (see Chapter 3). Furthermore, oestrogens are known liver carcinogens in the rat, and as tamoxifen has oestrogenic properties in rodents and humans this finding is not unexpected. A similar problem might be expected with oral contraceptives as their oestrogen component also induces rat liver tumours; however, although use in women for at least five years continuously increases the risk of hepatocellular carcinoma 10-fold, this risk is considered epidemiologically insignificant because this tumour is very rare in Western countries (five per 100 000) (Jordan, 1993b). Concerns about high doses of tamoxifen acting as a promoter of liver cancers in rats (only two cases of hepatocellular carcinoma have been reported in women receiving 40 mg of tamoxifen per day) or as a promoter of endometrial cancer in woman have not, as yet, been proved to be of great clinical relevance. It is relevant to note that the efficacy of oral contraceptives in preventing ovarian and endometrial cancer is well established, although their use is associated with increased risk of breast cancer in a duration-dependent manner (Bernstein *et al.*, 1992b).

Another point of concern is the effect of tamoxifen on ovarian function in pre-menopausal woman and the potential risks to the fetus if pregnancy does occur. Although there are no reports about the teratogenicity of tamoxifen in the human (see Chapter 3) it should not be used if the patient is pregnant and women should be counselled about the possible risk associated with pregnancy during tamoxifen treatment. Furthermore, in pre-menopausal women the use of an oral contraceptive with added benefit of breast cancer prevention is desirable and a trial, therefore, of the addition of the tamoxifen analogue toremifene (used in the treatment of tamoxifen-resistant cancer which does not form DNA adducts in rat liver; see Chapter 3) to the contraceptive pill is planned at the Royal Marsden Hospital with 200 young women with a family history of breast cancer. The use of prophylactic tamoxifen in younger women (aged up to 35), but only those with a strong family history of breast cancer, may be justified on the basis that some epidemiological and laboratory studies have shown breast tissue may be most susceptible to carcinogenic insult in early puberty, and that antihormone therapy is most effective closer to the time of insult (Jordan, 1993b). The beneficial effects on lipid levels and on bone density also support this potential usage in younger women.

The protection against CHD and other beneficial oestrogenic actions of tamoxifen, in addition to its likely preventive action against breast cancer, has led to the possibility of combining hormone replacement and tamoxifen therapy in women who have an increased risk of breast cancer and menopausal symptoms. This is of interest because many post-menopausal women receive hormone replacement therapy (HRT; with oestrogens) and the exact impact of this HRT on the incidence of breast cancer is not clear. Oestrogen replacement therapy has many benefits, including the prevention of CHD, in addition to the prevention of osteoporosis and vasomotor symptoms. Unfortunately HRT can be a cause of endometrial cancer and its use requires the careful monitoring recommended for tamoxifen use. It would appear that the use of particular oestrogens especially with the addition of a progestin is not associated with an increased risk of breast cancer. Furthermore, it has been suggested that patients who have already undergone successful treatment for oestrogen-dependent tumours, including endometrial carcinoma, should not necessarily be excluded from receiving oestrogen replacement therapy (Gelety and Judd, 1992).

In conclusion, it is clear that a full evaluation of the safety of tamoxifen can only be determined in large-scale randomised trials. The vast genetic and biochemical differences and thus differing responses that are evident among individuals in a population necessitate the maintenance of reasonable care in health monitoring, and in observation and reporting adverse reactions to the prophylactic and therapeutic use of tamoxifen.

REFERENCES

A'Hern, R.P., Baum, M., Dowsett, M. (1991) *Lancet* **337**, 439.

Andersson, M., Storm, H.H., Mouridsen, H.T. (1991) *Journal of the National Cancer Institute* **83**, 1013–1016.

Andersson, M., Storm, H.H., Mouridsen, H.T. (1992) *Acta Oncologica* **31**, 259–264.

Arevalo, J.H., Taussig, M.J., Wilson, I.A. (1993) *Nature* **365**, 859–863.

Badwe, R.A., Gregory, W.H., Chaudary, M.A., Richards, M.A., Bentley, A.E., Rubens, R.D., Fentiman, I.S. (1991) *Lancet* **337**, 1261–1264.

Baltuch, G., Schenouda, G., Langleben, A., Villemire, J.G. (1993) *Canadian Journal of Neurological Science* **20**, 168–174.

Barkai, U., Kidron, T., Kraicer, P.F. (1992) *Biology of Reproduction* **46**, 733–739.

Barraclough, J., Osmond, C., Taylor, I., Perry, M., Collins, P. (1993) *British Medical Journal* **25**, 1563.

Bates, T., Riley, D.L., Houghton, J., Fallowfield, L., Baum, M. (1991) *British Journal of Surgery* **78**, 591–594.

Baum, M., Houghton, J., Riley, D. (1991a) *Lancet* **338**, 114.

Baum, M., Ziv, Y., Colletta, A.A. (1991b) *British Journal of Cancer* **64**, 205–207.

Benson, J.R., Baum, M. (1993) *Lancet* **341**, 836.

Bentley, C.R., Davies, G., Aclimandos, W.A. (1992) *British Medical Journal* **304**, 495–496.

Bernstein, L., Ross, R.K., Henderson, B.E. (1992a) *Monographs of the National Cancer Institute* **12**, 137–147.

Bernstein, L., Ross, R.K., Henderson, B.E. (1992b) *American Journal of Epidemiology* **135**, 142–152.

Boccardo, F., Rubagotti, A., Amoroso, D., Sismondi, P., Genta, F., Nenci, I., Piffanelli, A. (1992) *European Journal of Cancer* **28**, 673–680.

Broulik, P.D. (1991) *Endocrinology and Regulation* **25**, 217–219.

Bush, T.L., Helzlsouer, K.J. (1993) *Epidemiologic Reviews* **15**, 233–243.

Busse, E., Bartsch, O., Kornhuber, B. (1991) *Journal of Cancer Research and Clinical Oncology* **117**, 449–453.

Buzaid, A.C., Murren, J.R (1992) *International Journal of Clinical Laboratory Research* **21**, 205–209.

Buzaid, A.C., Murren, J.R., Durivage, H.J. (1991) *Cancer* **68**, 1238–1241.

Buzdar, A.U., Hortobagyi, G.N., Frye, D., Ho, D., Booser, D. J., Valero, V., Holmes, F.A., Birmingham, B.K., Bui, K., Yeh, C. (1994) *Journal of Clinical Oncology* **12**, 50–54.

Cantrill, R.C., Ellis, G., Chisholm, K., Horrobin, D.F. (1993) *Cancer Letters* **72**, 99–102.

Cathcart, C.K., Jones, S.E., Pumroy, C.S., Peters, G.N., Knox, S.M. (1993) *Breast Cancer Research and Treatment* **27**, 277–282.

Chander, C.L., Desa, F.M. (1991) *Agents and Actions* **34**, 282–284.

Chang, T., Gonder, J.R., Ventresca, M.R. (1992) *Canadian Journal of Ophthalmology* **27**, 148–149.

Chevalier, S., Tuchweber, B., Bhat P.V., Lacroix, A. (1993) *Nutritional Cancer* **20**, 187–191.

Chlebowski, R.J., Butler, J., Nelson, A., Lillington, L. (1993) *Cancer* **72** (suppl. Aug. 1), 1032–1037.

Clark, S. (1993) *Lancet* **342**, 168.

Cobleigh, M.A., Dowlatshahi, K., Deutsch, T.A., Mehta, R.G., Moon, R.C., Minn, F., Benson, A.B., Rademaker, A.W., Ashenhurst, J.B., Wade, J.L. (1993) *Journal of Clinical Oncology* **11**, 474–477.

Coccini, G., Bella, M., Calabrein, F., Tonato, M., Canaletti, R., Boni, C., Buzzi, F., Ceci, G., Corgna, E., Costa, P. (1992) *New England Journal of Medicine* **327**, 516–523.
Cohen, I. (1993) *British Journal of Obstetrics and Gynaecology* **100**, 705.
Cohen, I., Shapira, J., Altaras, M.M., Cordoba, M., Rosen, D., Beyth, Y. (1992) *British Journal of Obstetrics and Gynaecology* **99**, 773–774.
Cohen, I., Rosen, D.J.D., Shapira, J., Cordoba, M., Gilboa, S., Altaras, M.M., Yigael, D., Beyth, Y. (1993) *British Journal of Obstetrics and Gynaecology* **100**, 567–570.
Corley, D., Rowe, J., Curtis, M.T., Hogan, W.M, Noumoff, J.S., Livolsi, V.A. (1992) *Obstetrics and Gynecology* **79**, 111–116.
Costa, A. (1993) *Lancet* **342**, 444.
Costa, A., Sacchini, V., Pecensi, A. (1993) *International Journal of Clinical and Laboratory Research* **23**, 53–55.
Couldwell, W.T., Weiss, M.H., DeGiorgio, C.M., Weiner, L.P., Hinton, D.R., Erresmann, G.R., Conti, P.S., Apuzzo, M.L.J., Kornblith, P., Detriboler, W. (1993) *Neurosurgery* **32**, 485–490.
Culliton, B.J. (1993) *Nature* **366**, 11.
Cummings, F.J., Gray, R., Tormy, D.C., Davis, T.E., Volks, H., Harris, J., Falkson, G., Bennett, J.M. (1993) *Journal of Clinical Oncology* **11**, 29–35.
Cuzick, J. (1992) *Cancer Detection and Prevention* **16**, 81–85.
Cuzick, J., Allen, D., Baum, M., Barrett, J., Clark, G., Kakkar, V., Melissari, E., Moniz, C., Mlooe, J., Parsons, V. (1993) *European Journal of Cancer* **29A**, 15–20.
de Takats, P.G., Dunn, J.A., Kerr, D.J., Morrison, J.M. (1993) *Cancer Treatments Review* **19** (suppl. B), 11–19.
Devillee, P., Cornelisse, C.J. (1990) *Cancer Surveys* **9**, 605–630.
Dewar, J.A., Horobin, J.M., Preece, P.E., Tavendale, R., Tunstallpedoe, H., Wood, R.A.B. (1992) *British Medical Journal* **305**, 225.
Dixon, J.M. (1992) *British Medical Journal* **304**, 996–997.
Dreicer, R., Wiliding, G. (1992) *Cancer Investigation* **10**, 27–42.
Facundus, M., Lifsey, D., Kardinal C.G. (1993) *Journal of the Louisiana State Medical Society* **145**, 147–149.
Farinati, F., Salvagnini, M., DeMaria, N., Fornasiero, A., Chiaramonte, M., Rossaro, L., Naccarato, R. (1990) *Journal of Hepatology* **11**, 297–301.
Farinati, F., DeMaria, N., Fornasiero, A., Salvagnini, M., Fagiuoli, S., Chiaramonte, M., Naccarato, R. (1992) *Digestive Diseases and Sciences* **37**, 659–662.
Fentiman, I.S., Saad, Z., Caleffi, M., Chaudary, M.A., Fogelman, I. (1992) *European Journal of Cancer* **28**, 684–685.
Fisher, B., Redmond, C. (1991) *Journal of the National Cancer Institute* **83**, 1278–1281.
Fornander, T., Hellstrom, A.C., Mobersi, B. (1993) *Journal of the National Cancer Institute* **85**, 1850–1855.
Foudraine, N.A., Verhoef, L.C.G., Burghouts, J.T.M. (1992) *European Journal of Cancer* **28A**, 900–903.
Freedman, L.S., Prentice, R.L., Clifford, C., Harlan, W., Henderson, M., Rossoulo, J. (1993) *Journal of the National Cancer Institute* **85**, 764–765.
Frei, E. (1993) *Lancet* **342**, 665–669.
Fukutomi, T., Adachi, I., Watanabe, T., Nanasawa, T., Yamamoto, H. (1993) *Acta Oncologica* **32**, 573.
Gale, K.E., Andersen, J.W., Tormey, D.C., Mansour, E.G., Davis, J.E., Horton, J., Wolter, J.M., Smith, T.J. Cummings, F.J. (1994) *Cancer* **73**, 354–361.
Garcia-Giralt, E., Ayme, Y., Carton, M., Daban, A., Delozier, T., Fargeot, P., Fumoleau, P., Gorins, A., Guerin, D., Guerin, R. (1993) *Breast Cancer Research and Treatment* **24**, 139–145.

Gelety, T.J., Judd, H.L. (1992) *Current Opinions in Obstetrics and Gynecology* **4**, 346–353.
Goldstein, S.R. (1994) *American Journal of Obstetrics and Gynecology* **170**, 447–451.
Goulding, A., Gold, E., Fey, W. (1992) *Bone and Mineral* **18**, 143–152.
Gundersen, S. (1991) *European Cancer News* **4**, 1–2.
Hajjar, L.R., Kim, W.S., Nolm, G.H., Turner, S., Raju, U.R. (1993) *Obstetrics and Gynecology* **82**, 642–643.
Hatch, K.D., Beecham, J.B., Blessing, J.A., Creasman, W.T. (1991) *Cancer* **68**, 269–271.
Henderson, B.E., Ross, R.K., Pike, M.C. (1993) *Science* **259**, 633–638.
Hulka, C.A., Hall, D.A. (1993) *American Journal of Roentgenology* **160**, 809–812.
Hunter, D.J., Manson, J.E., Colditz, G.A., Stampfer, M.J., Rosner, B., Hennekens, C.H., Speizer, F.E., Willett, W.C. (1993) *New England Journal of Medicine* **329**, 234–240.
Jones, A.L., Powles, T.J. (1992) In *Introducing New Treatments for Cancer: Practical, Ethical and Legal Problems* (ed. C.J. Williams), John Wiley & Sons, Chichester, pp. 323–339.
Jones, A.L., Powles, T.J., Treleaven, J.G., Burman, J.F., Nicolson, M.C., Chung, H.I., Ashley, S.E. (1992) *British Journal of Cancer* **66**, 744–747.
Jordan, V.C. (1992a) *Current Problems in Cancer* **16**, 129–176.
Jordan, V.C. (1992b) *Journal of the National Cancer Institute* **84**, 231–234.
Jordan, V.C. (1993a) *British Journal of Pharmacology* **110**, 507–518.
Jordan, V.C. (1993b) *British Medical Journal* **307**, 1371–1372.
Kalef-Ezra, J., Glaros, D., Klouvas, G., Hatzikonstantinou, J., Karantanas, A., Siamopoulos, K.C., Pavlidis, N. (1992) *British Journal of Radiology* **65**, 417–420.
Kantorowitz, D.A., Thompson, H.J., Furmanski P. (1993) *International Journal of Radiation Oncology Biology and Physics* **26**, 89–94.
Kaufmann, M., Jonat, W., Abel, U., Hilfrich, J., Caffier, H., Kreienberb, R., Trams, G., Brunnert, K., Schermann, J., Kleine, W. (1993) *Journal of Clinical Oncology* **11**, 454–460.
Kedar, R.P., Bourne, T.H., Powles, T.J., Collins, W.P., Ashley, S.E., Cosgrove, D.O. (1994) *Lancet* **343**, 1318–1321.
Keen, J.C., Miller, E.P., Bellamy, C., Dixon, J.M., Miller, W.R. (1994) *Lancet* **343**, 1047–1048.
King, R.J.B. (1991) *Journal of Steroid Biochemistry and Molecular Biology* **39**, 811–818.
King, R.J.B. (1993) *Breast Cancer Research and Treatment* **27**, 3–15.
Kinzler, K.W., Vogelstein, B. (1993) *Nature* **363**, 495.
Kulcsar, A., Kulcsar-Gergely, J. (1991) *Arzneimittelforschung* **41**, 1298–1301
Kumar, K., Sachdanandam, P., Arivazhagan, R. (1991) *Biochemistry International* **23**, 581–589.
Kurz, C., Scholten, C., Zielinski, C., Czerwenka, K., Kubista, E., Spona, J., Sevelda, P. (1992) *Deutsche Medizinische Wochenschrift* **117**, 1943–1946.
Lahti, E., Blanco, G., Kauppila, A., Apaja-Sarkkinen, M., Taskinen, P.J., Laatikainen, T. (1993) *Obstetrics and Gynecology* **81**, 660–664.
Lalle, P., Bignon, Y.J., Stoppalyonnert, D., Narod, S.A., Rio, P., Courjal, F., Bartholin, P., Sobel, H., Powles, T.J., Baum, M. (1993) *Lancet* **341**, 1422.
Lang-Averous, G., Rupp, K., Wehner, H., Dallenbach-Hellweg, G. (1991) *Verhlag Deutsche Gerschalt Pathologie* **75**, 366–369.
Leake, R.E. (1991) *British Medical Journal* **303**, 1061.
Leis, H.P. Jr (1993) *International Surgery* **78**, 176–182.
Loffeld, R.J.L.F., Vanweel, T.F. (1993) *Lancet* **341**, 382.

Lonn, Y., Lonn, S., Stenkvist, B. (1993) *International Journal of Cancer* **53**, 574–578.
Love, R.R. (1992a) *Cancer Investigation* **10**, 587–594.
Love, R.R. (1992b) In *Introducing New Treatments for Cancer: Practical, Ethical and Legal Problems* (ed. C.J. Williams), John Wiley & Sons, Chichester, pp. 342–356.
Love, R.R., Feyzi, J.M. (1993) *Journal of the National Cancer Institute* **85**, 673.
Love, R.R., Cameron, L., Connell, B.L., Leventhal, H. (1991a) *Archives of Internal Medicine* **151**, 1842–1850.
Love, R.R., Wiebe, D.A., Newcombe, P.A., Cameron, L., Leventhal, H., Jordan, V.C., Feyzi, J., DeMets, D.L. (1991b) *Annals of Internal Medicine* **115**, 860–864.
Love, R.R., Mazess, R.B., Barden, H.S., Epstein, S., Newcombe, P.A., Jordan, V.C., Carbone, P.P., DeMets, D.L. (1992a) *New England Journal of Medicine* **326** 852–856.
Love, R.R., Surawicz, T.S., Williams, E.C. (1992b) *Archives of Internal Medicine*, **152**, 317–320.
Love, R.R., Mamby, C.C., Feyzi, J.M. (1993) *Journal of the National Cancer Institute* **85**, 1344–1346.
Macheledt, J.E., Buzdar, A.U., Hortobagyi, G.N., Frye, D.K., Gutterman, J.U., Holmes, F.A. (1991) *Breast Cancer Research and Treatment* **18**, 165–170.
Maenpaa, J., Dooley, T., Wurz, G., Vandenberg, J., Robinson, E., Emshoff, V., Sipila, P., Wiebe, V., Day, C., DeGregorio, M. (1993) *Cancer Chemotherapy and Pharmacology* **32**, 392–395.
Malfetano, J.H. (1990) *Gynecological Oncology* **39**, 82–84.
Martelli, G., Moglia, D., Boracchi, P., Delprato, I., Galante, E., Depato, G. (1993) *European Journal of Cancer* **29A**, 2080–2082.
McAuliffe, F.M., Foley, M.E. (1993) *Lancet* **342**, 1124.
McClay, E.F., McClay, M.E.T. (1994) *Journal of Clinical Oncology* **12**, 617–620.
McDonald, C.C., Stewart, H.J. (1991) *British Medical Journal* **303**, 435–437.
McKeage, M.J., Lorentzos, A., Gore, M.E. (1993) *New England Journal of Medicine* **328**, 140.
Mohapatro, S.K., Dandapat, M.C., Padhi, N.C. (1992) *Journal of the Indian Medical Association* **90**, 39–42.
Montes, A., Powles, T.J., Obrien, M.E.R., Ashley, S.E., Luckit, J., Treleaven, J. (1993) *European Journal of Cancer* **29A**, 1854–1857.
Morris, D.L. (1993) *British Journal of Surgery* **80**, 1083.
Nayfield, S.G., Karp, S.E., Ford, L.G., Dorr, F.A., Kramer, B.S. (1991) *Journal of the National Cancer Institute* **83**, 1450–1459.
Neal, A.J., Evans, K., Hoskin, P.J. (1993) *European Journal of Cancer* **29A**, 1971–1972.
Neven, P. (1993) *Lancet* **342**, 452.
Neven, P., Shepherd, J.H., Lowe, D.G. (1993) *British Journal of Obstetrics and Gynaecology* **100**, 893–897.
O'Connell, G., Arnold, A. (1993) *Canadian Medical Association Journal* **148**, 2113.
Papac, R.J., Keohane, M.F. (1993) *European Journal of Cancer* **29A**, 997–999.
Parazzini, F., Colli, E., Scatigna, M., Tozzi, L. (1993) *Oncology* **50**, 483–489.
Parry, B.R. (1992) *Lancet* **340**, 49.
Paterson, A.H.G., Geggie, P.H.S. (1993a) *Canadian Medical Association Journal* **148**, 141–144.
Paterson, A.H.G., Geggie, P.H.S. (1993b) *Canadian Medical Association Journal* **148**, 2114.
Pavlidis, N.A., Petris, C., Briassoulis, E., Klouvas, G., Psilas, C., Rempapis, J., Petroutsos, G. (1992) *Cancer* **69**, 2961–2964.
Plowman, P.N. (1993) *Drugs* **46**, 819–833.

Polubiec, A., Pietrzak, J., Pniewska, I., Freisleben, G. (1991) *Acta Medica Austriaca* **18**, 130–132.

Potischman, N., Byers, T., Houghton, L., Root, M., Nemoto, T., Campbell, T.C. (1992) *Cancer Epidemiology, Biomarkers and Prevention* **1**, 555–559.

Powles, T.J. (1992) *Lancet* **340**, 1145–1146.

Powles, T.J., Baum, M. (1993) *Lancet* **341**, 1422.

Powles, T.J., Tillyer, C.R., Jones, A.L., Ashley, S.E., Treleaven, J., Daveyt, J.B., McKinna, J.A. (1990) *European Journal of Cancer* **6**, 680–684.

Ramirez, A.J., Craig, T.J.K., Watson, J.P., Fentiman, I.S., North, W.R.S., Rubens, R.D. (1989) *British Medical Journal* **289**, 291–293.

Ramirez, A.J., Richards, M.A., Gregory, W.M., Craig, T.J.K., Watson, J.P., Fentiman, I.S. (1992) *British Medical Journal* **304**, 1632.

Rayter, Z., Shepherd, J., Gazet, J.C., Trott, P., Svensson, W., A'Hern, R. (1993) *Lancet* **342**, 1124.

Reed, M.J., Chrisodoulides, A., Koistinen, R., Seppala, M., Teale, J.D., Ghilchik, M.W. (1992) *International Journal of Cancer* **52**, 200–212.

Ribeiro, G., Swindell, R. (1992) *British Journal of Cancer* **65**, 252–254.

Riley, D., Baum, M., MacIntyre, J., Berstock, D., Mckinna, A., Jackson, I., Sainsbury, J.R.C. (1992) *European Journal of Cancer* **28A**, 904–907.

Rohan, T.E., Hillers, J.E., Mcmichael, A.J. (1993) *Nutritional Cancer* **20**, 167–178.

Rohen, C., Bonk, U., Staats, B., Barnitzke, S., Bullerdiek, J. (1993) *Cancer Genetics and Cytogenetics* **69**, 68–71.

Rose, D.P., Chlebowski, R.J., Connolly, J.M., Jones, L.A., Wynder, E.L. (1992) *Cancer Research* **52**, 5386–5390.

Rose, D.P., Connolly, J.M., Chelbowski, R.T., Buzzard, I.M., Wynder, E.L. (1993) *Breast Cancer Research and Treatment* **27**, 253–262.

Rouleau, G.A., Mere, P., Lutchman, M., Sanson, M., Zucman, J., Marineau, C., Hoang-Xuan, K., Demczuk, S., Demaze, C., Plougastel, B., Pulst, S.M., Lenoir, G., Bijlsma, E., Fashold, R., Dumanski, J., de Jong, P., Parry, D., Eldrige, R., Aurias, A., Delattre, O., Thomas, G. (1993) *Nature* **363**, 515–521.

Rutqvist, L.E. (1991) *Medical Oncology and Tumour Pharmacotherapeutics* **8**, 163–168.

Rutqvist, L.E., Mattsson, A. (1993) *Journal of the National Cancer Institute* **85**, 1398–1406.

Schapira, D.V., Kumar, N.B., Lyman, G.H. (1990) *Breast Cancer Research and Treatment* **17**, 3–7.

Schifeling, D.J., Jackson, D.V., Zekan, P.J., Muss, H.B. (1992) *American Journal of Clinical Oncology* **15**, 233–235.

Schomburg, A., Kirchner, H., Fenner, M., Menzel, T., Poliwoda, H., Atzpodien, J. (1993) *European Journal of Cancer* **29A**, 737–740.

Seoud, M.A.F., Johnson, J., Weed, J.C. (1993) *Obstetrics and Gynecology* **82**, 165–169.

Smith, T.J., Hillner, B.E. (1993) *Journal of Clinical Oncology* **11**, 771–776.

Smith, I.E., Talbot, D.C. (1992) *British Journal of Cancer* **65**, 787–793.

Spinelli, G., Bardazzi, N., Citernesi, A., Fontanarosa, M., Curiel, P. (1991) *Journal of Chemotherapy* **3**, 267–270.

Stahl, M., Schmoll, E., Becker, H., Schicter, A., Hoffmann, L., Wagner, H., Possinger, K., Muller, W., Kollermann, M., Weidenhammer, W. (1991) *Seminars in Oncology* **18** (suppl. 4), 33–37.

Swarovsky, B., Wolf, M., Havemann, K., Arnold, R. (1993) *Oncology* **50**, 226–229.

Taylor, O.M., Benson, E.A., Mcmahon, M.J. (1993) *British Journal of Surgery* **80**, 384–386.

Toi, M., Hattori, T., Agkagi, M., Inokuchi, K., Orita, K., Sugimachi, K., Dohi, K., Nomura, Y., Monden, Y., Hamada, Y. (1992) *Cancer* **70**, 2475–2483.
Trump, D.L., Smith, D.L., Ellis, P.G., Rogers, M.P., Schold, S.C., Winer, E.P., Panella, T.J., Jordan, V.C., Fine, R.L. (1992) *Journal of the National Cancer Institute* **84**, 1811–1815.
Tsai, C.L., Liu, T.K. (1992) *Life Sciences* **50**, 1943–1951.
Uchino, J. Samejima, N., Tanable, T., Hayasaka, H., Mito, M., Hata, Y., Asaishi, K., Sasaki, M., Ogita, M., Saito, T. (1994) *British Journal of Cancer* **69**, 767–771.
Ugwumadu, A.H.N. (1993) *British Journal of Obstetrics and Gynaecology* **100**, 704.
Ugwumadu, A.H.N., Bower, D., Ho, P.K.H. (1993) *British Journal of Obstetrics and Gynaecology* **100**, 386–387.
Uziely, B., Lewin, A., Brufman, G., Dorembus, D. (1993) *Breast Cancer Research and Treatment* **26**, 101–106.
Vanchien, C. (1993) *Journal of the National Cancer Institute* **85**, 1450.
Vanderstappen, D., Bonte, J. (1992) *European Journal of Gynaecological Oncology* **13**, 113–123.
Van Leeuwen, F., Benraadt, J., Coebergh, J.W.W., Kiemeney, L.A.L.M., Gimbrère, C.H.F., Otter, R., Schouten, L.J., Damhuis, R.A.M., Bontenbal, M., Diepenhorst, F.W., van den Belt-Dusebout, A.W., van Tinteren, H. (1994) *Lancet* **343**, 448–452.
Veronesi, U., Maltoni, C., DePalo, G., Costa, A., D'Aiuto, G., Boyle, P., Audisio, R., Zurrida, S. (1992) In *Progress and Perspectives in Chemoprevention of Cancer* (eds G. DePalo, M. Sporn, U. Veronesi), Raven Press, New York, pp. 267–277.
Vertosick, F.T., Selker, R.G., Pollack, I.F., Arena, V. (1992) *Neurosurgery* **30**, 897–903.
Vishnevsky, A.S., Bokhman, Ya.V., Loutfi, G. (1993) *European Journal of Gynaecological Oncology* **14**, 150–153.
Ward, R.L., Morgan, G., Dalley, D., Kelley, P.J. (1993) *Bone and Mineral* **22**, 87–94.
Whittemore, A.S., Henderson, B.E. (1993) *Journal of the National Cancer Institute* **85**, 762–763.
Williams, D.C., Paul, D.C., Black, L.J. (1991) *Bone and Mineral* **14**, 205–220.
Wiseman, H. (1994) *Lancet* **343**, 598.
Wiseman, H., Rice-Evans, C., Halliwell, B. (1994) *Breast Cancer Research and Treatment* **29**, 307.
Wolf, D.M., Jordan, V.C. (1992) *Gynecology and Oncology* **45**, 118–128.
Wong, A., Chan, A. (1993) *Cancer* **71**, 2200–2203.
Wright, C.D.P., Mansell, R.E., Gazet, J.C., Compston, J.E. (1993) *British Medical Journal* **306**, 429.
Zumoff, B. (1993) *Steroids* **58**, 196–204.

5

Oestrogen Receptor-mediated Mechanisms of Anticancer Action of Tamoxifen

FEATURES OF HUMAN BREAST CANCER CELLS

Human breast cancer cell lines such as the oestrogen receptor-positive MCF-7 cell line have been widely used in the study of the oestrogen receptor-dependent mode of action of tamoxifen. The MCF-7 cell line was cultivated from an effusion derived from a patient with breast cancer, whose disease was previously controlled by radiotherapy and hormone therapy; this cell line has a tendency to undergo spontaneous genetic variations in culture as shown by karyotypic analysis. MCF-7 cells, which are fully transformed according to the criteria of immortalised growth, anchorage independence, aneuploidy and a lack of serum requirement, have been found to possess progesterone and glucocorticoid receptors (in addition to the oestrogen receptor).

Another oestrogen-responsive breast cancer cell line, EFF-3 that may be of use in investigating the oestrogen receptor-dependent mechanism of action of tamoxifen, has been isolated and characterised (Healicon *et al.*, 1993). The heterogeneity of progesterone content, analysed by quantitative dual-parameter flow cytometry, has been used to characterise subpopulations of cultured human breast cancer cells (Graham *et al.*, 1992). It is also of interest that subtypes of non-transformed human mammary epithelial cells cultured *in vitro* can now be identified and that histo blood group antigen-H type 2 defines basal cell-derived cells (Karsten *et al.*, 1993). Furthermore, a myoepithelial cell line has been derived from normal human breast (Seitz *et al.*, 1993). The effects of tamoxifen on the morphology and evolution of the non-cancerous mouse mammary gland have also been studied (Kotoula and Karkavelas, 1993).

ACTION OF TAMOXIFEN ON CANCER CELL GROWTH

A direct mitogenic effect of exogenous 17β-oestradiol on MCF-7 cell growth, and the ability to prevent the growth inhibitory effects of low concentrations of tamoxifen (i.e., 1 μM), has been demonstrated for this cell line (Furuya *et al.*, 1989) (see Figure 5.1). The inhibitory effect of tamoxifen on MCF-7 cell growth at low concentrations of tamoxifen (0.1–2.5 μM) can be reversed by the addition of oestradiol to the culture medium. Between 2.5 and 7.5 μM of tamoxifen, more marked growth inhibition was observed. At concentrations over 10 μM, tamoxifen had a cytotoxic effect on MCF-7 and other breast cancer cell lines and caused cell death within 48 h. Furthermore, at concentrations above 10 μM, tamoxifen has been reported to have an oestrogen-irreversible effect on MCF-7 and other breast cancer cell lines. Similar studies have been carried out using oestrogen receptor-positive and receptor-negative ovarian cancer cell lines (Langdon *et al.*, 1990). In other oestrogen receptor-negative cell lines such as the BT-20 cell line, tamoxifen was found to inhibit growth at identical concentrations to those at which it inhibited the growth of MCF-7 cells.

A novel series of cycloproyl antioestrogens have been demonstrated to have an antiproliferative activity on MCF-7 human breast cancer cells in culture (Jain *et al.*, 1991). In addition the phenanthrenes produced by exposure of tamoxifen to ultraviolet (UV) irradiation suppressed MCF-7 cell growth in a dose-dependent manner, but these were not as effective

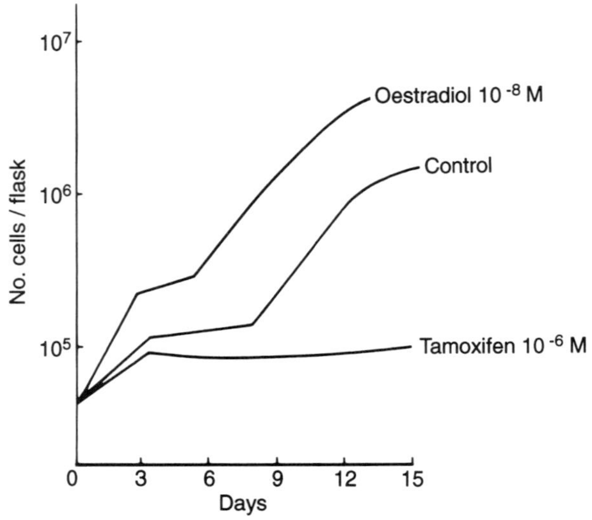

Figure 5.1. Simplified scheme for the stimulation of growth of MCF-7 breast cancer cells by oestradiol and inhibition by tamoxifen

as tamoxifen and, in contrast to treatment with tamoxifen, growth could not be restored by simultaneous exposure to oestradiol (Wilson and Reunitz, 1993). Retinoic acid has also been shown to have an anti-oestrogenic effect in MCF-7 cells (Demirpence *et al.*, 1992) and the interactive effects of interleukin-6, 17β-oestradiol and progesterone on growth in human breast carcinoma cells have been studied (Speirs *et al.*, 1993).

The ability of tissue culture conditions to determine the effects of oestrogen and growth factors on the anchorage-independent growth of human breast cancer cell lines has been reported (Zugmaier *et al.*, 1991). Commercial preparations of charcoal-stripped (to remove steroids) adult bovine serum, which can be used to replace calf serum (which has to be charcoal stripped in the laboratory) have been used in the study of oestrogenic responses and the control of proliferation MCF-7 cells (Welshons *et al.*, 1992). In another study, although tamoxifen inhibited the growth of rapidly growing MCF-7 cells (i.e., supplemented with oestradiol) and pre-incubation with tamoxifen prevented subsequent oestradiol-stimulated growth, it did not inhibit the growth of MCF-7 cells in the dormant or slow growth phase i.e. in oestradiol-free medium (Tanino *et al.*, 1993).

In the soft agar clonogenic assay, which has been used to study the hormone dependency of the MCF-7 cell line under conditions of anchorage-independent growth in serum-free media, physiologically relevant concentrations of oestradiol, progesterone and prolactin were found similarly to stimulate MCF-7 cell colony formation even in the absence of serum (Manni *et al.*, 1991). Furthermore, addition of an antibody against insulin-like growth factor 1 (IGF-1) inhibited the ability of oestradiol and progesterone, but not prolactin, to stimulate growth. Antibodies against transforming growth factor α (TGF-α) or epidermal growth factor inhibited only oestradiol-stimulated growth in soft agar. TGF-β1, -β2 and -β3 suppressed cell colony formation to an extent comparable to that observed with 4-hydroxytamoxifen, and an antibody against TGF-β completely reversed the growth-inhibitory effect of 4-hydroxytamoxifen. These findings suggest that IGFs and TGF-α are important in the control of MCF-7 cells in soft agar and that TGF-β plays a role in mediating the growth-inhibitory action of antioestrogens. In addition, these growth factors do not appear to modulate the action of prolactin, whereas IGFs may be involved in the action of progesterone. Growth factors are discussed further in Chapter 6.

Tamoxifen and 4-hydroxytamoxifen demonstrated a good ability to suppress the anchorage-independent growth of MCF-7 cells (73% and 90%, respectively). These cells exhibited linear cell-proliferative kinetics with a 41 h population doubling time and a 15% colony-forming efficiency in 0.33% agar (Suto *et al.*, 1993). In addition, 4-hydroxytamoxifen induced a 1.3-fold increase in the extent of 2-hydroxylation of oestradiol. This may contribute to the growth-inhibitory ability of 4-hydroxytamoxifen because the metabolic ability of cells to biotransform oestradiol may modulate growth.

Progestins have been shown to influence the proliferation of oestrogen-dependent breast cancer cells in liquid culture under growth factor-defined conditions (Vanderburg *et al.*, 1992), and the mechanisms of growth inhibition by antioestrogens and progestins have been studied in human breast and endometrial cancer cells (Murphy *et al.*, 1992). The stimulation of breast cancer cell growth by norgestrol and gestodene has been reported to occur through an oestrogen receptor-mediated mechanism (Catherino *et al.*, 1993).

An outline of the action of tamoxifen on cell cycle parameters

The effects of 17β-oestradiol and its metabolites (Lottering *et al.*, 1992) and of tamoxifen and derivatives (Suzuki, 1992; Tominaga *et al.*, 1993) on the cell cycle in MCF-7 cells have been studied. It has been found that tamoxifen reduced the proportion of cells in S phase and increased the number of cells in G_0/G_1, probably by arresting the cells in this early G_0/G_1 phase of the cell cycle. Furthermore, combined effects of tamoxifen and RU486 on the MCF-7 cell cycle have been reported (Thomas and Monet, 1992). A tamoxifen-induced increase in the potential doubling time of MCF-7 xenografts has been demonstrated by bromodeoxyuridine labelling and flow cytometry techniques (Sarkaria *et al.*, 1993). The role of signals, genes (Muller *et al.*, 1993) and epidermal growth factor (EGF) (Farnham *et al.*, 1993) in the control of the mammalian cell cycle has been extensively reviewed. Furthermore, oestradiol and EGF have been shown to be requirements for cell cycle progression in normal human mammary epithelial cells in culture (Coulomb *et al.*, 1991). It is of interest that the enzyme aromatase, which is involved in the biosynthesis of oestrogen (see Chapter 7), has been shown to contribute to DNA synthesis in MCF-7 cells (Kitawaki *et al.*, 1992). A 28 kDa protein has been identified in MCF-7 cells whose phosphorylation by protein kinase C is induced by protein kinase C activators such as the phorbol ester 12-*O*-tetradecanoyl phorbol-13-acetate (TPA), which has identity with both the oestrogen-regulated 24 kDa protein and the mammalian heat-shock protein 27 (see Chapter 6). It is thought that this protein may play a key role in the proliferation and differentiation of MCF-7 cells (Faucher *et al.*, 1993).

An oestrogen-irreversible concentration of tamoxifen (10 μM) inhibited proliferation of both T47D cells and MDA-MB-330 cells, which are oestrogen receptor negative, in an oestrogen-independent manner (Murphy and Sutherland, 1985). The cell cycle effects of tamoxifen in the MDA-MB-330 cell line were a decreased proportion of cells in the G_0/G_1 phase of the cell cycle and an increase in the proportion of cells in both the S phase and

$G_2 + M$ phase (Murphy and Sutherland, 1985); results are clearly different from those seen with the oestrogen receptor-positive MCF-7 cells. This observation is consistent with different mechanisms of action in the two cell lines, and suggests that the effects of tamoxifen on tumour growth should not be considered simply as an inhibition of oestrogen action; hence antioestrogens and oestrogens may be able to influence tumour cell growth in ways independent of the classical oestrogen receptor system. Apoptosis (programmed cell death) has also been studied in an oestrogen-independent human breast cancer cell line, MDA-MB-468 (Armstrong *et al.*, 1992), and this important area of cancer research should greatly increase our understanding of how to restore malignantly transformed cells to normal.

INTERACTIONS WITH THE OESTROGEN RECEPTOR AND OTHER STEROID RECEPTORS

Oestrogens acting via the oestrogen receptor are able to regulate nuclear events, including the activation of DNA polymerases, in the process leading to cell division. In this connection, there is evidence for the involvement of two different mechanisms in the oestrogenic and anti-oestrogenic down-regulation of oestrogen receptor levels (Gyling *et al.*, 1990). Differential interactions of oestrogens and antioestrogens at the 17β-hydroxy (or counterpart) moiety with the oestrogen receptor have been studied (Borgna and Scalia, 1991). A variety of monoclonal antibodies have been developed against the oestrogen receptor that recognise different antigenic determinants on the molecule and hence enable conformational changes induced by different ligands to be detected. The monoclonal antibody D547 developed against the oestrogen receptor from MCF-7 cells was able to discriminate between the activated and non-activated forms of the oestrogen receptor from fetal guinea-pig uterus.

It has been reported that antioestrogens such as tamoxifen can establish non-productive receptor complexes and thus alter chromatin structure at target enhancers (Pham *et al.*, 1991). However, although physicochemical and conformational differences between oestrogen receptor-tamoxifen and oestrogen receptor-oestradiol have been reported to exist, which underlie their differing nuclear interactions with chromatin that cause altered cellular proliferation (Green, 1990; Korach *et al.*, 1991; Ruth *et al.*, 1991), there is currently no overall hypothesis to explain the properties of the drug and to delineate its oestrogen-dependent mode of action at the molecular level. This is especially important because tamoxifen shows partial agonist action in addition to antagonistic action in some oestrogen-sensitive systems. A better understanding of this mode of action of tamoxifen may be possible through the use of pure oestrogen receptors, obtained by recombinant DNA technology. It is of considerable interest, therefore, that the human oestrogen receptor (Ricketts *et al.*, 1991) has been expressed in yeast (Metzger *et al.*, 1988). Clearly, the oestrogen receptor as a therapeutic target in breast cancer is attracting renewed interest.

Oestrogen receptor expression in normal and malignant breast tissue is heterogeneous (Walker *et al.*, 1992). Tamoxifen has been found to up-regulate the oestrogen receptor in human breast cancer (Noguchi *et al.*, 1993) and transcriptional control of the oestrogen receptor in oestrogen receptor-negative breast carcinoma has been examined (Weigel and Deconnide, 1993). The effects of oestrogenic and antioestrogenic triphenylethylene derivatives on oestrogen and progesterone receptor levels have been examined in MCF-7 cells (Legros *et al.*, 1991). Expression of the oestrogen receptor in MCF-7 cells appears to be a complex process that involves several steps subject to hormonal regulation by oestrogen: oestrogen suppresses oestrogen receptor mRNA by inhibition of oestrogen receptor gene transcription at early times and by a post-transcriptional effect on receptor mRNA at later times that is mediated through the oestrogen receptor, independent of protein synthesis (Martin *et al.*, 1993). The suppression of oestrogen receptor mRNA by oestrogen was blocked by 4-hydroxytamoxifen, which (as found for tamoxifen itself) is a competitive oestrogen antagonist. In addition, the expression of the oestrogen receptor and TGF-α has been studied in MCF-7 cells after exposure to fractionated irradiation (Schmidtullrich *et al.*, 1992). Variant messenger RNA for the oestrogen receptor lacking exon 4 has been reported in oestrogen-responsive breast cancer cell lines (Pfeffer *et al.*, 1993), while the acquisition of hormone-independent growth in MCF-7 cells is accompanied by increased expression of oestrogen-regulated genes but without detectable DNA amplifications (Brunner *et al.*, 1993).

The interaction of tamoxifen with oestrogen receptors from uterine myoma and unaltered myometrium has been described (Kareva and Kostyleva, 1993), and the effect of tamoxifen on oestrogen receptors during the luteal phase of the menstrual cycle has been studied using immunohistochemical techniques (Maentausta *et al.*, 1993). Recombinant human interferon-α_{2a} has been found to increase hormone receptor levels in a human breast carcinoma xenograft in nude mice and also enhances the antiproliferative action of tamoxifen (Josui *et al.*, 1992). Furthermore, recombinant interferon-α_{2b} alters proliferation, levels of steroid receptors and sensitivity to tamoxifen in cultured breast cancer cells (Sica *et al.*, 1992). The synergistic actions of tamoxifen and interferons are discussed in Chapter 6.

An important finding is that increased basement membrane invasiveness is associated with the absence of the oestrogen receptor and expression of vimentin in human breast cancer cells (Thompson *et al.*, 1992). It should be noted that the interaction with the basement membrane enables the growth and differentiation patterns of normal and malignant human breast epithelial cells to be rapidly distinguished (Petersen *et al.*, 1992). Studies of molecular mechanisms of metastasis should be facilitated by such investigations.

Molecular studies on the structure of the oestrogen receptor

The effect of ligand binding and DNA binding on the structure of the mouse oestrogen receptor has been reported: differences in DNA binding activity were found for oestradiol, 4-hydroxytamoxifen and a pure oestrogen antagonist (ICI 164, 384); however, no differences were detected in the cleavage pattern produced by proteases such as trypsin (Emmas *et al.*, 1992). Mutant mouse oestrogen receptors have been generated, which differ in their sensitivity to oestrogen and 4-hydroxytamoxifen (Danielian *et al.*, 1993). The ability of the oestrogen receptor to bind oestradiol and stimulate transcription is abolished by mutation of the glycine amino acid residue at position 525 in the oestrogen receptor protein and the methionine and/or serine at positions 521/522. However, these mutant receptors retained the partial agonist activity exhibited by the wild-type receptor in the presence of 4-hydroxytamoxifen. These mutations did not affect the expression and DNA binding ability of the receptor but prevented the oestrogen-induced increase in the mobility of the receptor-DNA complex observed with the wild-type receptor.

The structure of the DNA binding domain of the oestrogen receptor has now been solved (Schwabe *et al.*, 1990) and a minimal oestrogen receptor DNA binding domain has been defined (Mader *et al.*, 1993). Binding analysis of the oestrogen receptor to its specific DNA target site in human breast cancer has been carried out (Foster *et al.*, 1991), and characterisation of the DNA binding domain of the mouse uterine oestrogen receptor using site-specific polyclonal antibodies has been described (Ikeda *et al.*, 1993). A different reactivity of tamoxifen and 4-hydroxytamoxifen complexes with the monoclonal antibody H222 has also been found. The antigenic determinant recognised by this antibody appeared to be localised close to the steroid binding domain of the receptor. This domain was similarly affected by oestradiol and 4-hydroxytamoxifen, whereas tamoxifen induced a different conformation that could not be entirely recognised by the antibody. It has been reported that 16α-hydroxyoestrone (a physiological metabolite of 17β-oestradiol), in MCF-7 cells in long-term culture, formed covalent associations with the oestrogen receptor (in contrast to the classical reversible oestrogen binding). This resulted in decreased levels of oestrogen and progesterone receptors but did not inhibit the proliferative action of the hormone (Swaneck and Fishman, 1991). This suggests that the covalently bound oestrogen receptor is able to perform some but not all of the functions of the reversible complex (Swaneck and Fishman, 1991).

The human oestrogen receptor becomes phosphorylated in the presence of oestradiol or 4-hydroxytamoxifen or the pure oestrogen antagonist, ICI 164 384, although less efficiently than with oestradiol (Ali *et al.*, 1993). One of the multiple sites of phosphorylation of the human oestrogen receptor has been mapped using deletion and point mutants to the N-terminal A/B region at serine 118. In a number of cell types, mutation of this serine to alanine causes a reduction in transcriptional activation by the human oestrogen receptor of reporter genes containing an oestrogen response element. However, it does not affect the DNA binding properties or the nuclear localisation of the human oestrogen receptor. It appears likely that phosphorylation of serine 118 modulates the transcriptional activation function 1 (AF-1) located in the A/B region of the oestrogen receptor. Human oestrogen receptor mutants with altered oestrogen and antioestrogen ligand discrimination have been described (Pakdel and Katzenellenbogen, 1992).

Growth regulation of oestrogen receptor-negative breast cancer cells transfected with complementary DNAs for the oestrogen receptor has been demonstrated (Jiang and Jordan, 1992). In addition, a point mutation of the oestrogen receptor in the ligand binding domain has been found that changes the pharmacology of antioestrogens in oestrogen receptor-negative breast cancer cells stably expressing complementary DNAs for the oestrogen receptor (Jiang *et al.*, 1992) Indeed. radiation has been found to inactivate the oestrogen receptor in intact MCF-7 cells, possibly because of a subsequent lack of energy transfer to the oestradiol binding domain (Toulas *et al.*, 1991). In MCF-7 cells treated with 4-hydroxytamoxifen, accumulation of a non-binding form of the oestrogen receptor has been found (Leclercq *et al.*, 1992) and transcriptionally active non-ligand binding oestrogen receptors can occur in breast cancer (Marsigliante *et al.*, 1992). Altered folding of the MCF-7 oestrogen receptor protein or altered phosphorylation of its hormone binding domain are possible explanations for these non-binding oestrogen receptor molecules, which may have a physiological role such as competing with the unaltered oestrogen receptor molecules for the oestrogen-responsive elements on the DNA (Leclercq *et al.*, 1992). The role of oestrogen receptor variants in the development of hormone resistance in breast cancer has been studied (Sluyser, 1992; Karnik *et al.*, 1994) and is discussed in Chapter 6.

Studies on the interaction of tamoxifen analogues with the oestrogen receptor

The structural components of tamoxifen (Murphy and Jordan, 1989) and hydroxylated metabolites of tamoxifen (Murphy *et al.*, 1990) necessary for their antioestrogenic activity have been investigated and it is possible that the lone pair of electrons within the side-chain of the tamoxifen molecule is responsible for the antioestrogenic (rather than oestrogenic) activity of tamoxifen observed when it binds to the oestrogen receptor. The introduction of a single *para*-hydroxyl into tamoxifen (to give 4-hydroxytamoxifen) has been shown to increase the affinity of the ligand for the oestrogen receptor, and addition of a further hydroxyl group in the *meta* position also increased the oestrogen receptor affinity of the ligand in comparison to tamoxifen. Conversely, methylation of the free phenol group of 4-hydroxytamoxifen (to produce the methyl ether derivative) decreased its affinity for the oestrogen receptor. In comparison, substitution of tamoxifen at the *para* position in the phenyl ring with methyl, fluorine or chlorine does not greatly affect the affinity of the molecule for the oestrogen receptor. The following modifications to the side-chain of tamoxifen—removal of a single methyl group (*N*-desmethyltamoxifen), removal of the dimethylamine and replacement with a hydroxyl (metabolite Y) or removal of the whole side-chain to produce a phenol (metabolite E) (Murphy and Sutherland, 1985)—all reduce the affinity of the ligand for the oestrogen receptor. Additionally introduction of methyl groups, particularly two such groups *ortho* to the aminoethoxy side-chain of tamoxifen, restricts the number of conformations that the side chain can adopt in space, and hence reduces the affinity for the mouse uterine oestrogen receptor, and the MCF-7 cell line oestrogen receptor (Murphy and Sutherland, 1985). Studies with other tamoxifen analogues substituted with various side-chains (to form the compounds quaternary tamoxifen, piperazinyltamoxifen and chlorotamoxifen) have shown that their oestrogen antagonism in immature rat uterus was enhanced by the presence of the *β*-*tert*-nitrogen (Agarwal and Bindal, 1991).

The affinity of triarylethylene carboxylic acids related to tamoxifen for the oestrogen receptor and their ability to inhibit MCF-7 cell growth has been described (Wilson *et al.*, 1992). DP-TAT-59, an active metabolite of a new triphenylethylene derivative (TAT-59), has been reported to interact with the oestrogen receptor (Toko *et al.*, 1992). Halogenated analogues of tamoxifen have been synthesised, and their ability to bind to the oestrogen receptor and inhibit the growth of MCF-7 cells has been investigated (Chander *et al.*, 1991; Yang *et al.*, 1992). Pyrrolidino-4-iodotamoxifen and 4-iodotamoxifen have both been shown to have 2.5-fold higher affinities for the oestrogen receptor compared with tamoxifen. In addition, pyrrolidino-4-iodotamoxifen was 1.5-fold more effective in causing inhibition of oestrogen-induced growth of MCF-7 cells compared with tamoxifen. These compounds also have antiproliferative activities in the nitrosomethylurea-induced rat mammary tumour model (see below).

Novel oestrogen derivatives, oestrogen-*cis*-dichloroethylene diamene-platinum-(II) complexes (Spyriounis *et al.*, 1992) and also ^{125}I-iodinated oestrogen derivatives (Souttou *et al.*, 1993) have been evaluated for affinity for the oestrogen receptor and ability to inhibit the growth of MCF-7 cells. Amino acid and peptide derivatives of oestradiol have been synthesised and their binding affinities for the oestrogen receptor determined (Ye *et al.*, 1993). The comparative effect of synthetic amino-oestrogens and oestradiol on platelet aggregation has also been studied (Delapena *et al.*, 1993). It is of interest that the growth inhibitory action of melatonin on human breast cancer cells has been reported to be linked to the oestrogen response system (Hill *et al.*, 1992). The oestrogenic activity of the dietary isoflavonoids (phyto-oestrogens) coumestrol, genistein and daidzein was found to be as great as that of oestradiol when assayed by oestrogen-specific enhancement of alkaline phosphatase activity through binding to the oestrogen receptor, and was suppressed by 4-hydroxytamoxifen (Markiewicz *et al.*, 1993).

Interaction of oestrogen and tamoxifen with the vitamin D receptor

There is evidence that 1,25-dihydroxyvitamin D3 exerts an antiproliferative effect on breast cancer cells through binding to the vitamin D receptor (VDR). Exposure of cells which contain VDR receptors to oestradiol or dihydrotestosterone (10^{-7} M) resulted in a significant increase in VDR levels and this up-regulation was completely suppressed by tamoxifen (10^{-6} M) (Escaleira *et al.*, 1993). However, tamoxifen treatment alone produced a significant dose-dependent increase in VDR content. It appears likely that the up-regulation of VDR by oestradiol or dihydrotestosterone occurs via an oestrogen receptor-mediated mechanism. In addition, similar effects of tamoxifen on VDR expression have been reported in the ROS 17/2.8 osteoblast cell line (Liel *et al.*, 1992). In T47D human breast cancer cells oestradiol enhanced growth and progesterone receptor expression; this action was antagonised by tamoxifen, whereas dihydrotestosterone did not alter growth but down-regulated the progesterone receptor (Liberato *et al.*, 1993).

Retinoic acid is known to inhibit proliferation in human breast cancer cells; the interaction between 4-hydroxytamoxifen, retinoic acid and 1,25-dihydroxyvitamin D3 in T47D cells (Koga and Sutherland, 1991) and the expression and regulation of retinoic acid receptors in human breast cancer cells (Roman *et al.*, 1992) have been investigated. Retinoic acid and 1,25-dihydroxyvitamin D3 showed a synergistic inhibitory effect on the growth of T47D cells and retinoic acid also enhanced the growth inhibitory effect of 4-hydroxytamoxifen. However, retinoic acid did not affect oestrogen-induced growth stimulation and did not alter VDR and oestrogen receptor levels. The synergistic effects of retinoic acid appear to involve interactions with steroid hormone action that are distinct from alterations in receptor levels. The regulation of androgen receptor gene expression by steroids and retinoic acid in human breast cancer cells has also been studied (Hall *et al.*, 1992).

OESTROGEN RECEPTOR ASSAYS: USE IN TREATMENT

The presence of steroid hormone receptors can be considered to be an independent prognostic factor as well as a predictive factor for hormonal manipulation in the clinical management of breast cancer. However, the exact contribution of each receptor or combinations of different receptors remains unclear. In advanced breast cancer the oestrogen receptor (but not progesterone receptor) level was found to correlate with response to tamoxifen (Bezwoda *et al.*, 1991). In addition, the influence of tamoxifen on oestrogen receptor concentration has to be taken into consideration when assessing results in tamoxifen-treated patients, and the measurement of steroid hormone receptors in breast cancer patients treated with tamoxifen has been reported (Encarnacion *et al.*, 1993). Changes in the oestrogen receptor status of breast cancer have been shown to change with age (Gaskell *et al.*, 1992), and determination of oestrogen receptor content allows selection of elderly patients with breast cancer for conservative tamoxifen treatment (Low *et al.*, 1992). In a study of 326 primary breast carcinomas a negative correlation was found between oestrogen receptor and epidermal growth factor receptor (see Chapter 6) status: 69% of epidermal growth factor receptor-negative tumours were oestrogen receptor positive (Zeillinger *et al.*, 1993). Furthermore, a combination of oestrogen receptor-negative and epidermal growth factor receptor-positive was more frequent in poorly differentiated tumours; however, patient outcome did not show statistically significant differences in relation to the epidermal growth factor receptor status.

The prognostic significance of progesterone receptor levels has also been evaluated in oestrogen receptor-positive metastatic breast cancer treated with tamoxifen (Ravdin *et al.*, 1992). In one study the oestrogen receptor, progesterone receptor and androgen receptor content in the cytosols of cells from patients with operable breast cancer (stages I and II) were measured, and androgen receptor category was an independent predictor of axillary metastases; and in patients with a low androgen receptor content the progesterone receptor status was a single independent prognostic factor of relapse-free survival (Soreide *et al.*, 1992). The variations in oestrogen and progesterone receptor levels after short-term tamoxifen treatment in breast carcinoma have been examined (Montoya *et al.*, 1992).

Oestrogen receptor analysis in early carcinoma of the breast is thought to be of importance in long-term prognosis (Winstanley *et al.*, 1991). Techniques for the determination and standardisation of oestrogen receptors are clearly important (Chapman *et al.*, 1993) and a study comparing different oestrogen receptor assays in the clinical course of patients with advanced breast cancer has been reported (Robertson *et al.*, 1992a). It is also of interest that a failure to detect gonodotrophin-releasing hormone receptors in human benign and malignant breast tissue and in MCF-7 and MDA-MB-231 cancer cells has been reported (Mullen *et al.*, 1993; Zeillinger *et al.*, 1993).

In cancer-associated normal tissue, tamoxifen therapy was not found to influence the expression of progesterone receptors and epidermal growth factor receptors measured using immunochemical assays or Ki_{67} antibody immunostaining, but it was found significantly to increase oestrogen receptor positivity in ductal tissue (Walker *et al.*, 1991). The cellular effects of tamoxifen in primary breast cancer have also been studied (Robertson *et al.*, 1992b). The effect of tamoxifen on the Ki_{67} labelling index (LI) in human breast tumours has been measured and related to oestrogen and progesterone receptor status (Clarke *et al.*, 1993). Tamoxifen treatment reduced the Ki_{67} LI in human breast tumours *in vivo* and may be useful in monitoring response to tamoxifen therapy. However, this decrease in Ki_{67} LI did not correlate with oestrogen or progesterone receptor status and did not predict recurrence over a short follow-up period.

An assay which measures displacement by tamoxifen of oestradiol from the oestradiol–oestrogen receptor complex (Levin *et al.*, 1990) and an immunobiochemical assay for the determination of nuclear steroid receptors during tamoxifen treatment have been described (Vering *et al.*, 1993). In the immunobiochemical assay the receptor modulation of tumours xenotransplanted into nude mice after injection of 50 μg of tamoxifen per mouse was studied, and unoccupied and occupied determinations were done by enzyme immunoassay for the oestrogen receptor under low and high salt extraction. A comparison has been made of tritiated oestradiol and aziridine tamoxifen for the measurement of oestrogen receptors in human breast cancer cell cytosols (Piccart *et al.*, 1991). The *in vivo* uptake of 16α-[^{18}F]fluorooestradiol by target tissues in the rat and competition by tamoxifen has been reported in a study that has implications both for quantitating oestrogen receptors *in vivo* and for the use of animal models in the development of radiopharmaceuticals that bind to receptors (Katzenellenbogen *et al.*, 1993). Oxohexestral derivatives labelled with [^{18}F]fluorine have been reported to have potential as breast tumour imaging agents (Bergmann *et al.*, 1994).

ACTION ON OESTROGEN-REGULATED GENE TRANSCRIPTION AND PROTEIN SYNTHESIS

Tamoxifen has been found to stimulate both RNA polymerase I and II: a transient rise in RNA polymerase II was observed followed by increased activity of RNA polymerase I, and finally a secondary rise in RNA polymerase II activity occurred. However, the secondary stimulation of RNA polymerase II was not sustained by the tamoxifen receptor complex, as it was by oestradiol, even though the tamoxifen receptor complex was found in the nucleus. Although these observations are consistent with the partial agonist properties of tamoxifen, it is not known why the tamoxifen receptor complex is defective in this respect. In the MCF-7 cell-line, tamoxifen and 4-hydroxytamoxifen (at oestrogen-reversible concentrations) have been shown to have a complicated antagonist/partial agonist effect on gene transcription. They were found to increase the level of the oestrogen-regulated pNR-1 mRNA to about 80% of the oestradiol-induced level, and its induction by oestradiol was not significantly antagonised by either antioestrogen. In contrast, however, the pNR-2 mRNA was only increased to about 10% of the oestradiol-induced level and its induction by oestradiol was antagonised by both tamoxifen and 4-hydroxytamoxifen (May and Westley, 1987). Hence these two antioestrogen-regulated mRNAs respond in vastly different ways to these compounds. Although 4-hydroxytamoxifen and oestradiol have similar affinities for the oestrogen receptor ($K_d \simeq 2 \times 10^{-10}$ M), the induction of both mRNAs by 4-hydroxytamoxifen required a 10-fold higher concentration than oestradiol for maximum agonist activity, and a 500-fold molar excess was required to antagonise the induction by oestradiol. In the case of tamoxifen, which has a 20 to 100-fold lower affinity than oestradiol for the oestrogen receptor, a 200-fold higher concentration was required for maximum agonist activity and a 10 000-fold molar excess to antagonise the induction by oestradiol (May and Westley, 1987).

Similarly in the EFM-19 breast cancer cell line, where oestrogen receptor mRNA levels are higher than in other oestrogen-responsive cell lines, the levels of four oestrogen-inducible mRNAs (pNR-1, pNR-2, pNR-25 and pNR-100) were measured (Westley *et al.*, 1989). It was found that oestradiol treatment increased the levels of the four regulated mRNAs between three-fold (pNR-100) and >100-fold (pNR-2) and the induction was half-maximal between 1.5×10^{-11} and 1.5×10^{-10} M oestradiol. Tamoxifen was found to be a partial oestrogen agonist for the induction of the pNR-1 (induction was about 70% of the level obtained with oestradiol) and the pNR-25 RNAs but had very little effect on the pNR-2 and pNR-100 mRNA levels (Wesley *et al.*, 1989). The pNR-2 mRNA levels were less induced by tamoxifen in EFM-19 cells (Westley *et al.*, 1989) than in MCF-7 cells (May and Westley, 1987). Additionally, the oestrogen-induced levels of the four mRNAs were reduced by tamoxifen to the mRNA levels present in cells treated with tamoxifen alone (Westley *et al.*, 1989).

It is of interest, therefore, that the pNR-2 mRNA was expressed in only a subset of oestrogen receptor-positive tumours taken from breast cancer patients, and that the presence of pNR-2 levels was associated with response to primary tamoxifen therapy (Henry *et al.*, 1989). It has been proposed that pNR-2 mRNA may be useful as a predictive marker of response to tamoxifen in primary breast cancer (Henry *et al.*, 1989).

The effects of tamoxifen on protein synthesis in oestrogen-responsive tissues have provided an insight into gene regulation. Tamoxifen increased the production of progesterone receptors in MCF-7 cells, which is a typically oestrogenic effect. However, in GH4C1 pituitary tumour cells tamoxifen acts as a classical antioestrogen by partially blocking the induction of progesterone receptors (Shull *et al.*, 1992). Furthermore, dissociated effects of tamoxifen on growth and on progesterone receptor induction in quail oviduct have been reported (Laugier *et al.*, 1991). Tamoxifen also selectively increased the production of an M_r 37 000 secreted protein (but not in the oestrogen receptor-negative MDA-MB231 cell-line) and the production of this protein was inhibited by concomitant oestradiol treatment. Conversely, tamoxifen inhibited the response to oestrogen of a 46 kDa glycoprotein and a plasminogen activator protein. Tamoxifen also inhibited the production of a 32 kDa secreted protein (in MCF-7 cells) that is stimulated by oestradiol.

EFFECT IN ANIMAL MODELS

Rat mammary tumour models

The dimethylbenz(*a*)anthracene (DMBA)-induced rat mammary carcinoma model has been widely used to investigate hormone-dependent cancer and hence to evaluate potential treatments for breast cancer. The growth of established DMBA-induced tumours can be inhibited by tamoxifen and the mechanism of action in this model system is thought to be by the direct blocking of the binding of oestrogen to the tumour oestrogen receptor. The simultaneous administration of a large dose of tamoxifen (5 mg × 2 subcutaneously) with the DMBA almost completely inhibited the appearance of tumours. Although 4-hydroxytamoxifen is more potent as an antioestrogen in classical pharmacological models it was less effective than tamoxifen when given for 30 days in the DMBA-induced tumour model, which may be due to its shorter half-life. The effect of intermittent progesterone on inhibition of tumour growth in the DMBA tumour model by tamoxifen has been studied (Gibson *et al.*, 1993). The antitumour effect of the angiogenesis inhibitor AGM-1470 and its effect in combination with tamoxifen have been studied in DMBA-induced mammary tumours in rats (Toi *et al.*, 1993) and the inhibitory effect of combined treatment with the aromatase inhibitor exemestane and tamoxifen on these tumours has been reported (Zaccheo *et al.*, 1993). The combined treatment of tamoxifen (1 mg/kg per day) and exemestane (20 mg/kg per day) resulted in a higher antitumour effect than either single treatment and suggests that oestrogen deprivation through aromatase inhibition and oestrogen receptor antagonism results in a more effective inhibition of DMBA-induced mammary tumours than either form of treatment alone. The effect of coconut and corn oils on DMBA-induced mammary tumours in mice has also been studied (Gaigschmidt *et al.*, 1993). The role of tamoxifen in the induction of hormone-independent rat mammary tumours has also been investigated in this model (Fendl and Zimniski 1992). Tamoxifen was administered either with the DMBA or after initial tumour formation and, while fewer tumours were found after co-administration of tamoxifen and DMBA and tamoxifen treatment caused regression of existing tumours, new tumours developed in the presence of tamoxifen in both studies, which were hormone independent because regression was not observed following ovariectomy.

N-Nitroso-*N*-methylurea (NMU) is a carcinogen used to induce mammary carcinoma in the rat. The tamoxifen derivative droloxifene (3-hydroxytamoxifen) has been found to inhibit the growth of NMU-induced rat mammary tumours and influence oestrogen receptor content in this model (Winterfeld *et al.*, 1992; Gorlich *et al.*, 1992). The therapeutic response to tamoxifen in NMU-induced rat mammary tumours has been monitored using ^{31}P magnetic resonance spectroscopy (MRS) (Baluch *et al.*, 1991). Chemopreventive effects of tamoxifen in NMU-induced (Moon *et al.*, 1992; Osborne *et al.*, 1992) and ethylmethanesulphonate-induced (Ueo *et al.*, 1990) rat mammary carcinogenesis have been demonstrated. Tamoxifen was effective in suppressing NMU-induced mammary tumour incidence and frequency; and NMU-induced hyperproliferation, an intermediate stage in NMU carcinogenesis, is also suppressed by tamoxifen. Pyrrolidino-4-iodotamoxifen caused regression in 92% of rats in the NMU-induced mammary tumour model, whereas tamoxifen caused regression in only 75% of rats (Chander *et al.*, 1991).

Mammary adenocarcinomas were found to develop in Sprague–Dawley rats following irradiation with [^{137}Cs] γ-rays. These tumours were responsive to hormonal manipulation, and tamoxifen given around the time of irradiation or for 60 days starting 30 days after irradiation reduced the incidence of tumours. In the EnDA endometrial adenocarcinoma, which is an oestrogen-sensitive metastasising *in vivo* tumour model in the rat, the growth of the primary tumour was inhibited by medroxyprogesterone acetate and by tamoxifen (Horn *et al.*, 1993). However, tamoxifen treatment did not alter the number of lung metastases, whereas medroxyprogesterone acetate or ovariectomy produced a significant reduction in the number of lung metastases. The EnDA endometrial carcinoma of the DA/Han rat resembles a typical endometrial adenocarcinoma with respect to its oestrogen sensitivity, oestrogen receptor expression, morphology and metastatic growth and is a useful experimental model.

Athymic mice for the transplantation and study of human breast tumours

Human tumours can be transplanted into the immune-deficient athymic or 'nude' mouse for laboratory investigation. In addition, transgenic mouse models are likely to provide molecular insights into human breast cancer (Dickson *et al.*, 1991). The athymic mouse system is sufficiently standardised to enable detailed testing of the sensitivity of human tumour biopsy samples to chemotherapeutic agents, and there is evidence that tamoxifen suppressed the growth of the oestrogen receptor-positive human breast tumour transplant Br-10 but not the receptor-negative transplant MX-1. MCF-7 cells injected into athymic mice can develop into solid tumours, provided oestrogen is administered to the mouse. Tamoxifen has been shown to reversibly control the oestradiol-stimulated growth of MCF-7 tumours in this system (Lino *et al.*, 1991). Effects of tamoxifen, oestradiol and medroxyprogesterone acetate on tumour growth and oncogene expression in MCF-7 cells transplanted into nude mice have been reported (Mizukami *et al.*, 1991). Oestradiol increased the growth of MCF-7 tumours, and the proportion of [^{3}H]thymidine-labelled cells was increased. The converse was found for tamoxifen: the tumour content of IGF-1 and the occurrence of IGF-1-positive cells were lower in the oestradiol-treated group but higher in the tamoxifen-treated group (Noguchi *et al.*, 1991). It would appear that the tumour content of IGF-1 and the proportion of IGF-1-positive cells are inversely related to tumour growth and the [^{3}H]-thymidine labelling index.

Studies have been made *in vivo* by magnetic resonance imaging and spectroscopy of the response to tamoxifen of MCF-7 human breast cancer cells implanted in nude mice (Furman *et al.*, 1991). Tumours have been monitored by this method during oestrogen-dependent growth and tamoxifen-induced remission. Enhanced tumour necrosis developed early after tamoxifen administration and extended to most of the tumour volume, which was followed by tumour regression and the growth of repair tissue. Tamoxifen treatment also increased the nucleoside triphosphate/inorganic phosphate ratio probably as a result of the growth of reparative tissue.

It is also of interest that tamoxifen exhibited paradoxical oestrogen-like effects on human endometrial carcinomas (the most common malignancy of the female genital tract) grown in ovariectomised nude mice. The growth rate of the oestrogen receptor-positive, well-differentiated endometrial carcinoma EnCa-X in nude mice was increased in the presence of 17β-oestradiol or tamoxifen (both at a concentration of 20 ng/ml). However, combination treatment with tamoxifen and progestin was superior to progestin alone in controlling tumour growth. This is thought to be because the presence of progesterone receptors may be a prerequisite for eliciting progestin response, and tamoxifen has been shown to increase the concentrations of progesterone receptors in endometrial carcinoma.

The growth of the transplantable Shionoyi mouse mammary tumour Sc115 is inhibited by tamoxifen (0.5–50 mg/kg daily). The cytosol oestrogen receptor was found to be depleted after tamoxifen treatment, suggesting a direct effect of tamoxifen on the oestrogen receptor system. In addition, clonal cell lines with heterogeneic properties have been derived from canine mammary carcinomas and their sensitivity to tamoxifen has been determined (Sartin *et al.*, 1993). The culture of tumour explants has not been widely used, even though it has been recommended as a system for the determination of hormone dependency. A highly significant inhibition of the thymidine labelling index has been observed for breast cancer explants treated with tamoxifen. Tamoxifen was found to be effective only in explants possessing high levels of oestrogen receptors and was without effect in tumours where the receptor was either absent or present only at low levels. This system, therefore, has potential for the selection of patients for antioestrogen therapy, but is likely to be more difficult to develop than the oestrogen receptor assay procedures.

REFERENCES

Ali, S., Metzger, D., Bornert, J.M., Chambon, P. (1993) *European Molecular Biology Organization Journal* **12**, 1153–1160.

Argwal, A.K., Bindal, R.D. (1991) *Steroids* **56**, 486–488.

Armstrong, D.K., Isaacs, J.T., Ottaviano, Y.L., Davidson, N.E. (1992) *Cancer Research* **52**, 3418–3424.

Baluch, S., Midwood, C.J., Griffiths, J.R., Stubbs, M., Coombes, R.C. (1991) *British Journal of Cancer* **63**, 901–904.

Bergmann, K.E., Landvatter, S.W., Rocque, P.G., Carlson, K.E., Welch, M.J., Katzenellenbogen, J.A. (1994) *Nuclear Medicine and Biology* **21**, 25–40.

Bezwoda, W.R., Esser, J.D., Dansey, R., Kessel, I., Lange, M. (1991) *Cancer* **68**, 867–872.

Borgna, J.L., Scalia, J. (1991) *European Journal of Biochemistry* **199**, 575–586.

Brunner, N., Bouley, V., Fojo, A., Fretter, C.E., Lippman, M.E., Clarke, R. (1993) *Cancer Research* **53**, 283–290.

Catherino, W.H., Jeng, M.H., Jordan, V.C. (1993) *British Journal of Cancer* **67**, 945–952.

Chander, S.K., McCague, R., Luqmai, Y., Newton, C., Dowsett, M., Jarman, M., Coombes, R.C. (1991) *Cancer Research* **51**, 5851–5858.

Chapman, J.A.W., Mobbs, B.G., Hanna, W.M., Sawka, C.A., Pritchard, K.J., Lickley, H.L., Trudeau, M.E. (1993) *Journal of Steroid Biochemistry and Molecular Biology* **45**, 367–374.

Clarke, R.B., Laidlaw, I.J., Jones, L.J., Howell, A., Anderson, E. (1993) *British Journal of Cancer* **67**, 606–611.

Colomb, E., Berthon, P., Dussert, C., Calvo, F., Martu, P.M. (1991) *International Journal of Cancer* **49**, 932–937.

Danielian, P.S., White, R., Hoare, S.A., Fawell, S.E., Parker, M.G. (1993) *Molecular Endocrinology* **7**, 232–240.
Delapena, A., Bano, G., Izaguire, R., Mandoki, J.J., Fernandez, J.M. (1993) *Steroids* **58**, 407–409.
Demirpence, G., Pons, M., Balaguer, P., Gagne, D. (1992) Biochemical and Biophysical Research Communications **183**, 100–106.
Dickson, R.B., Gottardis, M.M. Merlino, G.T. (1991) *Bioessays* **13**, 591–596.
Emmas, C.E., Fawell, S.E., Hoare, S.A., Parker, M.G. (1992) *Journal of Steroid Biochemistry and Molecular Biology* **41**, 291–299.
Encarnacion, C.A., Ciocca, D.R., McGuire,W.L., Clark, G.M., Fuqua, S.A.W.M., Osborne, C.K. (1993) *Breast Cancer Research and Treatment* **26**, 237–246.
Escaleira, M.T., Sonohara, S., Brentani, M.M., (1993) *Journal of Steroid Biochemistry and Molecular Biology* **45**, 257–263.
Farnham, R.J., Slansky, J.E., Kollmar, R. (1993) *Biochimica et Biophysica Acta* **115**, 125–132.
Faucher, C., Capdevielle, J., Canal, I., Ferrara, P., Mazarguil, H., McGuire, W.L., Darbon, J.M. (1993) *Journal of Biological Chemistry* **268**, 15168–15173.
Fendl, K.C., Zimniski, S.J. (1992) *Cancer Research* **52**, 235–237.
Foster, B.D., Cavener, D.R., Pagl, F.F. (1991) *Cancer Research* **51**, 3405–3410.
Furman, E., Margalit, R., Bendel, P., Horowitz, A., Degani, H. (1991) *Cancer Communications* **3**, 287–297.
Furuya, Y., Kohno, N., Fujiwara, Y. and Saitoh, Y. (1989) *Cancer Research* **49**, 6670–6674.
Gaigschmidt, M., White, M.J., Teer, P., Johnson, J., Wilance, H. (1993) *Nutritional Cancer*, **20**, 99–106.
Gaskell, D.J., Sangster, K., Tesdale, A.L., Carson, D., Hawkins, R.A. (1992) *Breast Cancer Research and Treatment* **66**, 610–613.
Gibson, D.F.C., Johnson, D.A., Langan-Fahey, S.M., Lababidi, M.K., Wolberg, W.H., Jordan, V.C. (1993) *Breast Cancer Research and Treatment* **27**, 283–287.
Gorlich, M., Winterfeld, W., Hauff, P., Arnold, W., Fichtner, I., Staab, H.J. (1992) *Journal of Cancer Research and Clinical Oncology* **119**, 97–101.
Graham, M.L., Smith, J.A., Jewett, P.B., Horowitz, K.B. (1992) *Cancer Research* **52**, 593–602.
Green, S. (1990) *Journal of Steroid Biochemistry and Molecular Biology* **37**, 747–752.
Gyling, M., Leclercq, G., Heuson, J.C. (1990) *Journal of Receptor Research* **10**, 217–234.
Hall, R.E., Tilley, W.D., McPhaul, M.J., Sutherland, R.L. (1992) *International Journal of Cancer* **52**, 778–784.
Healicon, R.M., Westley, B.R., May, F.E.B. (1993) *International Journal of Cancer* **53**, 388–394.
Henry, J.A., Nicholson, S., Hennessy, C., Lennard, J.W.J., May, F.E.B., Westley, B.R. (1989) *British Journal of Cancer* **61**, 32–38.
Hill, S.M., Spriggs, L.L., Simon, M.A., Muraoka, H., Blask, D.E. (1992) *Cancer Letters* **64**, 249–256.
Horn, D.W., Vollmer, G., Deerberg, F., Schneider, M.R. (1993) *Journal of Cancer Research and Clinical Oncology* **119**, 450–456.
Ikeda, M., Ogata, F., Curtis, S.W., Lubahn, D.B., French, F.S., Wilson, E.M., Korach, K.S. (1993) *Journal of Biological Chemistry* **265**, 10296–10302.
Jain, P.T., Pento, J.T., Magarian, R.A., Graues, D.C. (1991) *Anticancer Drugs* **2**, 487–494.
Jiang, S.Y., Jordan, V.C. (1992) *Journal of the National Cancer Institute* **84**, 580–591.

Jiang, S.Y., Langan-Fahey, S.M., Stella, A.L., McCague, R., Jordan, V.C. (1992) *Molecular Endocrinology* **6**, 2167–2174.
Josui, K., Kubota, T., Kitajima, M. (1992) *Japanese Journal of Cancer Research* **83**, 1347–1353.
Kareva, E.N., Kostyleva, O.I. (1993) *Bulletin of Experimental Biology and Medicine* **115**, 280–281.
Karnik, P.S., Kulkarni, S., Liu, X.P., Budd, G.T., Bukowski, R.M. (1994) *Cancer Research* **54**, 349–353.
Karsten, U., Papsdorf, G., Pauly, A., Vojtesek, B., Moll, R., Lane, E.B., Clausen, H., Stosiek, P., Kasper, M. (1993) *Differentiation* **54**, 55–61.
Katzenellenbogen, J.A., Mathias, C.J., Vanbrocklin, H.F., Brodack, J.W., Welch, M.J. (1993) *Nuclear Medicine and Biology* **20**, 735–746.
Kitawaki, J., Fukuokay, M., Yamamoto, T., Honjo, H., Okada H. (1992) *Journal of Steroid Biochemistry and Molecular Biology* **42**, 267–278.
Koga, M., Sutherland, R.L. (1991) *Journal of Steroid Biochemistry and Molecular Biology* **39**, 455–460.
Korach, K.S., Chae, K., Gibson, M., Curtis, S. (1991) *Steroids* **56**, 263–270.
Kotoula, V., Karkavelas, G., (1993) *Histology and Histopathology* **8**, 627–636.
Langdon, S.P., Hawkes, M.M., Lawrie, S.S., Hawking, R.A., Tesdale A.L., Crew, A.J., Miller, W.R., Smyth, J.F. (1990) *British Journal of Cancer* **62**, 213–216.
Laugier, C., Fanidi, A., Dufrene, L., Fayard, J.M., Pageaux, J.F. (1991) *General and Comparative Endocrinology* **83**, 439–446.
Leclercq, G., Legros, N., Piccart, M.J. (1992) *Journal of Steroid Biochemistry and Molecular Biology* **41**, 545–552.
Legros, N., Leclercq, G., McCague, R. (1991) *Biochemical Pharmacology* **42**, 1837–1840.
Levin, E., Tomchinsky, S., Lopez, S. (1990) *Journal of Steroid Biochemistry and Molecular Biology* **37**, 681–686.
Liberato, M.H., Sonohara, S., Brentani, M.M. (1993) *Tumour Biology* **14**, 38–45.
Liel, Y., Kraus, S., Levy, J., Shany, S. (1992) *Endocrinology* **130**, 2597–2601.
Lino, Y., Wolf, D.M., Langan-Fahey, S.M., Johnson, D.A., Ricchio, M., Thompson, M.E., Jordan, V.C. (1991) *British Journal of Cancer* **64**, 1019–1024.
Lottering, M.L., Haug, M., Seegers, J.C. (1992) *Cancer Research* **52**, 5926–5932.
Low, J.C., Dixon, A.R., Bell, J., Ellis, I.O., Elston, C.W., Robertson, J.F.R., Blamey, R.W. (1992) *British Journal of Surgery* **79**, 1314–1316.
Mader, S., Chambon, P., White, J.H. (1993) *Nucleic Acids Research* **21**, 1125–1140.
Maentausta, O., Svalander, P., Danielsson, K.G., Bygdeman, M., Vihko, R. (1993) *Journal of Clinical Endocrinology and Metaboloism* **77**, 1913–1918.
Manni, A., Wright, C., Buck, H. (1991) *Breast Cancer Research and Treatment* **20**, 43–52.
Markiewicz, L., Garey, J., Aldercreutz, H., Gurpide, E. (1993) *Journal of Steroid Biochemistry and Molecular Biology* **45**, 399–405.
Marsigliante, S., Greco, S., Biscozzo, L., Barker, S., Baker, V., Giuseppes, L., Vinson, G.P., Storelli, C. (1992) *Cancer Letters* **66**, 183–192.
Martin, M.B., Saceda, M., Lindsey, R.K. (1993) *Advances in Experimental Medicine and Biology* **330**, 143–153.
May, F.E.B., Westley B.R. (1987) *Journal of Biological Chemistry* **262**, 15894–15899.
Metzger, D., White, J.H., Chambon, P. (1988) *Nature* **334**, 31–36.
Mizukami, Y., Taji, K., Nonomura, A., Noguchi, M., Taniya, T., Koyaski, N., Nakamura, S., Matsubara, F. (1991) *Anticancer Research* **11**, 1333–1338.
Montoya, F., Barbazan, M.J., Schneider, J., Matorras, R., Rodriguezescudero, F.J. (1992) *Oncology* **49**, 422–425.

Moon, R.C., Kelloff, G.J., Detrisac, C.J., Steele, V.E., Thomas, C.F., Sigman, C.L. (1992) *Anticancer Research* **12**, 1147–1154.

Mullen, P., Bramley, T.,Menzie, G.A., Miller, B. (1993) *European Journal of Cancer* **29A**, 248–251.

Muller, R., Mumberg, D., Lucibello, F.C. (1993) *Biochimica Biophysica Acta* **115**, 151–180.

Murphy, L.C., Dotzlaw, H., Alkhalaf, M., Coutts, A., Miller, T., Wong, M.S., Gens, Y., Murphy, L.J. (1992) *Journal of Steroid Biochemistry and Molecular Biology* **43**, 117–122.

Murphy, C.S., Jordan, V.C. (1989) *Journal of Steroid Biochemistry* **34**, 407–411.

Murphy, C.S., Langan-Fahey, S.M., McCague, R., Jordan, V.C. (1990) *Molecular Pharmacology* **38**, 737–743.

Murphy, L.C., Sutherland, R.L. (1985) *Endocrinology* **116**, 1071–1078.

Noguchi, M., Koyasaki, N., Miyzaki, I., Mizukami, Y. (1991) *Japanese Journal of Cancer Research* **82**, 1199–1202.

Noguchi, S., Motomura, K., Inaji, H., Imaoka, S., Koyamoa, H. (1993) *Cancer* **71**, 1266–1272.

Osborne, M.P., Ruperto, J.F., Crowe, J.P., Rosen, P.P., Telang, N.R. (1992) *Cancer Research* **52**, 1477–1480.

Pakdel, F., Katzenellenbogen, B.S. (1992) *Journal of Biological Chemistry* **267**, 3429–3437.

Petersen, O.W., Ronnovjessen, I., Howlett, A.R., Bisseu, M.J. (1992) *Proceedings of the National Academy of Sciences USA* **89**, 9054–9069.

Pfeffer, U., Fecarotta, E., Castagnetta, L., Vidali, G. (1993) *Cancer Research* **53**, 741–743.

Pham, T.A., Elliston, J.F., Nawaz, Z., Mcdonnell, D.P., Tsai, M.J., Omalley, B.W. (1991) *Proceedings of the National Academy of Sciences USA* **88**, 3125–3129.

Piccart, M.J., Muquardt, C., Bosman, C., Pirotte, P., Veenstra, S., Grillo, F., Leclercq, G. (1991) *Journal of the National Cancer Institute* **83**, 1553–1559.

Ravdin, P.M. Green, S., Dorr, T.M., McGuire, W.L., Fabian, C., Pugh, R.P., Carter, R.D. (1992) *Journal of Clinical Oncology* **10**, 1284–1291.

Ricketts, D., Turnbull, L., Ryall, G., Bakhshi, R., Rawson, N.S.B., Gazet, J.C., Nolan, C., Coombes, R.C. (1991) *Cancer Research* **51**, 1817–1822.

Robertson, J.F., Bates, K., Pearson, D., Blaney, R.W., Nicholson, R.I. (1992a) *British Journal of Cancer 65*, 727–730.

Robertson, J.F.R., Ellis, I.O., Nicholson,R.I., Robins, A., Bell, J., Blamey, R.W. (1992b) *Breast Cancer Research and Treatment* **20**, 117–124.

Roman, S.D., Clarke, C.L., Hall, R.E., Alexander, I.E., Sutherland, R.L. (1992) *Cancer Research* **52**, 2236–2242.

Ruh, T.S., Turner, J.W., Ruh, M.F. (1991) In *Antihormones in Health and Disease* (ed. M.K. Agarwal), Karger, Basel, pp. 73–86.

Sarkaria, J.N., Gibson, D.F.C., Jordan, V.C., Fowler, J.F., Lindstrom, M.J., Mulcaly, R.T. (1993) *Cancer Research* **53**, 4413–4417.

Sartin, E.A., Barnes, S., Toiviokinnuran, M., Wright, J.C., Wolfe, L.E. (1993) *Anticancer Research* **13**, 229–236.

Schmidtullrich, R.K., Valerie, K., Chan, W., Wazer, D.E., Lin, P.S. (1992) *International Journal of Radiation Biology* **61**, 405–416.

Schwabe, J.W.R., Neuhaus, D., Rhodes, D. (1990) *Nature* **348**, 458–461.

Seitz, P.K., Cooper, K.M, Ives, K.L., Ishizuka, J., Townsend, C.M., Rajaraman, S., Cooper, C.W. (1993) *Endocrinology* **133**, 1116–1124.

Shull, J.D., Beams, F.E., Baldwin,T.M., Gilchrist, C.A., Hrbek, M.J. (1992) *Molecular Endocrinology* **6**, 529–535.

Sica, G., Iacopino, F., Dellacunu, G.R., Marchetti, P. (1992) *Anticancer Drugs* **3**, 147–154.

Sluyser, M. (1992) *Clinical Biochemistry* **25**, 407–414.

Soreide, J.A., Lea, O.A., Varhaug, J.E., Skarstein, A., Kvinnsland, S. (1992) *European Journal of Surgical Oncology* **18**, 112–118.

Souttou, B., Moretti, J.L., Gross, J., Gilloteau, D., Circpin, M. (1993) *Journal of Steroid Biochemistry and Molecular Biology* **44**, 105–112.

Speirs, V., Adams, E.F., Rafferty, B., White, M.C. (1993) *Journal of Steroid Biochemistry and Molecular Biology* **46**, 11–18.

Spyriounis, D.M., Demopoulos, V.J., Kouronakis, P.N., Kouretas, D., Kortsaris, A., Antonoglu, O. (1992) *European Journal of Medicinal Chemistry* **27**, 301–308.

Suto, A., Bradlow, H.L., Kubota, T., Kitajima, M., Wong, G.Y., Osborne, M.P., Telang, N.T. (1993) *Steroids* **58**, 215–219.

Suzuki, M. (1992) *Nippon Geka Gakkai Zasshi* **93**, 71–80.

Swaneck, G.E., Fishman, J. (1991) *Biochemical and Biophysical Research Communications* **174**, 276–281.

Tanino, H., Kubota, T., Saikawa, Y., Kuo, T.H., Takeuchi, T., Kase, S., Kurukawa, T. (1993) *Anticancer Research* **13**, 1219–1221.

Thomas, M., Monet, J.D. (1992) *Journal of Clinical Endocrinology and Metabolism* **75**, 865–870.

Thompson, E.W., Paik, S.M., Brunner, N., Sommers, C.L., Zugmaier, G., Clarke, R. (1992) *Journal of Cellular Physiology* **15**, 534–544.

Toi, M., Yamamoto, Y., Imazawa, T., Takayanagi, T., Akutsu, K., Tominaga, T. (1993) *International Journal of Oncology* **3**, 525–528.

Toko, T., Matsuo, K., Shibata, J., Wierzba, K., Nukatsuka, M., Takeda, S., Yamada, Y., Asao, T., Hirose, T., Sato, B. (1992) *Journal of Steroid Biochemistry and Molecular Biology* **43**, 507–514.

Tominaga, T., Yoshida, Y., Matsumoto, A., Hayashi, K., Kosaki, G. (1993) *Anticancer Research* **13**, 661–666.

Toulas, C., Beauregard, G, Delassus, F., Thauvette, L., Porter, M., Bayard, F., Faye, J.C. (1991) *Federation of European Biochemical Societies Letters* **285**, 28–30.

Ueo, H., Matsuoka, H., Honda, M., Inoeu, H., Takaki, R., Akiyoshi, T. (1990) *Cancer Letters* **71**, 19–24.

Vanderburg, B., Kalkhoven, E., Isbrucker, L., Delaat, S.W. (1992) *Journal of Steroid Biochemistry and Molecular Biology* **42**, 457–466.

Vering, A., Vockel, A., Stegmuller, M., Bender, H.G. (1993) *Journal of Cancer Research and Clinical Oncology* **119**, 415–420.

Walker, K.J., Price-Thomas, J.M., Candlish, W., Nicholson, R.I. (1991) *Breast Cancer Research and Treatment* **64**, 764–768.

Walker, K.J., McClelland, R.A., Candlish, W., Blamey, R.W., Nicholson, R.I. (1992) *European Journal of Cancer* **28**, 34–36.

Weigel, R.J., Deconnide, E.C. (1993) *Cancer Research* **53**, 3472–3474.

Welshons, W.V., Grady, L.H., Engler, K.S.M., Judy, B.M. (1992) *Breast Cancer Research and Treatment* **23**, 97–104.

Westley, B.R., Holzel, F., May, F.E.B. (1989) *Journal of Steroid Biochemistry* **32**, 365–372.

Wilson, S., Reunitz, P.C. (1993) *Journal of Pharmaceutical Sciences* **82**, 571–574.

Wilson, S., Reunitz, P.C., Ruzicki, R.A. (1992) *Journal of Steroid Biochemistry and Molecular Biology* **42**, 613–616.

Winstanley, J., Cooke, J., George, W.D., Murray, G., Holt, S., Croton, R., Griffiths, K., Nicholson, R. (1991) *British Journal of Cancer* **64**, 99–101.

Winterfeld, G., Hauff, P., Goirlich, M., Arnold, W., Fichtner, I., Staab, H.J. (1992) *Journal of Cancer Research and Clinical Oncology* **119**, 91–96.

Yang, D.J., Tewson, T., Tansey, W., Kaung, L.R., Reger, G., Cherif, A., Wright, K.C. (1992) *Journal of Pharmaceutical Sciences* **81**, 622–625.

Ye, Y.H., Huang, Y.S., Wang, Z.Q., Chen, S.M., Ying, T. (1993) *Steroids* **58**, 35–39.

Zaccheo, T., Giudici, D., Disalle, E. (1993) *Journal of Steroid Biochemistry and Molecular Biology* **44**, 677–680.

Zeillinger, R., Kury, F., Speiser, P., Sliutz, G., Czerwenka, K., Kubista, E. (1993) *Clinical Biochemistry* **26**, 221–227.

Zugmaier, G., Knabbe, C., Fritsch, C., Simpson, S., Ennis, B., Lippman, M.E., Dickson, R.B. (1991) *Journal of Steroid Biochemistry and Molecular Biology* **39**, 681–686.

6

Modulation by Tamoxifen of Oncogenes and Growth Factors and the Problem of Tamoxifen Resistance in Breast Cancer

ACTION OF TAMOXIFEN ON ONCOGENES AND SIGNAL TRANSDUCTION IN BREAST CANCER

A brief overview of the role of proto-oncogenes and oncogenes in breast cancer

Oncogenes (genes involved in malignant progression; see Figures 6.1 and 6.2) play an important role in breast cancer (Carney and Sikora, 1990; Sluyser, 1990; MacDonald and Ford, 1991; Vile, 1992; Dickson and Lippman, 1992). Proto-oncogenes are the original cellular genes, which have the potential to be activated to oncogenes and are involved in basic functions such as the regulation of cell growth and differentiation. The protein products of these proto-oncogenes are found at a number of different cellular locations and a mutation in any of these genes could modulate the ability of the cell to respond to growth-regulatory signals. Proto-oncogenes can be classified according to cellular function into one of four groups.

The first group of proto-oncogenes comprises those involved in the control of gene expression via their action on DNA: this is the level at which cell growth and proliferation are controlled and modulated by the messages sent by growth factors. The protein products of the proto-oncogenes *myc*, *fos* and *jun* have been shown to bind to DNA and are thought to control gene transcription. Expression of the *myc* gene is

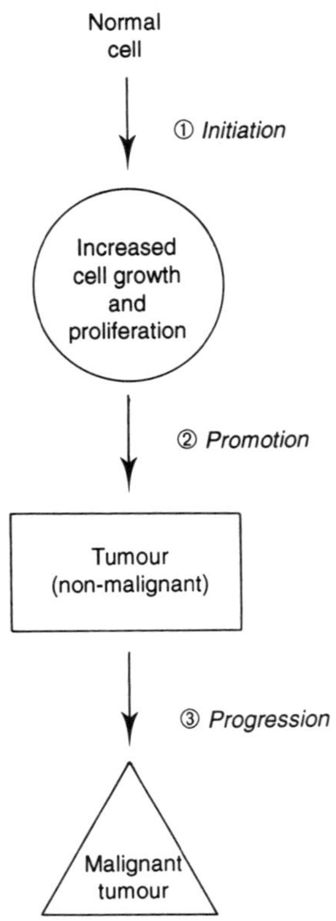

Figure 6.1. A simplified model for carcinogenesis.

(1) Initiation: caused by DNA damage by carcinogens, free radicals and lipid peroxidation products; also proto-oncogene activation and inactivation of tumour suppressor genes
(2) Promotion: induced by tumour promoters, altered signal transduction and secondary genetic damage produces cells with a growth advantage (growth is independent of a requirement for tumour promoters)
(3) Progression: results from further genetic alterations to produce highly malignant metastatic cells

thought to be involved in entry and exit from the cell cycle and its product, the p62 protein, is likely to be important in cell proliferation and differentiation: p62 may play a role in DNA replication by binding to the initiation sites for the biosynthesis of DNA. Furthermore, the protein product of the *jun* gene is a transcription factor involved in the formation of the RNA polymerase-related complex: mutations in these genes will therefore affect transcription of essential cellular genes. A second group of proto-oncogenes comprises the signal transducers and the *ras* gene family code for the protein p21, which can bind GTP and exhibit GTPase activity.

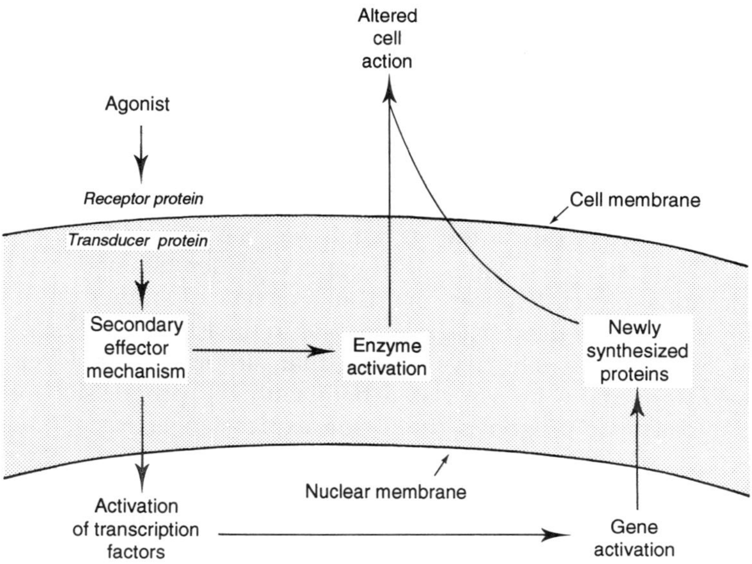

Figure 6.2. A simple overview of cellular signal transduction

The *ras* oncogene is discussed in further detail in the next section. The third group of proto-oncogenes encodes either growth factor receptors or proteins with a homologous function; for example, the product of the *erb-B* gene is homologous to the epidermal growth factor (see below). The final group of proto-oncogenes comprises those that encode growth factors; for example, the *sis* oncogene codes for a protein that is homologous to a subunit of platelet-derived growth factor.

Proto-oncogenes can be activated to produce a gene with oncogenic potential (the oncogene) and there are three main mechanisms of proto-oncogene activation. The first mechanism of activation is amplification of the proto-oncogene, resulting in over-production of the normal product. In breast cancer amplification of the *myc* gene and the *erbB-2* gene has been reported (see below) and the *ras* oncogene (activated by point mutation) has also been found to be amplified in some tumours. The second mechanism of oncogene activation involves loss of control mechanisms: insertional mutagenesis results in transcriptional activation. The final mechanism involves the production of abnormal products, which can occur by point mutations, for example in the *ras* gene, leading to amino acid substitutions which alter the structure of the protein, resulting in abnormal activity. Oncogeneic forms of *ras* produce a protein with decreased GTPase activity which prevents deactivation of the Ras–GTP complex and therefore causing prolonged stimulation from growth factor receptors (see below). Oncogenes have also been detected as a result of chromosomal translocation, which can for example result in formation of a fusion protein with an abnormal tyrosine kinase activity with transforming ability. In addition, truncation of the protein is another oncogenic mutation of proto-oncogenes (e.g. loss of the C-terminus of *v-src*, resulting in increased protein kinase activity). The result of oncogene activation is therefore the production of a protein that can contribute to abnormal cell growth.

Oncogene expression has been extensively studied in breast cancer and either *myc*, *erbB-2* or one of the *ras* family has been found to be expressed in over 60% of samples. Although there is considerable evidence for *myc* amplifications in breast cancer, the results of several studies do not show a clear prognostic or diagnostic role for *myc* in breast cancer. Furthermore, studies of the *ras* family have shown that although high levels of *ras* expression appear to be associated both with the progression of breast cancer and a poor prognosis (increased expression of *ras* p21 has been detected in 63–86% of malignant breast tumours), there is no clear evidence for point mutations or structural alterations in this gene family. The amplification of *erbB-2* in breast cancer has been found to correlate with a poor prognosis in lymph node-positive and lymph node-negative patients in some but not all the studies in this area, and further work is required to establish the role of *erbB-2* as a prognostic indicator in breast cancer. It is of interest that *erbB-2* overexpression has been reported to be an independent predictive factor in subsets of breast cancer patients with a probable poor prognosis, such as those indicating lymph node involvement (Schönborn *et al.*, 1994).

Introduction to the *ras* oncogene

Signal transduction involving the Ras protein, an oncogene product, has been found to be of great importance in cell and tumour biology (reviewed by Egan and Weinberg, 1993). The normal products of the *ras* gene are members of a family of proteins (the p21 proteins) known to bind guanine nucleotides. These Ras proteins bind the nucleoside diphosphate GDP at the inner surface of the cell membrane pending an incoming activating signal. When such a molecular signal is received Ras releases GDP and binds the triphosphate form GTP instead, enabling it briefly to send growth-stimulatory signals into the cell in the form of phosphorylated proteins. However, the GTP is rapidly hydrolysed to GDP by activation of the intrinsic GTPase activity of Ras and this switches off Ras activity. It is of interest in this connection that 17β-oestradiol up-regulates the expression of the stimulatory GTP-binding protein in the MCF-7 cell line (Yasutomo *et al.*, 1993).

The oncogenic form of Ras proteins is found in many cancers; they act in a different way in part because they have a reduced GTPase activity, enabling them to remain switched on for long periods and thus swamp the cell with growth-stimulatory signals. In addition, a defect is likely in the

GTPase-activating proteins (GAPs) normally associated with Ras proteins and thereby switching them off. A number of distinct Ras exchange factors (also known as guanine nucleotide-releasing factors) are known to activate Ras by causing it to release its old GDP and thus take on a new GTP molecule. Upstream gene controllers of Ras exchange factors have been found and these are known as Grb2. The protein made by the *raf* oncogene has been found to be associated with Ras forming a bimolecular complex, and Ras appears to be passing signals down to the Raf protein. Once activated, the Raf protein phosphorylates a second kinase known as MAP kinase kinase, which controls a third kinase termed MAP kinase (MAPK). MAPK, and other kinases further down the cascade, phosphorylate transcription factors including oncogene products and thus send signal molecules into the cell nucleus. In addition, the action of G protein-coupled receptor kinases has been extensively reviewed (e.g., Lefkowitz, 1993). It is of interest that *ras* oncogene-transformed mouse mammary epithelial cells demonstrate persistent responsiveness to oestrogen (Suto *et al.*, 1992).

Protein tyrosine kinases in breast cancer: a brief overview

Other oncogene products, in addition to Ras, have been identified that can transform normal cells into tumour cells and these have been demonstrated to possess a wide range of enzymic activities. Some of these oncogenes encode kinases able to phosphorylate specific threonine and serine amino acid residues of target proteins, while others encode a protein tyrosine kinase that phosphorylates specific tyrosine residues of other proteins. The cell surface receptor for epidermal growth factor also has a tyrosine kinase activity; protein tyrosine kinases have been characterised from human breast cancer cells, and the involvement of the *c-src* oncogene product (see below) has been investigated (Ottenhoffkalff *et al.*, 1992). Elevated expression has been reported of protein tyrosine kinase *c-yes* but not *c-src* in human malignant melanoma (Lognazo *et al.*, 1993). The *her-4/erbB-4* gene encodes a transmembrane protein (structurally related to the product of the *her-2/erbB-2* proto-oncogene), which possesses an intrinsic tyrosine kinase activity that is specifically activated by a glycoprotein (p45) and also heregulin (a family of proteins isolated as specific ligands for Her-2—a protein kinase). Both of these ligands can induce differentiation of breast cancer cells and activation of tyrosine phosphorylation in MDA-MB453 cells (Plowman *et al.*, 1993). Heregulin requires the presence of Her-4 in order to induce phosphorylation of Her-2 and most breast cancer cells that over-express Her-2 (and co-express Her-4) are responsive to heregulin. Furthermore, a tyrosine kinase inhibitor has been shown to inhibit the growth of breast cancer cell growth *in vitro* (Reddy *et al.*, 1992), and cell-signalling targets for the development of new anticancer drugs are currently of great interest (Brunton and Workman, 1993).

In addition, the interferon-induced nuclear signalling is mediated by Jak protein tyrosine kinases (Silvennoinen *et al.*, 1993; Shual *et al.*, 1993): protein tyrosine kinase Jak-1 complements defects in interferon-α/β and γ signal transduction (Muller *et al.*, 1993), and protein tyrosine kinase Jak-2 has been reported to complement a mutant cell line defective in the interferon-γ signal transduction pathway (Watling *et al.*, 1993). Another potent class of growth-regulating signalling proteins are the steroid receptors including, the *erbA* oncoprotein, which recognise signals in the form of steroid hormones and eventually alter gene expression by modulating transcription.

Tamoxifen and oncogene expression

Tamoxifen has been found to increase the steady-state mRNA level of *c-jun*, a proto-oncogene coding for a component of the AP-1 transcription factor complex that regulates the expression of many unlinked genes. This *c-jun* mRNA level in the oviducts of 17β-oestradiol-treated chickens is decreased by 17β-oestradiol in 17β-oestradiol-withdrawn chickens. In contrast, tamoxifen had the opposite effect in the liver (Lau *et al.*, 1991). It has been found that this regulation of steady-state *c-jun* mRNA levels by tamoxifen and 17β-oestradiol occurs at both the transcriptional and post-transcriptional steps, although the role of the product of this proto-oncogene in relation to the growth-inhibitory ability of tamoxifen is unknown (Lau *et al.*, 1991). Furthermore, oestrogen is known to regulate the expression of the *jun* family of proto-oncogenes in the uterus (Chiapetta *et al.*, 1992).

Oestrogens regulate the expression of the *c-fos* proto-oncogene at the transcriptional level, and tamoxifen has been reported to stimulate the expression of *c-fos* in immature rat uterus; *c-fos* transcript levels were monitored by blot analysis, and the response was similar in magnitude to that observed with oestradiol (Kirkland *et al.*, 1993). This induction of *c-fos* by both tamoxifen and oestradiol can be blocked by the progestin medroxy-progesterone acetate. In this study tamoxifen also increased uterine levels of *c-jun, jun-B* and *c-myc* mRNAs and it has been suggested that tamoxifen acts as an oestrogen agonist *in vivo* by activating expression of cellular oncogenes in normal uterine tissue. It has also been found that both 17β-oestradiol and tamoxifen can induce *c-fos* but not *c-jun* or *c-myc* proto-oncogene mRNA expression in human endometrial carcinoma grown in nude mice, and this is thought to be consistent with the oestrogen-like effect of tamoxifen on endometrial carcinoma growth (Sakakibara *et al.*, 1992). In another study tamoxifen was found to induce *c-fos* and *jun-B* but not *c-jun* or *jun-D* proto-oncogenes in adult ovariectomised rat uterus *in vivo* (Nephew *et al.*, 1993). These immediate early-response genes are regulatory factors that can regulate the expression of genes containing an AP-1 recognition site. Northern blotting analysis of total uterine RNA revealed that tamoxifen elevated levels of *c-fos* and *jun-B* mRNA but only slight induction of *c-jun* and *jun-D* expression was observed. However, the pattern of tamoxifen-induced expression of these genes was very different from that reported for oestrogen. Activation of immediate early-response genes by tamoxifen may be important in the uterotrophic actions of tamoxifen, and indeed tamoxifen is less effective at transcriptional activation of oncogenes than oestrogen. The effect of tamoxifen on proto-oncogene expression in immature rat uterus has also been studied (Bhattacharyya *et al.*, 1994).

The hormonal regulation of *c-erbB-2* oncogene expression has been studied in breast cancer cells (Debortoli *et al.*, 1992) and in primary human breast cancers (Delvenne *et al.*, 1992). Furthermore, the role of *erbB-2* and its ligands in the control of the growth of malignant breast epithelium has been investigated (Lupu *et al.*, 1992). Tamoxifen has been reported both to up-regulate *c-erbB-2* expression in oestrogen-responsive breast cancer cells *in vitro* (Antoniotti *et al.*, 1992) and also to decrease levels of *c-erbB-2 and c-myc* in tamoxifen-treated breast cancer (Leroy *et al.*, 1991). The differential regulation of *c-myc* by progestins and antioestrogens in T47D human breast cancer cells has also been reported (Wong and Murphy, 1991). Although in breast cancer cell lines *c-myc* amplification is often associated with a loss of oestrogen responsiveness, it has been reported that in the oestrogen-responsive cell line VHB1, which displayed *c-myc* amplification and over-expression, 17β-oestradiol was still able to stimulate *c-myc* expression while 4-hydroxytamoxifen equally decreased expression (Collyn-d'Hooghe *et al.*, 1991). The role of *c-myc* proto-oncogene expression is thus of importance in oestrogen-dependent and oestrogen-independent breast cancer (Shiu *et al.*, 1993). The relationship of *int-2* amplification in breast cancer to amplification of *c-erbB-2* and *c-myc* has been studied and has been found to be associated with decreased survival of patients (Henry *et al.*, 1993). Activation of expression of *c-myc* promotes cell proliferation and blocks differentiation.

It is of interest that *c-myc*, but not *EJ-ras*, *c-fos* or *c-jun*, appears to functionally antagonise the ability of the retinoblastoma protein to arrest the cell cycle but does not inhibit the activity of the p53 tumour suppressor protein (Goodrich and Lee, 1992). The biological role of p53 has been discussed (Selter and Montenarh, 1994). Retinoblastoma protein is a negative regulator of cell growth, and inactivating mutations of the retinoblastoma gene are found in many tumor cells. Furthermore, loss of function of the p53 protein appears to be central to the development of human cancers because both gene alleles for this protein are often found to be mutated in a range of tumour types. The prognostic significance of p53 gene alteration in node-negative breast cancer has been noted (Elledge *et al.*, 1993). In addition, wild-type p53 gene expression can inhibit transformation by viral and cellular oncogenes *in vitro* and p53 is classified as a tumour suppressor. The normal functions of p53 could involve the activation of gene expression through the binding of specific DNA-regulatory sequences, and over-expression of p53 can result in growth inhibition. It specifically interferes with the onset of S phase and can repress transcription at a variety of promoters. It has been demonstrated that wild-type p53 specifically represses the activity of promoters whose initiation is dependent on the presence of a TATA box (Mack *et al.*, 1993). In addition, p53 interacts with and inhibits the function of a cellular DNA replication factor, the single-stranded DNA-binding protein complex RPA (replication protein A) (see also Chapter 9), and this may contribute to the growth-suppressing action of p53 (Dutta *et al.*, 1993). In aggressive breast cancer p53 mutations have been shown to occur (Mazars *et al.*, 1992). In addition, two distinct mechanisms have been shown to alter p53 in breast cancer, mutation and nuclear exclusion: some breast cancers that contain the wild-type form of p53 may inactivate the tumour-suppressing activity of this protein by sequestering it in the cytoplasm (a mechanism employed in normal lactating breast tissue to permit transient cell proliferation), thereby preventing it reaching its site of action in the nucleus and this could explain how some breast cancer tissues inactivate p53 function without mutation (Moll *et al.*, 1992). The genetic basis for p53 over-expression in breast cancer has been investigated (Davidoff *et al.*, 1991). The immune response to p53 in breast cancer patients is directed against immunodominant epitopes that are unrelated to the mutational hot spot (Schlichtholtz *et al.*, 1992). The gene for the p53-binding protein Mdm-2 has been shown to be differentially expressed in human breast carcinoma (Sheikh *et al.*, 1993). The tumour suppressor protein p53 has been found to have a role in apoptosis (Sen and P'Incalci, 1992) and this p53-dependent apoptosis has been suggested to modulate the cytotoxicity of anticancer agents (Lowe *et al.*, 1993).

MODULATION OF GROWTH FACTORS IN BREAST CANCER

The role of growth factors in breast cancer and in particular their involvement in the cellular processes from mitogenesis to transformation (Dickson and Lippman, 1992) is a subject of considerable interest. The modulation by oestrogens of the proliferative response of breast cancer cells to growth factors has been studied (Stewart *et al.*, 1992). Indeed, growth factor regulation by tamoxifen has been reported in patients with breast cancer (Jordan, 1993). The transforming growth factors β (TGF-β) are a family of peptide growth factors that play a role in the regulation of cell growth and differentiation. Although loss of sensitivity to these peptides may contribute to epithelial carcinogenesis, many breast cancer cells remain sensitive to their growth-inhibitory effects, and the local induction of TGF-β by tamoxifen, synthetic progestins and retinoids offers a pharmacological approach to chemoprevention (Dickens and Colletta, 1993). Tamoxifen has been found to induce the hormonally regulated negative growth factor TGF-β in MCF-7 cells (Knabbe *et al.*, 1991). TGF-β also inhibits the growth of MDA-MB-231 and MDA-MB-468 cells in culture (Toi *et al.*, 1992). Furthermore, induction of TGF-β_1 in human breast cancer *in vivo* following tamoxifen treatment has been reported (Butta *et al.*, 1992). Immunohistochemical techniques showed that three months of tamoxifen treatment resulted in a consistent induction of extracellular TGF-β_1 in breast cancer biopsies and occurred in both oestrogen receptor-positive and oestrogen receptor-negative tumours (Butta *et al.*, 1992). It has been suggested that this is a novel oestrogen receptor-independent mechanism of action of tamoxifen that involves the stromal induction of a potent growth inhibitor for epithelial cells.

The ability of tamoxifen to decrease the rate of proliferation of vascular smooth muscle in cells in culture has been found to be through the induction of TGF-β (Grainger *et al.*, 1993). It is of interest also that RRR-α-tocopheryl succinate inhibits the growth of oestrogen receptor-positive and receptor-negative human breast cancer cells and that this was established to be through enhanced secretion of TGF-β (Charpentier *et al.*, 1993). Tamoxifen has been found to down-regulate TGF-α levels in oestrogen receptor-positive and progesterone receptor-positive breast cancers through the oestrogen receptor (Noguchi *et al.*, 1993). In addition, TGF-α levels in oestrogen receptor-negative and progesterone receptor-negative breast cancer were not affected by tamoxifen treatment. Furthermore, positivity of epidermal growth factor (EGF) receptor was 60% in oestrogen receptor-negative and progesterone receptor-negative breast cancer and only 30% in oestrogen receptor-positive and progesterone receptor-positive breast cancer. TGF-α appears to be more important as an autocrine growth factor in oestrogen receptor-negative and progesterone receptor-negative breast cancer than in oestrogen receptor-positive and progesterone receptor-positive breast cancers. It is of associated interest that immunoreactivity to TGF-α has been reported in a variety of epithelial tissues (Alison *et al.*, 1993). The effect of 17β-oestradiol, and also TGF-α, on polyphosphoinositide metabolism has been reported in MCF-7 cells (Etindi *et al.*, 1992). Furthermore, tamoxifen and vanadate synergistically caused the accumulation of polyphosphoinositides in cell membranes (Friedman, 1993).

It is somewhat paradoxical, therefore, that TGF-β_1 can also induce oestrogen-independent tumorigenicity of human breast cancer cells in athymic mice (Arteaga *et al.*, 1993). Although TGF-β inhibited the growth of Ishikawa cells, it stimulated the proliferation of HEC–50 human endometrial adenocarcinoma cells (Murphy *et al.*, 1992). 4-Hydroxytamoxifen had no effect on HEC-50 growth and under some conditions had growth-stimulating effects on Ishikawa cells (Gong *et al.*, 1992). In addition, TGF-β and fibroblast growth factor (see below) have both been reported to be promoters of tumour progression to malignancy (Wright *et al.*, 1993). TGF-β appears to have a role in resistance to inhibition of cell growth and oncogenesis (Fynan and Reiss, 1993) in addition to its antiproliferative action. The role of TGF-β and the cell surface in tumour progression has also been considered (Newman, 1993). Fibroblast growth factor 4 (FGF-4) transfection of MCF-7 cells has been shown to produce cell lines that are tumorigenic and metastatic in ovariectomised or tamoxifen-treated athymic mice (Mcleskey *et al.*, 1993). Furthermore, a qualitative demonstration has been made of spontaneous metastasis by MCF-7 cells co-transfected with FGF-4 and *lacZ* (Kurebayshi *et al.*, 1993).

Tamoxifen and its metabolite 4-hydroxytamoxifen have been reported to block the mitogenic activity of EGF and insulin-like growth factor (IGF) (see below). EGF is a protein kinase considered to be an important target site for breast cancer therapy (Modjtahedi *et al.*, 1993). Secretion of EGF by the macrophages associated with breast carcinoma has been reported: these tumour-associated macrophages may enhance tumour growth and may be associated with a poor prognosis (O'Sullivan *et al.*, 1993). A study has been made of EGF receptors and steroid receptors in breast cancer in terms of tumour grading, tumour size, lymph involvement and age (Zeillinger *et al.*, 1993); an inverse correlation was found between oestrogen receptor and EGF receptor status (see Chapter 5). The EGF receptor has also been studied in breast cancer tissue and a comparison made with non-malignant breast tissue (Dittadi *et al.*, 1993). EGF has been shown to disrupt gap junctional communication and induces phosphorylation of connexin on serine 43 (Lau *et al.*, 1992). Cell-to-cell communication can be inhibited by methimazole (Asakawa *et al.*, 1992) and gap junctional communication in neoplastic transformation is of considerable interest (Hotzwagenblatt and Shalloway, 1993). The ability of antioestrogens to inhibit growth factor-activated proliferation and to alter early gene expression in MCF-7 cells has been evaluated (Wosikowski *et al.*, 1993). Antioestrogens antagonise (and oestradiol increases) the growth factor-induced activator protein 1 activity but without altering *c-fos* and *c-jun* synthesis in MCF-7 cells (Philips *et al.*, 1993).

The expression of the IGF-1 receptor in human breast cancer, in contrast to the EGF receptor, has been reported to correlate directly with oestrogen receptor status (Figueroa *et al.*, 1993). Furthermore, an elevated IGF-1 receptor content has been reported in most human breast cancers compared with normal tissue, and an elevated IGF-1 receptor content is a favourable prognostic indicator (Papa *et al.*, 1993). Tamoxifen inhibits the action of IGF-1 in the MCF-7 cell line (Freiss *et al.*, 1990), and of IFG-1 in patients with stage I breast cancer (Pollak *et al.*, 1990; Rosen *et al.*, 1991; Lien *et al.*, 1992). Suppression of serum IGF-1 levels in breast cancer patients has been reported during adjuvant tamoxifen therapy (Pollak, *et al.*, 1992; Lonning, *et al.*, 1992; Friedl *et al.*, 1993). In the MCF-7 cell line this is thought to occur both by modulation of the concentration of growth factor binding sites and by alteration of growth factor receptor function

(Freiss *et al.*, 1990). A decrease in IGF-1 binding sites was also found, which may explain the inhibition of the mitogenic action of IGf-1 by tamoxifen (Freiss *et al.*, 1990). In addition, the binding proteins for IGF have now been identified in breast cancer cells such as the MCF-7 cell line (Yee *et al.*, 1991). Tamoxifen has also been reported to inhibit IGF-1 gene expression in an *in vivo* experimental system and it has been demonstrated that this is in part a consequence of a pituitary-independent action of tamoxifen (Huynh *et al.*, 1993). It is likely that tamoxifen and 4-hydroxytamoxifen can interfere with the initial steps of growth factor binding and action in oestrogen receptor-negative as well as in oestrogen receptor-positive cells.

ACTION AS A GROWTH MODULATOR OF CANCER CELLS IN COMBINATION WITH OTHER COMPOUNDS

Tamoxifen has been used in combination with interferon in the treatment of advanced breast cancer, and the biological effects of these two growth modulators has been assessed *in vivo* (Buzzi *et al.*, 1992; Seymour and Bezwoda, *et al.*, 1993). The early events in signalling by interferons have been discussed (Pellegrini and Schindler, 1993). Tamoxifen modulates the antiproliferative action of interferon-α in U937 cells (Balint *et al.*, 1992) and cytoxicity in MCF-7 cells has been augmented by using combinations of tamoxifen, interferons (type I and type II) and tumour necrosis factor α (Tiwari *et al.*, 1991). Furthermore, synergistic cytotoxic effects of tamoxifen, tumour necrosis factor and interferon-γ have been reported in breast cancer cell lines (Matsuo *et al.*, 1992). Tamoxifen used in combination with human recombinant interferon-β SER (rIFN-β SER) inhibited the growth of the MCF-7 and the MDA-MB-231 cell lines and was totally growth suppressive for the MCF-7 xenografts in nude mice (see Chapter 5; Gibson *et al.*, 1993). This combination of tamoxifen plus interferon has been suggested to be useful in the prevention of disease recurrence that occurs as a result of the development of resistance to tamoxifen, and consequent relapse (see below).

Tamoxifen has been shown to attenuate pulsatile growth hormone secretion—an effect mediated in part by somatostatin (Tannenbaum *et al.*, 1992)—and to have a direct effect on growth hormone secretion by pituitary cells *in vitro* (Malaab *et al.*, 1992). Tamoxifen inhibited the proliferation of human pituitary adenomas *in vitro* and this was independent of oestrogen receptor expression, whereas 17β-oestradiol stimulated and progesterone inhibited cell growth and this correlated with specific receptor expression (Caronti *et al.*, 1993). A non-calcaemic analogue of calcitrol, 22-oxa-calcitrol, has been shown to have an antitumour effect on both oestrogen receptor-positive (MCF-7 and ZR-75-1) and -negative (MX-1) breast cancer tumours, in athymic mice (see Chapter 5) implanted with human breast carcinoma; this effect was enhanced by tamoxifen in oestrogen receptor-positive tumours (Abe-Hashimoto *et al.*, 1993).

The antitumour effect of ionidamine has been studied in combination with tamoxifen in human breast cancer cells (Sica *et al.*, 1991). It is of interest also that suramin has been shown to antagonise the ability of 4-hydroxytamoxifen to inhibit the growth of MCF-7 cells (Berthosis *et al.*, 1992). Tamoxifen has a synergistic antiproliferative activity with cisplatin on primary ovarian tumours (Scambia *et al.*, 1992) and increases the response rate of human malignant melanoma cells to treatment with cisplatin, carmustine and dacarbazine (McClay *et al.*, 1993a, 1993b; McClay and McClay, 1994). Investigations have shown that the synergy between tamoxifen and cisplatin is not mediated by the effects of tamoxifen on the oestrogen receptor, calmodulin, protein kinase C, or cell cycle regulation, although the factors that determine cellular sensitivity to tamoxifen also determine whether tamoxifen interacts synergistically with cisplatin (McClay *et al.*, 1993a). Furthermore, an *in vitro* synergism between a novel amphibian oocytic ribonuclease and tamoxifen, lovastatin and cisplatin has been reported in the human OVCAR-3 ovarian carcinoma cell line (Mikulski *et al.*, 1992).

A synergistic action of tamoxifen and pre-activated photofrin-II in killing breast cancer cells has been reported (Chang *et al.*, 1991). Tamoxifen can enhance the radiosensitivity of C6 glioma cells (Wei *et al.*, 1992); the use of tamoxifen in the treatment of malignant gliomas is discussed in Chapter 4. The inhibitory effects of tamoxifen on the growth of rat mammary tumours (see Chapter 5) can be potentiated by the use of krestin (Lino *et al.*, 1992). Furthermore, 4-hydroxytamoxifen prevents the stimulatory effects of L-triiodothyronine on MCF-7 cell proliferation (Zhou-Li *et al.*, 1992). Tamoxifen also enhanced the ability of doxorubicin to inhibit the growth of the ovarian GZL-8 cell line, which had unusual characteristics, including chromosomal alterations, rapid growth and the accumulation of lipids; a new compound related to doxorubicin, ruboxyl (a nitroxyl derivative of daunorubicin), has been synthesised that has an acute toxicity and antitumour effect in animals (Leonetti *et al.*, 1993).

Angiogenesis can be assessed by use of antibodies to the platelet endothelium cell adhesion molecule, and this is considered to be an indicator of node metastases and survival in breast cancer (Horak *et al.*, 1992). Tumour growth and angiogenesis can be inhibited using tamoxifen in combination with a bacterial polysaccharide (Tanuka *et al.*, 1991). Tamoxifen inhibits angiogenesis in the chick egg chorioallantoic membrane and this angiostatic activity is not altered in the presence of excess 17β-oestradiol (Gagliardi and Collins, 1993). This finding suggests that this activity is exerted via mechanisms independent of the oestrogen receptor, and it may contribute to the therapeutic effect of tamoxifen in some oestrogen receptor-negative tumours.

MODULATION OF THE IMMUNE SYSTEM AND ROLE IN CYTOKINE ACTION ON BREAST CANCER CELLS

In human carcinomas there is often an infiltration of lymphocytes and other cells of the immune system that are able to produce a range of cytokines, which may affect the growth of the tumour epithelium. Indeed, the cytokine interleukin-4 (IL-4) inhibited the growth of MCF-7, MDA-MB-231 and MDA-MB-468 breast cancer cells in culture, and combined treatment with tamoxifen resulted in additive inhibition (Toi *et al..*, 1992). Furthermore, IL-4 inhibited 90% of the 17β-oestradiol-stimulated growth of MCF-7 cells in a dose-dependent manner but without a change in expression of the oestrogen receptor, and growth inhibition by IL-4 was less in the absence of oestrogens (Toi *et al.*, 1992). Tamoxifen has been reported to potentiate the antitumour activity of IL-2 (Kim *et al.*, 1990) and also P-30, which is a protein possessing antitumour activity (Mikulski *et al.*, 1990). Furthermore, IL-1 has been found to inhibit the growth of the ovarian cancer cell line NIH-OVCAR-3 (Kilian *et al.*, 1991).

The effects of tamoxifen and oestradiol on mixed lymphocyte reactions have been examined in the rat (Baral *et al.*, 1991). Tamoxifen exerted a constant inhibitory effect over the concentration range 0.4–400 ng/ml. Although oestradiol was ineffective at physiological concentrations (0.4 ng/ml), at pharmacological levels (400 ng/ml) some inhibitory effects were observed. An evaluation has been made of ADP ribosylation as an indicator of mononuclear leucocyte responsiveness in breast cancer patients treated with tamoxifen (Pero *et al.*, 1992) and poly(ADP-ribosylation) has been proposed as a target for cancer chemotherapy (Judson and Threadgill, 1993). The influence of oestradiol and tamoxifen on the susceptibility of human breast cancer cells to lysis by lymphokine-activated killer cells in breast cancer patients treated with tamoxifen has been reported (Albertini *et al.*, 1992). Tamoxifen has been shown to modulate natural killer (NK) cell activity *in vivo* in patients with bilateral primary breast cancer (BBC): lymphocytes derived from 10 BBC patients treated with tamoxifen exhibited NK cell activity that was comparable to that of normal controls and patients with single-breast cancer, but was reduced compared to the pre-treatment period (Robinson *et al.*, 1993; Lukač *et al.*, 1994). Furthermore, patients with BBC also showed a reduction in the proportion of CD4+ T cells and in autologous mixed lymphocyte reaction proliferative responses compared to normal controls. Tamoxifen has been reported to assist the recovery of lymphocyte populations in breast cancer patients that are decreased as a result of radiotherapy (Lukač *et al.*, 1994). In patients with breast cancer elevated prostaglandin E_2 production by monocytes is thought to be responsible for the depressed levels of NK and lymphokine-activated killer cell function (Baxevanis *et al.*, 1993). It is of related interest that in patients with stage II breast cancer adjuvant chemotherapy but not tamoxifen therapy has been reported to cause a prolonged decrease in mitogenic stimulation of peripheral blood mononuclear cells (Knogler *et al.*, 1992). Antioestrogens are known to modulate the immune responses of normal human mononuclear cells: tamoxifen was shown to be immunosuppressive; however, it additionally stimulated the production of tumour necrosis factor, which may be beneficial (Tedorczyk-Injeyan *et al.*, 1993). 17β-Oestradiol when added to human peripheral blood mononuclear cells (PBMC) stimulated by sheep red blood cells (SRBC) was found to augment the antigen-specific primary antibody response *in vitro* (Clerici *et al.*, 1991). However, PBMC incubated with tamoxifen prior to culture were no longer stimulated to produce an increased number of anti-SRBC antibodies compared to control cultures. 17β-Oestradiol augments the immune response to SRBC by inhibiting CD8+ T suppressor cells, and this effect is reversed by the binding of tamoxifen to the CD8+ oestrogen receptors. In addition, oestradiol has been shown to augment whilst tamoxifen inhibits mast cell secretion in rats (Vliagoftis *et al.*, 1992). Tamoxifen has been reported to induce an immune system-mediated destruction of platelets (Candido *et al.*, 1993).

RESISTANCE OF BREAST CANCER CELLS

Antioestrogen resistance is an important mechanism by which breast cancer cells can prevent endocrine therapy being effective (Katzenellenbogen, 1991). Tamoxifen resistance is a major cause of treatment failure in breast cancer, and molecular mechanisms of resistance to tamoxifen therapy in breast cancer have been considered (Morrow and Jordan, 1993) and strategies for controlling tamoxifen-resistant breast cancer have been discussed (Jiang and Jordan, 1992.) Acquired tamoxifen resistance has been correlated with reduced tumour levels of tamoxifen and isomerisation of *trans*-4-hydroxytamoxifen (Osborne *et al.*, 1991). When oestrogen receptor-positive MCF-7 cells were implanted in athymic nude BALB/c mice it was found that after four to six months of tumour growth suppression by *trans*-tamoxifen, tumour progression was observed. This acquired resistance was not due to loss of oestrogen receptors or to alterations in serum or tumour oestrogen levels, or even to changes in tamoxifen or its major metabolites in serum. Indeed, tamoxifen-resistant tumours remained oestrogen dependent *in vivo*. However, resistant tumours did have significantly lower intracellular tamoxifen levels and there was a high level of isomerisation of the potent antioestrogenic metabolite *trans*-4-hydroxytamoxifen to the less potent *cis* form. The mechanism of this tamoxifen-stimulated breast tumour growth has now been investigated with non-isomerisable analogues of tamoxifen and its metabolites. It was found that metabolism and isomerisation of tamoxifen to oestrogenic compounds was not the mechanism of tamoxifen-stimulated growth in athymic mice (Wolf *et al.*, 1993). Other potential mechanisms for tamoxifen-stimulated growth such as oestrogen receptor mutation (see Chapter 5) may appear more likely. However, mutations in the oestrogen receptor have been found to occur at such low frequency that it is unlikely that they account for most oestrogen-independent tamoxifen-resistant breast cancer (Karnik *et al.*, 1994).

The levels of tamoxifen and isomers of 4-hydroxytamoxifen have been measured by high-performance liquid chromatography (HPLC) (see Chapter 4) in tamoxifen-resistant tumours from breast cancer patients, and a wide range of tumour tamoxifen levels and accumulation of the less antioestrogenic *cis* isomer of 4-hydroxytamoxifen were found (Osborne *et al.*, 1992). However, it was not entirely clear from these findings whether this profile was indeed related to the development of tamoxifen resistance. The occurrence of oestrogenic tamoxifen metabolites in tamoxifen-resistant human breast tumours have been measured by HPLC and mass spectrometry, and metabolite E (a known oestrogenic metabolite of tamoxifen) and another oestrogenic metabolite, bisphenol, were identified (Wiebe *et al.*, 1992). These oestrogenic metabolites may contribute to the stimulation of growth of oestrogen-responsive tumours during prolonged exposure to tamoxifen. It is clear that further study of the relationship between metabolism (see Chapter 3) and acquired tamoxifen resistance is required.

Progression from a hormone-sensitive to -insensitive tumour can take place by a number of independent pathways, some of which involve loss of receptors, whereas others may be because of the presence of abnormal receptors (King, 1992). Hormonal insensitivity has been reported in cells in the presence of apparently normal receptors and it is likely that such cells are generated either by spontaneous changes or by steroid deprivation. Oestrogen receptor variants have been implicated in the development of hormone resistance in breast cancer (Sluyser, 1992). It has been proposed that it is the molecular heterogeneity of oestrogen receptors in breast cancer cells, characterised by the presence of mutant receptor forms, that generates the cellular heterogeneity evident when progesterone receptors or DNA ploidy are analysed in cell subpopulations. It is this cellular heterogeneity that is likely to lead to the lack of uniformity in response to tamoxifen (Horwitz, 1993). This is because of the existence of mixed subpopulations of breast cancer cells, reflected in heterogeneity of progesterone receptors and DNA ploidy, which are being modulated under the influence of tamoxifen. Furthermore, it is possible that rather than being resistant, different subsets of cells can be inhibited or stimulated by tamoxifen, and their suppression or outgrowth alters the phenotype of the tumour. This mixed and potentially dangerous response to tamoxifen treatment may perhaps be predicted by progesterone-receptor heterogeneity.

Unusual expression and localisation of particular heat-shock proteins (HSP) have been reported in human tumour cells (Ferrarini *et al.*, 1992). It is thought that under physiological conditions the synthesis of HSP27 (a substrate for protein kinase C; see Chapter 7) is regulated by oestrogen in oestrogen-responsive human breast cancer cell lines. Although high levels of HSP27 in breast tumours are associated with a poor prognosis in early breast cancer, this appears to switch to being a good prognostic factor in advanced breast cancer; the biological explanation for this has not yet been identified (Love and King, 1994). HSP27 may play an important role in the growth and progression of the human breast cancer cell and, in particular, over-expression of HSP27 in drug-sensitive cells appears to confer resistance to cytotoxic drugs (multidrug resistance). Radiation damage to drug-resistant sublines of a human breast cancer cell line has been reported (Alaouijamali *et al.*, 1992). It is of interest that occurrence of HSP27 has been reported to correlate with growth and drug resistance in human breast cancer cell lines (Oesterreich *et al.*, 1993). Furthermore, the relationship of HSP27 and the oestrogen receptor in hormone-sensitive and -insensitive cell lines has been investigated and it appears that there is a good correlation between the presence of the oestrogen receptor and high amounts of HSP27, but that low amounts of HSP27 are present in many oestrogen receptor-negative cells (Dunn *et al.*, 1993). This important area of investigation shows considerable promise for understanding the interaction between different receptors and important proteins such as the HSP in breast cancer.

Although combined treatment with tamoxifen and progestin effectively controlled human endometrial tumour growth in the nude mouse, after this initial response the tumours became resistant to continuous progestin administration (Satyaswaroop *et al.*, 1992). Although the characteristic progesterone receptor proteins were detected by Western blot analysis in tamoxifen-treated tumours, the tumours treated with both tamoxifen and progestin were devoid of such receptors. This observed resistance to combination treatment with tamoxifen and progestin in human endometrial carcinoma may, therefore, result from desensitisation to progestin following down-regulation of progesterone receptors.

Tamoxifen can stimulate the growth *in vivo* of the multidrug-resistant oestrogen receptor-negative MDA-MB-A1 human breast cancer cell line (Maenpaa *et al.*, 1993). Although no inhibitory or stimulatory effect of tamoxifen was observed *in vitro,* tamoxifen had a clear tumour growth-stimulating effect when tamoxifen-treated and control cells were inoculated into nude mice, some of which were then treated with tamoxifen. The most pronounced stimulatory effects were observed in cells that had been cultured with tamoxifen, and these results suggest that prolonged *in vitro* exposure to tamoxifen induces cellular changes that result in tumours that are stimulated to grow faster in mice following treatment with tamoxifen. An oestrogen receptor-positive MCF-7 clone has been developed that is resistant to both antioestrogens and to oestradiol (Jiang *et al.*, 1992). Transfection of MCF-7 cells with the *her-2/neu* gene has been shown to result in oestrogen-dependent, tamoxifen-resistant tumorigenic growth (Benz *et al.*, 1992). Prolonged exposure to tamoxifen has been reported to result in the selection of a stable breast cancer clone (Sipila *et al.*, 1993). Resistance to tamoxifen with persisting sensitivity to oestrogen has also been reported (Pavlik *et al.*, 1992) and this may be mediated by excessive antioestrogen binding site activity (see Chapter 7). TGF-β_1 (see above) has been implicated in the failure of tamoxifen therapy in human breast cancer (Thompson *et al.*, 1991).

A tamoxifen-resistant variant (ZR-75-9a1) has been obtained from the ZR-75-1 cell line, which does not contain detectable levels of oestrogen receptors and progesterone receptors, and has a longer cell number doubling time than the parent line. Tamoxifen-resistance in ZR-75-9a1 cells was found to be reversed by the absence of tamoxifen (unless the medium was also devoid of oestrogenic activity) and this may have a clinical parallel among those patients who initially relapse while undergoing antioestrogen therapy but later respond to challenge with tamoxifen. Changes in EGF expression and response to ligand are both associated with acquired tamoxifen resistance or oestrogen independence in the ZR-75-1 cell line (Long *et al.*, 1992). The synthesis of secreted proteins has been studied in the tamoxifen resistant variant subline of the MCF-7 cell line, the AL-1 cell line (Lykkesfeld and Sorensen, 1992. A combination of tamoxifen and interferon-β is being tested as a way of overcoming clinical resistance to tamoxifen in advanced breast cancer (Buzzi *et al.*, 1992). The ability of retinoic acid to inhibit the growth of both tamoxifen-sensitive and tamoxifen-resistant MCF-7 sublines has been investigated (Butler and Fontana, 1992). A 4-hydroxytamoxifen-resistant human breast cancer variant (MCF-7/LCC2) has been identified that retains sensitivity to the pure steroidal antioestrogen ICI 182 780 (Brunner *et al.*, 1993). Indeed use of ICI 182 780 has been suggested as a strategy for overcoming resistance to tamoxifen (Hu *et al.*, 1993), and the potential importance of such pure antioestrogens in the treatment of patients who have become resistant to tamoxifen therapy (Wakeling, 1993) is discussed in Chapter 10. The tamoxifen analogue toremifene has also been found to be useful in the treatment of some breast cancer patients with tamoxifen-resistant breast cancer who have relapsed during tamoxifen therapy (Pyrhönen *et al.*, 1994.)

REFERENCES

Abe-Hashimoto, J., Kikuchi, T., Matsumoto, T., Nishii, Y., Ogata, E., Ikeda, K. (1993) *Cancer Research* **53**, 2534–2537.

Alaouijamali, M.A., Batist, G., Lehnert, S. (1992) *Radiation Research* **129**, 37–42.
Albertini, M.R., Gibson, D.F.C., Robinson, S.P., Howard, S.P., Tans, K., Lindstrom, M.J., Robinson, R.R., Tormey, D.C., Jordan, V.C., Sondel, P.M. (1992) *Journal of Immunotherapy* **11**, 30–39.
Alison, M.R., Nasim, M.M., Anikumar, T.V., Sarraf, C.E. (1993) *Cell Proliferation* **26**, 449–461.
Antoniotti, S., Maggiora, P., Dati, C., Debotoli, M. (1992) *European Journal of Cancer* **28A**, 318–321.
Arteaga, C.L., Cartydugger, T., Moses, H.L., Hurd, S.D., Pietenpol, J.A. (1993) *Cell Growth and Differentiation* **4**, 193–202.
Asakawa, H., Yamasaki, H., Hanafusa, T., Kono, N., Tarui, S. (1992) *Research Communications in Chemical Pathology and Pharmacology* **77**, 131–146.
Balint, E., Grimley, P.M., Michalic, R., Aszalos, A. (1992) *Cancer Letters* **67**, 13–20.
Baral, E., Kwok, S., Berczi, I. (1991) *Immunopharmacology* **21**, 191–197.
Baxevanis, C.N., Redos, G.J., Gritzapis, A.D., Dedousis, G.V.Z., Missitzis, I., Papamichail, M. (1993) *Cancer* **72**, 491–501.
Benz, C.C., Scott, G.K., Sarup, J.C., Johnson, R.M., Tripathy, D., Coronadao, E., Shepard, H.M., Osborne, C.K. (1992) *Breast Cancer Research and Treatment* **24**, 85–96.
Berthois, Y., Dong, X.F., Martin, P.M., Cvitkovic, E. (1992) *Journal of the National Cancer Institute* **84**, 1438–1443.
Bhattacharyya, N., Ramsammy, R., Eatman, E., Hollis, V.W., Anderson, W.A. (1994) *Journal of Submicroscopic Cytology and Pathology* **26**, 147–162.
Brunner, N., Frandsen, T.L., Holsthansen, C., Bei, M., Thompson, E.W., Wakeling, A.E., Lippman, M.E., Clarke, R. (1993) *Cancer Research* **53**, 3229–3232.
Brunton, V.G., Workman, P. (1993) *Cancer Chemotherapy and Pharmacology* **32**, 1–19.
Butler, W.B., Fontana, J.A. (1992) *Cancer Research* **52**, 6164–6167.
Butta, A., MacLennan, K., Flanders, K.C., Sacks, N.P.M., Smith, I., Mckinna, A., Dowsett, M., Lalage, M., Wakefield, L.M., Sporn, M.B., Baum, M., Colletta, A.A. (1992) *Cancer Research* **52**, 4261–4264.
Buzzi, F., Brugia, M., Rossi, G., Giustini, L., Scoponi, C., Sica, G. (1992) *Anticancer Research* **12**, 869–872.
Candido, A., Bussa, S., Tartaglione, R., Mancini, R., Rumi, C., Rossi, P., Bizzi, B. (1993) *Tumori* **79**, 231–237.
Carney, D., Sikora, K. (1990) *Genes and Cancer*, John Wiley & Sons, Chichester.
Caronti, B. Palladini, G., Bevilacqua, M.G., Petrangeli, E., Fraiolu, B., Cantore, G., Tamburrano, G., Carapella, C.M., Jaffain-Rea, M.J. (1993) *Tumour Biology* **14**, 59–68.
Chang, P.H., Pervaiz, S., Battaglino, M., Matthews, J.L., Clark,C., Day, J., Preskitt, J., Vanderpool, D., Gulliya, K.S. (1991) *European Journal of Cancer* **27**, 1034–1039.
Charpentier, A., Groves, S., Simmons-Menchaca, M., Turley, J., Zhao, B., Sanders, B.G., Kline, K. (1993) *Nutrition and Cancer* **19**, 225–239.
Chiapetta, C., Kirkland, J.L., Loosemitchell, D.S., Murphy, L., Stancel, G.M. (1992) *Journal of Steroid Biochemistry and Molecular Biology* **41**, 113–124.
Clerici, E., Bergamasco, E., Ferrario, E., Villa, M.L. (1991) *Journal of Clinical and Laboratory Immunology* **34**, 71–78.
Collyn-d'Hooghe, M., Vandewalle, B., Hornez, L., Lantoine, D., Revillion, F., Lefebvre, J., Kerckaert, J.P. (1991) *Anticancer Research* **11**, 2175–2179.
Davidoff, A.M., Humphrey, P.A., Iglehart, J.D., Marks, J.R. (1991) *Proceedings of the National Academy of Sciences USA* **88**, 5006–5010.

Delvenne, C.G., Winklergol, R.A., Piccart, M.J., Hustin, J., Michaux, D., Leclercq, G., Norgaret, J.M., Autier, P. (1992) *European Journal of Cancer* **28A**, 700–705.

Derbortoli, M., Dati, C., Antoniotti, S., Maggiora, P., Sapel, M.L. (1992) *Journal of Steroid Biochemistry and Molecular Biology* **43**, 21–26.

Dickens, T.A., Colletta, A.A. (1993) *Bioessays* **15**, 71–74.

Dickson, R.B., Lippman, M.E. (1992) *Genes, Oncogenes and Hormones: Advances in the Cellular and Molecular Biology of Breast Cancer*, Kluwer, Norwell.

Dittadi, R., Donisi, P.M., Brazzale, A., Cappellozza, L., Bruscagnin, G., Gion, M. (1993) *British Journal of Cancer* **67**, 7–9.

Dunn, D.K., Whelan, R.D.H., Hill, B., King, R.J.B. (1993) *Journal of Steroid Biochemistry and Molecular Biology* **46**, 469–480.

Dutta, A., Ruppert, J.M., Aster, J.C., Winchester, E. (1993) *Nature* **365**, 79–85.

Egan, S.E., Weinberg, R.A. (1993) *Nature* **365**, 781–783.

Elledge, R.M., Fuqua, S.A.W., Clark, G.M., Puyol, P., Allred, D.C., McGuire, W.L. (1993) *Breast Cancer Research and Treatment* **26**, 225–236.

Etindi, R.N., Manni, A., Martel, J. (1992) *Breast Cancer Research and Treatment* **24**, 61–70.

Ferrarini, M., Heltai, S., Zocchi, M.R., Rugarli, C. (1992) *International Journal of Cancer* **51**, 613–619.

Figueroa, J.A., Jackson, J.G., McGuire, W.L., Krywicki, R.F., Yee, D. (1993) *Journal of Cellular Biochemistry* **52**, 196–205.

Freiss, G., Rochefort, H., Vignon, F. (1990) *Biochemical Biophysical Research Communications* **173**, 919–926.

Friedl, A., Jordan, V.C., Pollak, M. (1993) *European Journal of Cancer* **29A**, 1368–1372.

Friedman, Z.Y. (1993) *Journal of Pharmacology and Experimental Therapeutics* **267**, 617–682.

Fynan, T.M., Reiss, M. (1993) *Critical Reviews in Oncogenesis* **4**, 493–540.

Gagliardi, A., Collins, D.C. (1993) *Cancer Research* **53**, 533–535.

Gibson, D.F., Johnson, D.A., Goldstein, D., Langanfahey, S.M., Borden, E.C., Jordan, V.C. (1993) *Breast Cancer Research and Treatment* **25**, 141–150.

Gong, Y., Ballejo, G., Murphy, L.C., Murphy, L.J. (1992) *Cancer Research* **52**, 1704–1709.

Goodrich, D.W., Lee, W.H. (1992) *Nature* **360**, 177–179.

Grainger, D.J., Weissberg, P.L., Metcalf, J.C. (1993) *Biochemical Journal* **294**, 109–136.

Henry, J.A., Hennessy, C., Levett, D.L., Lennard, T.W.J., Westley, B.R., May, F.E.B. (1993) *International Journal of Cancer* **53**, 774–780.

Horak, E.R., Leck, R., Klenk, N., Lejeune, S., Smith, K., Stuart, N., Greenall, M., Stepniewska, K., Harris, A.L. (1992) *Lancet* **340**, 1120–1123.

Horwitz, K.B. (1993) *Annals of the New York Academy of Sciences* **684**, 63–74.

Hotzwagenblatt, A., Shalloway, D. (1993) *Critical Reviews in Oncogenesis* **4**, 541–558.

Hu, X.F., Veroni, M., Deluise, M., Wakeling, A. Sutherland, R., Watts, C.K.W., Zalcberg, J.R. (1993) *International Journal of Cancer* **55**, 873–876.

Huynh, H.T., Tetenes, E., Wallace, L., Pollak, M. (1993) *Cancer Research* **53**, 1727–1730.

Jiang, S.Y., Jordan, V.C. (1992) *Cancer Surveys* **14**, 55–70.

Jiang, S.Y., Wolf, D.M., Yingling, J.M., Cheng, C., Jordan, V.C. (1992) *Molecular and Cellular Endocrinology* **90**, 77–86.

Jordan, V.C. (1993) *Cancer* **72**, 1–2.

Judson, I.R., Threadgill, M.D. (1993) *Lancet* **342**, 632.

Karnik, P.S., Kulkarni, S., Liu, X.P., Budd, G.T., Bukowski, R.M. (1994) *Cancer Research* **54**; 349–353.
Katzenellenbogen, B.S. (1991) *Journal of the National Cancer Institute* **83**, 1434–1435.
Kilian, P.L., Kaffka, K.L., Biondi, D.A., Lippman, J.M., Benjamin, W.R., Feldman, D., Campen C.A. (1991) *Cancer Research* **51**, 1823–1828.
Kim, B., Warnaka, P., Konard, C (1990) *Surgery* August, 139–145.
King, R.J.B. (1992) *Cancer Surveys* **14**, 131–146.
Kirkland, J.L., Murthy, L., Stamcel, G.M. (1993) *Molecular Pharmacology* **43**, 709–714.
Knabbe, C., Zugmaier, G., Schmahl, M., Dietel, M., Lippman, M.E., Dickson, R.B. (1991) *American Journal of Clinical Oncology* **14** (suppl. 2), S15–S20.
Knogler, W., Kubista, E., Zielinski, C.C. (1992) *Cancer Journal* **5**, 32–34.
Kurebayshi, J., Mclesky, S.W., Johnson, M.D., Lippman, M.E., Dickson, R.B., Kern, F.G. (1993) *Cancer Research* **53**, 2178–2188.
Lau, A.F., Kanemitsu, M.Y., Kurata, W.E., Danesh, S., Boynia, A.L. (1992) *Molecular Biology of the Cell* **3**, 865–874.
Lau, C.K., Subramanian, M., Rusmussen, K., Spelsburg, T.C. (1991) *Proceedings of the National Academy of Science USA* **88**, 829–833.
Lefkowitz, R.J. (1993) *Cell* **74**, 409–412.
Leonetti, C., Arcone, T., Konovalova, N., Diatchkovskaya, R., Shapiro, A., Franchi, F. (1993) *International Journal of Oncology* **3**, 615–618.
Leroy, X., Esrot, C., Brouillet, J.P., Theillet, C., Maudelonde, T., Simonylafontaine, J., Pujel, J., Rochefort, H. (1991) *Oncogene* **6**, 431–438.
Lien, E.A., Johannessen, D.C., Aakvaag, A., Lonning, P.E. (1992) *Journal of Steroid Biochemistry and Molecular Biology* **41**, 541–543.
Lino, Y., Takai, Y., Sugamata, N., Morishita, Y. (1992) *Anticancer Research* **12**, 2101–2104.
Loganzo, F., Dosik, J.S., Zhao, Y., Vidal, M.J., Nanus, D.M., Sudol, M., Albino, A.P. (1993) *Oncogene* **8**, 2637–2344.
Long, B., Mckibben, B.M., Lynch, M., Vandenberg, H.W. (1992) *British Journal of Cancer* **65**, 865–869.
Lonning, P.E., Hall, K., Aakvaag, A., Lien, E.A. (1992) *Cancer Research* **52**, 4719–4724.
Love, S., King, R.J.B. (1994) *British Journal of Cancer* **69**, 743–748.
Lowe, S.W., Ruley, H.E., Jacks, T., Houseman, D.E. (1993) *Cell* **74**, 957–968.
Lukač, J., Kusić, Z., Kordić, D., Končar, M., Bolanča, A. (1994) *Breast Cancer Research and Treatment* **29**, 279–285.
Lupu, R., Dickson, R.B., Lippman, M.E. (1992) *Journal of Steroid Biochemistry and Molecular Biology* **43**, 229–236.
Lykkesfeldt, A.E., Sorensen, G.K. (1992) *Acta Oncologica* **31**, 131–138.
McClay, E.F., Albright, K.D., Jones, J.A.M., Christen, R.D., Howell, S.B. (1993a) *Cancer Research* **53**, 1571–1576.
McClay, E.F. and McClay, M.E.T. (1994) *Journal of Clinical Oncology* **12**, 617–620.
McClay, E.F., McClay, M.E.T., Albright, K.D., Jones, J.A., Christen, R.D., Alcaraz, J., Holell, S.B. (1993b) *Cancer* **72**, 1914–1918.
MacDonald, F., Ford, C.H.J. (1991) *Oncogenes and Tumour Suppressor Genes*, BIOS Science Publishers, Oxford.
Mack, D.H., Vartikar, J., Pipas, J.M., Laimins, L.A. (1993) *Nature* **363**, 281–283.
Maenpaa, J., Wiebe, V., Koester, S., Wurz, G., Emshoff, V., Seymour, R., Sipila, P., DeGregorio, M. (1993) *Cancer Chemotherapy and Pharmacology* **32**, 396–398.
Malaab, S.A., Pollak, M.N., Goodyer, C.G. (1992) *European Journal of Cancer* **28A**, 788–793

Matsuo, S., Takano, S., Yamashita, J., Ogawa, M. (1992) *Anticancer Research* **12**, 1575–1580.

Mazars, R., Spinardu, L., Beniheikh, M., Simonylafontaine, J., Jeanteur, P., Theillet, C. (1992) *Cancer Research* **52**, 3918–3923.

Mcleskey, S.W., Kurebayshi, J., Honig, S.F., Zwiebel, J., Lippman, M.E., Dickson, R.B., Kern, F.G. (1993) *Cancer Research* **53**, 2168–2178.

Mikulski, S.M., Viera, A., Shogen, K. (1992) *International Journal of Oncology* **1**, 779–786.

Modjtahedi, H., Styles, J.M., Deen, C.J. (1993) *British Journal of Cancer* **67**, 247–253.

Moll, U.M., Riou, G., Levine, A.J. (1992) *Proceedings of the National Academy of Sciences USA* **89**, 7262–7266.

Morrow, M., Jordan, V.C. (1993) *Archives of Surgery* **128**, 1187–1191.

Muller, M., Briscoe, J., Laxton, C., Guschin, D., Ziemiecki, A., Silvennoinen, O., Harpur, A.G., Barbieri, G., Wittuhn, B.A., Schindler, C., Pellegrini, S., Wilks, A.F., Ihle, J.N., Stark, G.R., Kerr, I.M. (1993) *Nature* **366**, 129–135.

Murphy, L.J., Gong, Y., Murphy, L.C. (1992) *Journal of Steroid Biochemistry and Molecular Biology* **41**, 309–314.

Nephew, K.P., Polek, T.C., Akcali, K.C., Khan, S.A. (1993) *Endocrinology* **133**, 419–422.

Newman, M.J. (1993) *Cancer and Metastasis Reviews* **12**, 239–254.

Noguchi, S., Motomura, K., Inaji, H., Imaoka, S., Koyama, H. (1993) *Cancer* **72**, 131–136.

Oesterreich, S., Wong, C.N., Qui, M., Hilsenbeck, S.G., Osborne, C.K., Fuqua, S.A.W. (1993) *Cancer Research* **53**, 4443–4448.

Osborne, C.K., Coronado, E., Allred, D.C., Wiebe, V., DeGregorio, M. (1991) *Journal of the National Cancer Institute* **83**, 1477–1482.

Osborne, C.K., Wiebe, V.J., McGuire, W.L., Ciocca, D.R., DeGregorio, M.W. (1992) *Journal of Clinical Oncology* **10**, 304–310.

O'Sullivan, C., Lewis, C.E., Harris, A.L., Magee, J.O. (1993) *Lancet* **342**, 148–149.

Ottenhoffkalff, A.E., Rijksen, G., Vanbeurdang, E.A.C.M., Hennipnan, A., Michels, A.A., Staal, G.E.J. (1992) *Cancer Research* **52**, 4773–4778.

Papa, V., Gliozzo, B., Clark, G.M., McGuire, W.L., Fujita-Yamamguchi, Y., Vigneri, R., Goldfine, I.D. Pezzino, V. (1993) *Cancer Research* **53**, 3736–3740.

Pavlik, E.J., Nelson, K., Srinivasan, S., Powell, D.E., Kenady, D.E., Depriest, P.D., Gallion, H-H., Vannageli, J.R. (1992) *Cancer Research* **52**, 4106–4112.

Pellegrini, S., Schindler, C. (1993) *Trends in Biochemical Sciences* **18**, 338–342.

Pero, R.W., Olsson, H., Killander, F., Troll, W. (1992) *European Journal of Cancer* **28A**, 1803–1806.

Philips, A., Chalbos, D., Rochefort, H. (1993) *Journal of Biological Chemistry* **268**, 14103–14108.

Plowman, G.D., Green, J.M., Culouscou, J.M., Carlton, G.W., Rothwell, V.M., Buckley, S. (1993) *Nature* **366**, 473–475.

Pollak, M., Constantino, J., Polychronakos, C. (1990) *Journal of the National Cancer Institute* **82**, 1693–1697.

Pollak, M.N., Huynh, H., Lefebvre, S.P. (1992) *Breast Cancer Research and Treatment* **22**, 91–100.

Pyrhönen, S., Valavaara, R., Vuorinen, J., Hajba, A. (1994) *Breast Cancer Research and Treatment* **29**, 223–228.

Reddy, K.B., Mangold, G.L., Tandon, A.K., Konedea, T., Mundy, G.R., Ziberstein, A., Osborne, C.K. (1992) *Cancer Research* **52**, 3636–3641.

Robinson, E., Rubin, D., Mekori, T., Segal, R., Pollack, S., (1993) *Cancer Immunology and Immunotherapy* **37**, 209–212.

Rosen, N., Yee, D., Lippman, M.E., Paik, S., Cullen, K.J. (1991) *Breast Cancer Research and Treatment* **18** (suppl. 1), S55-S62.
Sakakibara, K., Kan, N.C., Satyaswaroop, P.G. (1992) *American Journal of Obstetrics and Gynecology* **166**, 206–212.
Satyaswaroop, P.G., Clarke, C.L., Ziano, R.J., Mortel, R. (1992) *Cancer Letters* **62**, 107–114.
Scambia, G., Ranelletti, F.O., Panici, P.B., Piantelli, M., Devincenzo, R., Bonanno, G., Ferrandina, G., Isola, G., Mancuso, S. (1992) *European Journal of Cancer* **28A**, 1885–1889.
Schönborn, I., Zschiesche, W., Spitzer, E., Minguillon, C., Möhner, M., Ebeling, K., Grosse, R. (1994) *Breast Cancer Research and Treatment* **29**, 287–295.
Schlichtholz, B., Legros, Y., Gillet, D., Gaillard, G., Marty, M., Lane, D., Calvo, F., Soussi, T. (1992) *Cancer Research* **52**, 6380–6384.
Selter, H., Montenarh, M. (1994) *International Journal of Biochemistry* **26**, 145–154.
Sen, S., P'Incalci, M. (1992) *Federation of European Biochemical Societies Letters* **307**, 122–127.
Seymour, L., Bezwoda, W.R. (1993) *British Journal of Cancer* **68**, 352–356.
Sheikh, M.S., Shao, Z.M., Hussalim, A., Fontana, J.A. (1993) *Cancer Research* **53**, 3226–3229.
Shiu, R.P., Watson, P.H., Dubik, D. (1993) *Clinical Chemistry* **39**, 353–362.
Shual, K., Ziemiecki, A., Wilks, A.F., Harpur, A.G., Sadowski, H.B., Gilman, M.Z., Darnell, J.E. (1993) *Nature* **366**, 580–583.
Sica, G., Lama, G., Iacopino, F., Angelucci, C., Dellacuna, G.R., Marchetti, P. (1991) *Anticancer Research* **11**, 2099–2102.
Silvennoinen, O., Ihle, J.N., Schlessinger, J., Levy, D.E. (1993) *Nature* **366**, 583–585.
Sipila, P.E.H., Wiebe, V.J., Hulbbard, G.B., Koester, S.K., Emshoff, V.D., Maenpaa, J.U., Wurz, R.C., Seymour, R.C., DeGregario, M.W. (1993) *European Journal of Cancer* **29A**, 2138–2143.
Sluyser, M. (1990) *Molecular Biology of Cancer Genes*, Ellis Horwood, Chichester.
Sluyser, M. (1992) *Clinical Biochemistry* **25**, 407–414.
Stewart, A.J., Westley, B.R., May, F.E.B. (1992) *British Journal of Cancer* **66**, 640–648.
Suto, A., Bradlow, H.L., Wong, G.Y., Osborne, M.P., Telang, N.T. (1992) *Steroids* **57**, 262–268.
Tannenbaum, G.S., Guard, W., Lapointe, M., Polak, M. (1992) *Endocrinology* **130**, 3395–3401.
Tanuka, N.K., Sakamoto, N., Korenaga, H., Inoue, K., Ogawa, H., Osada, Y. (1991) *International Journal of Radiation Biology* **60**, 79–84.
Tedorczyk-Injeyan, J., Cembrzynska-Nowak, M., Lalani, S., Kellen, J.A. (1993) *Anticancer Research* **13**, 279–283.
Thompson, A.M., Kerr, D.J., Steel, C.M. (1991) *British Journal of Cancer* **63**, 609–614.
Tiwari, R.K., Wong, G.Y., Liu, J., Miller, D., Osborne, M.P. (1991) *Cancer Letters* **61**, 45–52.
Toi, M., Bicknell, R., Harris, A.L. (1992) *Cancer Research* **52**, 275–279.
Vile, R.G. (1992) *Introduction to the Molecular Genetics of Cancer*, John Wiley & Sons, Chichester.
Vliagoftis, H., Dimitriadou, N., Boucher, W., Rozeniecki, J.J., Correia, I., Raam, S., Theoharides, T.C. (1992) *International Archives of Allergy and Immunology* **98**, 398–409.
Wakeling, A.E. (1993) *Breast Cancer Research and Treatment* **25**, 1–9 .
Watling, D., Guschin, D., Muller, M., Silvennoinen, O., Witthuhn, B.A., Quelle, F.W., Rogers, N.C., Schindler, C., Stark, G.R., Ihle, J.N. Kerr, I M. (1993) *Nature* **366**, 166–170.

Wei, Z., Yamada, H., Sakai, N., Nikawa, S., Nozawa, Y., Olsen, J., Vertosick, F.T. (1992) *Neurosurgery* **31**, 725–730.
Wiebe, V.J., Osborne, C.K., McGuire, W.L., DeGregorio, M.W. (1992) *Journal of Clinical Oncology* **10**, 990–994.
Wolf, D.M., Langanfahey, S.M., Parker, C.J., McCague, R., Jordan, V.C. (1993) *Journal of the National Cancer Institute* **85**, 806–812.
Wong, M.S.J., Murphy, L.C. (1991) *Journal of Steroid Biochemistry and Molecular Biology* **39**, 39–44.
Wosikowski, K., Kung, W., Hasmann, M., Loser, R., Eppenberger, U. (1993) *International Journal of Cancer* **53**, 290–297.
Wright, J.A., Turley, E.A., Greenberg, A.H. (1993) *Critical Reviews in Oncogenesis* **4**, 473–492.
Yasutomo, Y., Shimafda, N., Kimura, N., Nagata, N. (1993) *Federation of European Biochemical Societies Letters* **322**, 25–29.
Yee, D., Favoni, R.E., Lippman, M.E., Powell, D.R. (1991) *Breast Cancer Research and Treatment* **18**, 3–10.
Zeillinger, R., Kury, F., Speiser, P., Sliutz, G., Czerwenka, K., Kubista, E. (1993) *Clinical Biochemistry* **26**, 221–227.
Zhou-Li, F., Albaladejo, V., Joly-Pharaboz, M.D., Nicolas, B., Andre, J. (1992) *Endocrinology* **130**, 1145–1152.

7

Inhibitory Action of Tamoxifen on Enzymes Involved in the Synthesis of Oestrogens and in Signal Transduction: Importance to Anticancer Action?

INHIBITION OF ENZYMES INVOLVED IN OESTROGEN SYNTHESIS AND OESTROGEN-REGULATED ENZYMES

Oestrogen is an important mitogen for human breast cancer (see Chapter 4), and the enzymic regulation of 17β-oestradiol concentration in human breast cancer cells has been discussed (Adam, 1992). Aromatase is a key target enzyme in the pathway of oestrogen synthesis from cholesterol, and inhibition of this enzyme does not interfere with the synthesis of other steroids, particularly glucocorticoids. Aromatase inhibitors are often used for oestrogen suppression in breast cancer patients, and several aromatase inhibitors (e.g., aminoglutathiamide) are in clinical usage; the clinical effectiveness of these has been compared with tamoxifen (Dowsett, 1991). It is of interest that the role of the free radical scavenger system (see Chapter 8) of the human ovary has been reported (Okatani *et al.*, 1993).

Oestrone sulphate levels are 10-fold higher than the free oestrone and oestradiol levels in post-menopausal women, and potentially form a source from which free oestrogens could be synthesised *in situ* in breast cancer tissues. The enzymes catalysing conversion of oestrone sulphate to free oestrone and oestradiol are oestrone sulphatase and 17β-hydroxysteroid dehydrogenase (oestradiol dehydrogenase) respectively. The activity of oestrone sulphatase is modulated by both steroidal and non-steroidal therapeutic agents in both oestrogen-dependent and oestrogen-independent breast cancer cells (Purohit and Reed, 1992), and the selective inhibition of oestrone sulphatase and 17β-hydroxysteroid dehydrogenase may reduce tumour oestrogen levels and thus promote tumour regression. The regulation of 17β-hydroxysteroid dehydrogenase in a newly established breast carcinoma cell line has been reported (Mehta and Dasgupta, 1993). Tamoxifen has been shown to block the stimulatory effects of interleukin-6 on 17β-hydroxysteroid dehydrogenase activity in MCF-7 cells (Speirs *et al.*, 1993). Tamoxifen and its metabolites (4-hydroxytamoxifen and *N*-desmethyltamoxifen) inhibited the activity of oestrone sulphatase in rat breast tumours, and 4-hydroxytamoxifen also blocked 17β-hydroxysteroid dehydrogenase activity (Santner and Santen, 1993) (see Figure 7.1). In human breast tumours 4-hydroxytamoxifen and *N*-desmethyltamoxifen blocked oestrone sulphatase activity with IC_{50}s of 1–2 mM, i.e. at higher concentrations than in the rat. Inhibition of enzyme activity requires concentrations approximately 100-fold higher than those necessary for antioestrogenic effects. In another study, 4-hydroxytamoxifen and the pure antioestrogen ICI 164 384 inhibited oestrone sulphatase activity in T47D oestrogen-dependent and MDA-MB-231 oestrogen-independent human breast cancer cells, whereas tamoxifen had very little effect (Chetrite *et al.*, 1993). In addition, danzol has been shown

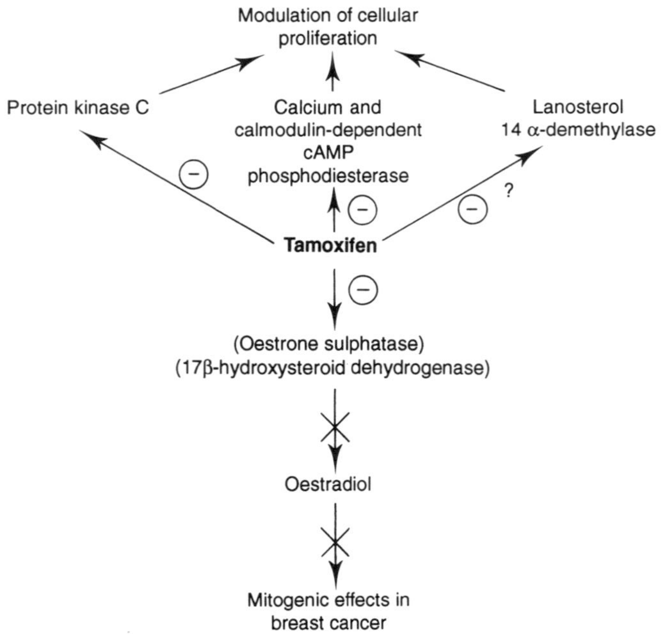

Figure 7.1. Inhibitory action of tamoxifen on enzymes

to affect the activity of this enzyme in MCF-7, T47D and MDA-MB-231 human breast cancer cells (Ngugen *et al.*, 1993). Intratumoral oestrone sulphatase activity may be useful as a prognostic marker in human breast carcinoma (Evans *et al.*, 1994).

17β-Oestradiol has been found to have rapid and long-term effects on the phosphatidylinositol 4,5-bisphosphate (PIP_2)-phospholipase C specific activity of MCF-7 cells (Graber *et al.*, 1993). Furthermore, oestrogen induces phospholipase A_2 activities in immature quail oviduct *in vivo*, which are blocked by tamoxifen (Fayard *et al.*, 1992). Tamoxifen also inhibited basal phospholipase A_2 activity. Tamoxifen has been shown to be a good inhibitor of collagenolytic activity in human leukaemic cells and this is thought to be related to its inhibitory action on plasmin and plasminogen activator (Akeli *et al.*, 1991). 4-Hydroxytamoxifen and *N*-desmethyltamoxifen were equally effective inhibitors of collagenolytic activity, but *cis*-tamoxifen was less effective. It has been reported that tamoxifen increased the level of 2′–5′ oligoadenylate synthetase in the oestrogen receptor-positive CG5 cell line but not in the oestrogen receptor-negative EVSA-T cell line (Viano *et al.*, 1989). Induction by tamoxifen of this enzyme (induced also by interferons), which polymerises adenosine triphosphate into the 2′–5′ oligoadenylate that inhibits cell growth by activation of a latent ribonuclease (degrades mRNA), may thus contribute to the oestrogen-dependent action of tamoxifen (Viano *et al.*, 1989). Conversely both 17β-oestradiol and tamoxifen stimulated the activity of the chloramphenicol acetyltransferase (CAT) reporter gene, fused to the 5′-flanking region of the brain-type isoenzyme of creatine kinase in order to study the induction mechanism of this enzyme and when given simultaneously tamoxifen and 17β-oestradiol acted synergistically (Spatz *et al.*, 1992).

INHIBITORY ACTION ON PROTEIN KINASE C AND OTHER CALCIUM-DEPENDENT ENZYMES AND ON CALCIUM CHANNELS

Inhibition of protein kinase C: an assessment of its significance

It has been reported that tamoxifen at micromolar concentrations inhibits the activity of protein kinase C from rat brain (Bignon *et al.*, 1990a) (see Figure 7.1). Protein kinase C (phospholipid/calcium-dependent protein kinase) is activated by phorbol esters such as 12-O-tetradecanoylphorbol-13-acetate (TPA) in addition to the endogenous second messengers calcium and diacylglycerol (DAG). It has been reported also that in addition to DAG, PIP_2 can activate protein kinase C in the presence of calcium and phosphatidylserine (Chauhan *et al.*, 1991). Protein kinase C is an important protein in the phosphorylation system and has been shown to play a key role in the transduction of membrane signals, cellular regulation and tumour promotion (Nishizuka, 1988; Bradshaw *et al.*, 1993).

Protein kinase C activities are known to be elevated in breast cancer compared to normal breast tissue (O'Brian *et al.*, 1989) and several studies have been made on protein kinase C in human breast cancer cell lines. Oestrogen receptor-negative cell lines have been shown to contain significantly higher levels of phorbol ester binding protein kinase C activity and protein than oestrogen receptor-positive cells, and this inverse relationship between oestrogen receptor levels and protein kinase C has also been observed in primary breast tumours (Borner and Fabbro, 1992). The c-protein kinase C-α appears to be the predominant isoform that contributes to the increased protein kinase C activities observed in oestrogen-independent and highly tumorigenic human breast cancer cells. However the absence of any tumour-specific expression levels of protein kinase C isoenzymes in human breast cancer cell cultures has also been reported (Imbi *et al.*, 1994).

The therapeutic potential of inhibitors of protein kinase C is well recognised (Bradshaw *et al.*, 1993) and both protein kinase C and adenylate cyclase have been identified as targets for the inhibition of the growth of human gastric cancer cells (Piontek *et al.*, 1993). Furthermore, tamoxifen and staurosporine (also a protein kinase C inhibitor) have been shown to suppress cell growth in established and low-passage glioma cell lines (Baltuch *et al.*, 1993).

Protein kinase C activation is thought to act as a stop signal for tumour cell locomotion. However, tamoxifen, unlike other protein kinase C inhibitors such as polymyxin B, which suppress cell polarity and locomotion, has no significant effect on shape changes and chemokinesis in Walker carcinosarcoma cells (Zimmermann and Keller, 1993).

Although an inhibitory action of tamoxifen on this enzyme could contribute to the antitumour action of this drug, tamoxifen did not, however, decrease TPA-induced protein kinase activity in intact MCF-7 cells (Issandou *et al.*, 1990). The activation of protein kinase C by TPA in human breast cancer cells has been shown to be associated with the phosphorylation of heat-shock protein (HSP) 27 (Borner and Fabbro, 1992). It has also been shown that phorbol esters such as TPA (and also DAG) inhibit the growth of MCF-7 cells (Darbon *et al.*, 1990; Issandou *et al.*, 1990). The signal transduction pathway mediating the effects of TPA on growth in human breast cancer cells is not yet clearly understood. Removal of TPA from growth-inhibited human breast cancer cells resulted in a gradual recovery of protein kinase C activity, which was associated with recovery of cell growth (Borner and Fabbro, 1992).

The mechanism by which tamoxifen inhibits the activity of calcium and phospholipid-dependent protein kinase C has been investigated (Edashige *et al.*, 1991). Tamoxifen was found to inhibit the protein kinase C-dependent phosphorylation of histone and r-annexin I *in vitro* and also phosphorylation of cytoplasmic proteins obtained from rat uterus and mammary gland by endogenous protein kinase C (Edashige *et al.*, 1991). This inhibitory effect of tamoxifen was dependent on the membrane–substrate protein interaction and thus interference with this interaction may be its mechanism of action. The influence of diphenylethylene and triphenylethylene structure on the mechanisms of protein kinase C inhibition by these compounds has been investigated using multivariate analysis (Bignon *et al.*, 1991). Furthermore, the relative involvement of protein kinase C and the oestrogen receptor in the ability of triphenylethylenes to inhibit the growth of MCF-7 cells has been determined by the use of correspondence factorial (CF) analysis (Ojasoo *et al.*, 1993).

Although tamoxifen has been found to inhibit protein kinase C activity *in vitro*, tamoxifen (at the micromolar concentrations reported to inhibit cell growth) did not significantly decrease TPA-induced protein kinase C activity in intact MCF-7 cells, as measured by protein phosphorylation (Issandou *et al.*, 1990). Furthermore, the inhibition observed *in vitro* was at low phospholipid concentrations, which probably do not correspond to the true environment of this enzyme in the cell (Issandou *et al.*, 1990). A further complication is that in the MCF-7 breast cancer cell line it has been demonstrated that activators of protein kinase C, such as DAG, and also tumour-promoting phorbol esters, completely inhibit cell proliferation (Darbon *et al.*, 1990;; Issandou *et al.*, 1990), in contrast to their usual role of stimulating cell proliferation (Nishizuka, 1988). This may relate to the different protein kinase C subspecies identified in oestrogen receptor-positive breast cancer cell lines and also in oestrogen receptor-negative breast cancer cell lines, although all of such subspecies have been found to be sensitive to triphenylethylenes such as tamoxifen (Bignon *et al.*, 1990b). If the anticancer action of tamoxifen is via inhibition of protein kinase C then it would be expected to stimulate MCF-7 cell growth, which it clearly does not. It seems to be unlikely that protein kinase C is a specific target site for tamoxifen in its ability to inhibit cell growth in either tumour cells (see above) or indeed yeast cells (see Chapter 9: a protein kinase C has been found in yeast but its properties are different from those of the mammalian enzyme; Ogita *et al.*, 1990).

Role of calmodulin binding in inhibition of calcium calmodulin-dependent enzymes and calcium channels by tamoxifen

Tamoxifen (at micromolar concentrations) has been shown to inhibit calcium calmodulin-dependent cAMP phosphodiesterase (see Figure 7.1), which catalyses the breakdown of the second messenger, cAMP, that plays an important role in the regulation of cell growth (Fanidi *et al.*, 1989, 1991, 1992; Rowlands *et al.*, 1990). The calcium-binding protein calmodulin is a regulatory protein of many cellular processes dependent on calcium, such as cell cycle progression. Molecular modelling techniques have been used to study the interactions between tamoxifen and derivatives and calmodulin (Edwards *et al.*, 1992). It is of interest that the oestrogen receptor from uterine cytosol can bind calmodulin and that tamoxifen antagonises this action (Bouhoute and Leclercq, 1992). Furthermore, derivatives of oestradiol that possess the side-chain of tamoxifen have been reported to antagonize the association between calmodulin and the oestrogen receptor (Bouhoute and Leclercq, 1994). Tamoxifen was found to be a potent antagonist of calmodulin in the activation of a purified bovine brain calcium calmodulin-dependent cAMP-phosphodiesterase. Calmodulin isolated from bovine brain has also been reported to bind tamoxifen in a calcium-dependent manner (Celeste *et al.*, 1990). Similar inhibitory results were obtained for tamoxifen using calcium calmodulin-dependent cAMP-phosphodiesterase from quail oviduct (Fanidi *et al.*, 1989, 1991, 1992) and beef heart (Rowlands *et al.*, 1990). Tamoxifen (at micromolar concentrations) has been found, however, to inhibit the action of both calmodulin-dependent and calmodulin-independent ($Ca^{2+} + Mg^{2+}$)-ATPase of synaptic plasma membranes and microsomal membranes, respectively, from sheep brain; these calcium transport proteins regulate the cytoplasmic calcium concentration in the nerve cells used in these experiments (Malva *et al.*, 1990). It would appear, therefore, from this lack of direct correspondence with calmodulin dependence that the interaction between tamoxifen and calmodulin is unlikely to be involved directly with the growth-inhibitory action of tamoxifen.

Tamoxifen has been shown to have calcium channel antagonistic properties in the PC-12 neurosecretory cell line (Greenburg *et al.*, 1987), and tamoxifen reduces calcium currents in a clonal pituitary cell line (Sartor *et al.*, 1988). The calcium antagonists, nicardipine and verapamil (1 μM for five days) were not as effective as tamoxifen in inhibiting the growth of MCF-7 cells. This suggests that any inhibitory effect of tamoxifen on calcium channels is not likely to be the sole cause of the ability of tamoxifen to inhibit tumour cell growth. In addition, in human prostatic cancer cells (DU 145) tamoxifen inhibited cell proliferation (IC_{50} of 5 μM compared to 55 μM for verapamil) but had no effect on ^{45}Ca uptake (verapamil paradoxically increased this uptake). It would appear that the inhibitory effect of tamoxifen on cell proliferation does not involve changes in transmembrane calcium movements in this system (Batra *et al.*, 1991).

ROLE OF THE ANTIOESTROGEN BINDING SITE IN ANTICANCER ACTION

[^{3}H]Tamoxifen binds to the antioestrogen binding site (AEBS) from chicken liver and from rat liver, in addition to that from human carcinomas (Lopes *et al.*, 1991) and from the MCF-7 cell line. Although the exact mechanisms involved are not clear, it is of interest that tamoxifen inhibited growth of MCF-7 cells with high concentrations of AEBS but was ineffective in a variant with fewer of these binding sites. Other studies have shown that these AEBS were present in equal amounts in three breast cancer lines (MCF-7, T47D and MDA-MB-231) that differed markedly in their oestrogen receptor content and their sensitivity to growth suppression by tamoxifen. Additionally, AEBS were found to be present in equal amounts in the MCF-7 clones R27 and R3-98, which were no longer growth inhibited by tamoxifen. However, tamoxifen resistance in the R27 cell line is due to its intensive metabolism of oestrone sulphate to oestradiol, thus blocking the antioestrogenic effects of tamoxifen. It has been shown also for tamoxifen and its derivatives, in MCF-7 cells, that the compounds with the highest affinity for the oestrogen receptor and the greatest antioestrogenic potency had the lowest affinities for these AEBS. Antioestrogenic potency correlated best with oestrogen receptor affinity and not with AEBS. It is of interest that *cis*-tamoxifen had an affinity for AEBS equal to that of *trans*-tamoxifen and that *cis*-tamoxifen acts as an oestrogen in MCF-7 cells. Furthermore, a hypothesis has been put forward for the interaction of antioestrogens with a site distinct from the oestrogen binding site (Berthois *et al.*, 1994).

The binding of tritiated 17β-oestradiol and 4-hydroxytamoxifen to the cytosol and microsomes of human breast tumours has been characterised (Lopes *et al.*, 1991). No correlation was found between the concentrations of oestrogen receptor and of AEBS in the tumours. The microsomal membranes were found to contain oestrogen binding sites that may be related to the cytosol oestrogen receptor recycling: in addition, specific AEBS were predominantly located in this membrane system (see below). It was found that the magnitude of the 17β-oestradiol binding to microsomes depends on the oestrogen receptor positivity of the tumours, whereas the magnitude of the antioestrogen binding to the microsomes was independent of the oestrogen receptor status of the tumour (Lopes *et al.*, 1991). The distinctly separate nature of the AEBS and the oestrogen receptor has been demonstrated by their respective differences in intracellular concentration, subcellular distribution, ligand specificity and thermal stability (Leo *et al.*, 1991). The location of AEBS has been shown to be predominantly microsomal and it is now known that AEBS are concentrated within the portion of the microsomal fraction that derives from the rough endoplasmic reticulum of MCF-7 cells and rat liver. The sensitivity of rat liver AEBS to enzyme treatment (phospholipases) is consistent with its being a membrane-bound protein. Purification of AEBS, however, has not yet been achieved. Studies have been carried out to determine the nature of the endogenous ligands for the AEBS, and the oxidation products of cholesterol, 7-ketocholestanol and 6-ketocholestanol have been indicated as possibilities for such ligands, although they were found to have much lower affinities for the AEBS than tamoxifen (Hwang, 1990). The comparative affinity of steroidal and non-steroidal antioestrogens, cholesterol derivatives and compounds with a dialkylamino side-chain for rat liver AEBS has been determined (Van den Koedijk *et al.*, 1992). Selective ligands for the AEBS, the 2-(*p*-chlorobenzyl)-3-aryl-6-methoxybenzofurans, have now been synthesised (Teo *et al.*, 1992). These benzofurans all bind to AEBS with equivalent or greater affinity than tamoxifen but display no significant interaction with the oestrogen receptor. These compounds decrease [^{3}H]thymidine incorporation in AEBS-containing EL-4 lymphoid cells and MCF-7 breast cancer cells and are generally more inhibitory than tamoxifen. Furthermore, they have no effect on cell growth in an AEBS MCF-7 variant (RTx6). These findings suggest a functional role for AEBS in mediating the growth-inhibitory action of these synthetic ligands (Teo *et al.*, 1992).

It has been concluded that the structural requirements of steroids for binding to AEBS are a hydrocarbon side-chain at C17, an oxygen function at C7, a hydroxyl group at C3 and the absence of a double bond between C5 and C6 (Hwang and Matin, 1989). The binding of tamoxifen-related compounds to the AEBS decreases with the removal of one methyl group from the dialkyl amino ethyl side-chain, and deletion of this side-chain causes an almost complete loss of activity (Van den Koedijk *et al.*, 1992). Addition of a hydroxyl group at R3 or R4 results in a decrease in the relative binding affinity, and replacement of the ethyl side-chain at R2 of tamoxifen by a cyano or ethyl chloride group causes a decrease in binding affinity, whereas derivatives with diethyl or pyrrolidino side-chains have a higher relative binding affinity for the AEBS than tamoxifen. Nafoxidine, which is structurally related to tamoxifen but possesses a pyrrolidino side-chain, has a two-fold higher binding affinity than tamoxifen.

The divergence between the ability of tamoxifen and its derivatives to bind to AEBS and their antioestrogenic activity, as assessed by antagonism of oestrogen-induced uterotrophic activity in the immature rat, suggests that AEBS are unlikely to play a functional role in mediating the antioestrogenic activity of tamoxifen. Although it was originally suggested that the AEBS might be cytochrome P-450 enzymes, these have now been shown to be different sites (Reidy and Murray, 1989). Initial suggestions that the AEBS was a histamine, dopamine or muscarinic-type receptor have now been discounted. It is possible that AEBS can facilitate the cellular uptake of its ligand and increase the intracellular concentration of tamoxifen, and thus increase its accessibility to the oestrogen receptor in oestrogen receptor-positive cells. Alternatively AEBS could modulate the ability of ligands to act via mechanisms unrelated to the oestrogen receptor in oestrogen receptor-negative cells.

It is of associated interest that tamoxifen inhibits the production of Moloney murine virions by fibroblastic A9 cells, which have no detectable oestrogen receptor. A specific ligand of the AEBS induced effects similar to those of tamoxifen, suggesting that tamoxifen may be acting to inhibit viral replication (the antiviral action of tamoxifen is discussed further in Chapter 9) through an oestrogen-independent pathway involving the AEBS (Chailleux *et al.*, 1993).

INHIBITION OF CYTOCHROME P-450-DEPENDENT ENZYMES INVOLVED IN CHOLESTEROL BIOSYNTHESIS: ROLE IN ANTICANCER ACTION?

Tamoxifen and 4-hydroxytamoxifen (at very low micromolar concentrations, e.g. 0.1 μM) have been shown to inhibit cholesterol synthesis in both oestrogen receptor-positive MCF-7 cells, where growth inhibition by tamoxifen at this concentration is oestrogen reversible, and in oestrogen receptor-negative BT-20 cells, where there is no growth inhibition by tamoxifen at this concentration (Cypriani *et al.*, 1988a, 1988b). Inhibition of cholesterol synthesis by tamoxifen and 4-hydroxytamoxifen was found to be mainly at the lanosterol demethylation step, and also at the conversion of C-27 sterol to cholesterol step (Cypriani *et al.*, 1988a). The cytochrome P-450-dependent enzyme lanosterol 14α-demethylase may thus be a key target site for tamoxifen in its inhibition of cholesterol synthesis (see Figure 7.1). Furthermore, tamoxifen and its metabolites were all inhibitors of rat hepatic cytochrome P-450-dependent mixed-function oxidation reactions, such as *N*-demethylation of ethylmorphine (see Chapter 3; Meltzer *et al.*, 1984) and four androstendione hydroxylase pathways (Reidy and Murray, 1989). It has been suggested that the inhibition of cholesterol synthesis by tamoxifen and 4-hydroxytamoxifen may involve the AEBS (see above), because in several cell lines some relationship was found between sensitivity to inhibition of cholesterol synthesis by 4-hydroxytamoxifen and AEBS content (Cypriani *et al.*, 1988b). Contraceptive steroids have also been shown to have an effect on hepatic cholesterol metabolism in the female rat (Kose *et al.*, 1993). Lanosterol 14α-demethylase is also found in fungi, such as in the ergosterol biosynthesis pathway in yeast (and in the cholesterol biosynthesis pathway). Cholesterol is a necessary component for the maintenance of membrane structural integrity and thus is required for the construction of new membranes during cellular proliferation. In the BT-20 cell line cultured in whole serum, however, it was found that synthesis of cholesterol was not limiting for cell growth (Cypriani *et al.*, 1988a). It appears, therefore, that inhibition of cholesterol biosynthesis by the low concentrations of 4-hydroxytamoxifen used in this study (Cypriani *et al.*, 1988a), which did not inhibit the growth of the BT-20 cells, is unlikely to be responsible for its antiproliferative ability in oestrogen receptor-negative cells. Benzofurans also have been shown to interfere with cholesterol biosynthesis and it has been suggested that this action may contribute to their ability to inhibit the growth of MCF-7 cells (Teo *et al.*, 1992).

Although it has been suggested that the microsomal AEBS is involved in this action of tamoxifen on cholesterol biosynthesis (Cypriani *et al.*, 1988b) and cell proliferation (Poirot *et al.*, 1990), no satisfactory overall hypothesis relating the nature of this binding protein to tamoxifen action has been made. In contrast to the initial suggestion that TABS might consist of cytochrome P-450 enzymes, it has now been shown that they are different sites (Reidy and Murray, 1989) despite the undoubted inhibition of the cytochrome P-450-dependent enzyme lanosterol α-demethylase by tamoxifen (see above). It is of interest also that oxygenated derivatives of cholesterol such as 7-ketocholestanol and 6-ketocholestanol bind to the TABS (Hwang, 1990) and this again is indicative of structural similarity between tamoxifen (and its derivatives) and cholesterol (and its derivatives). Furthermore, 6-ketocholestanol has been shown to modify membrane structure (Vasconcelles *et al.*, 1990), as found for cholesterol and tamoxifen (see Chapter 8). If changes in the AEBS can be demonstrated to play a role in the development of resistance to tamoxifen (see Chapter 6) then replacement of tamoxifen with an antioestrogen with affinity for the oestrogen receptor but without affinity for AEBS may cause tumour regression (see above section on AEBS).

REFERENCES

Adam, J.B. (1992) *Breast Cancer Research and Treatment* **20**, 145–154.

Akeli, M.G., Madoulet, C., Rallet, A., Jardillier, J.C. (1991) *Leukaemia Research* **15**, 1153–1157.

Baltuch, G.H., Coulwell, W.T., Villemure, J.G., Yong, V.W., Kornblith, P.L. (1993) *Neurosurgery* **33**, 495–501.

Batra, S., Popper, L.D., Hartley-Asp, B. (1991) *Prostate* **19**, 299–311.

Berthois, Y., Pons, M., Dussot, C., De Paulet, A.C., Martin, P.M. (1994) *Molecular and Cellular Endocrinology* **99**, 259–268.

Bignon, E., Pons, M., Gilbert, J., Nishizuka, Y. (1990a) *Federation of European Biochemical Societies Letters* **271**, 54–58.

Bignon, E., Ogita, K., Kishimoto, A., Nishizuka, Y. (1990b) *Biochemical and Biophysical Research Communications* **171**, 1071–1078.

Bignon, E., Pons, M., Dorc, J.C., Gilbert, J., Ojasoo, T., Miquel J.F., Rayanaud, J.P., Depaulet, A.C. (1991) *Biochemical Pharmacology* **42**, 1373–1384.

Borner, C., Fabbro, D. (1992) In *Protein Kinase C: Current Concepts and Future Perspectives* (eds D.S. Lester, R.M. Epand), Ellis Horwood, Chichester, pp. 297–354.

Bouhoute, A., Leclercq, G. (1992) *Biochemical and Biophysical Research Communications* **184**, 1432–1440.

Bouhoute, A., Leclercq, G. (1994) *Biochemical Pharmacology* **47**, 748–751.

Bradshaw, D., Hill, C.H., Nixon, J.S., Wilkinson, S.E. (1993) *Agents and Actions* **38**, 135–147.

Celeste, M., Lopes, F., Giaca, M., Vale, P., Carvalho, A.P. (1990) *Cancer Research* **50**, 2753–2758.
Chailleux, C., Mesange, F., Bayard, F., Prats, A.C., Faye, J.C. (1993) *Molecular Pharmacology* **44**, 324–327.
Chauhan, A., Chauhan, V.P.S., Erockerhoff, H. (1991) *Biochemical and Biophysical Research Communications* **175**, 852–857.
Chetrite, G., Varin, C., Delalonde, L., Pasqualini, J.R. (1993) *Anticancer Research* **13**, 931–934.
Cypriani, B., Tabacik, C., Descomps, B. (1988a) *Biochimica Biophysica Acta* **972**, 167–178.
Cypriani, B., Tabacik, C., Descomps, B., Crastes de Paulet, A. (1988b) *Journal of Steroid Biochemistry* **31**, 763–771.
Darbon, J.M., Valette, A., Jozan, S., Issandou, M., Bayard, F. (1990) *Biochemical Pharmacology* **40**, 1785–1792.
Dowsett, M. (1991) *Journal of Steroid Biochemistry and Molecular Biology* **39**, 805–809.
Edashige, K., Sato, E.F., Akimaru, K., Yoshioka, T., Utsumi, K. (1991) *Cell Structure and Function* **16**, 273–281.
Edwards, K.J., Laughton, C.A., Neidle, S. (1992) *Journal of Medicinal Chemistry* **35**, 2753–2760.
Evans, T.R.J., Rowlands, M.G., Law, M., Coombs, R.C. (1994) *British Journal of Cancer* **69**, 555–561.
Fanidi, A., Courion-Guichardaz, C., Fayard, J., Pageaux, J., Laugier, C. (1989) *Endocrinology* **125**, 1187–1193.
Fanidi, A., Pageaux, J.F., Courion, C., Fayard, J.M., Laugier, C. (1991) *Biology of the Cell* **72**, 181–186.
Fanidi, A., Ahnadi, C., Fayard, J.M., Pageaux, J.F., Laugier, C. (1992) *Journal of Steroid Biochemistry and Molecular Biology* **41**, 571–577.
Fayard, J.M., Chanal, S., Fanidi, A., Pageaux, J.F., Lagarde, M., Laugier, C. (1992) *European Journal of Pharmacology* **216**, 127–130.
Graber, R., Sumida, C., Valette, G.A., Nunoz, E.A. (1993) *Cellular Signalling* **5**, 181–186.
Greenburg, D.A., Carpenter, C.L , Messing, R.O. (1987) *Cancer Research* **47**, 70–74.
Hwang, P.L.H. (1990) *Biochimica et Biophysica Acta* **1033**, 154–161.
Hwang, P.H.L., Matin, A. (1989) *Journal of Lipid Research* **30**, 239–245.
Imbi, R., Haberthur, F., Meier, F., Filipuzzi, I., Almendral, A.C. (1994) *Carcinogenesis* **15**, 359–364.
Issandou, M., Faucher, C., Bayard, F., Darbon, J.M. (1990) *Cancer Research* **50**, 5845–5850.
Kose, K., Dogan, P., Czesmi, C. (1993) *Biochemistry and Molecular Biology International* **30**, 237–244.
Leo, G., Cappiello, G., Poltronieri, P., Giardina, C., Manca, C., Storelli, C., Marsigliante, S. (1991) *European Journal of Cancer* **27**, 452–455.
Lopes, M.C., Tavares, M.C., Vale, M.G., Carvalho, A.P. (1991) *Journal of Steroid Biochemistry and Molecular Biology* **39**, 343–352.
Malva, J.O., Celeste, M., Lopes, F., Graca, M., Vale, P., Carvalho, A.P. (1990) *Biochemical Pharmacology* **40**, 1877–1884.
Mehta, R.R., Dasgupta, T.K. (1993) *Journal of Steroid Biochemistry and Molecular Biology* **46**, 623–630.
Meltzer N.M., Stang, P., Sternson, L.A. (1984) *Biochemical Pharmacology* **33**, 115–123.
Ngugen, B.L., Ferne, I., Chetrilte, G., Pasqualini, J.R. (1993) *Journal of Steroid Biochemistry and Molecular Biology* **46**, 17–24.
Nishizuka, Y. (1988) *Nature* **334**, 661–665.

O'Brian, C.A., Vogel, V.G., Singletary, S.E., Ward, N.E. (1989) *Cancer Research* **49**, 3215–3217.
Ogita, K., Migamoto, S., Koide, H., Iwai, I., Oka, M., Ando, K., Kishimoto, H., Ikeda, K., Fukami, Y., Nishizuka, Y. (1990) *Proceedings of the National Academy of Sciences USA* **87**, 5011–5015.
Ojasoo, T., Bignon, E., Depaulet, A.C., Dore, J.C., Gilbert, J., Miquel, J.F., Pons, M., Raynaud, J.P. (1993) *Journal of Steroid Biochemistry and Molecular Biology* **44**, 239–250.
Okatani, Y., Morioka, N., Wakatsuki, A., Nakano, Y., Sagara, Y. (1993) *Hormone Research* **39** (suppl. 1), 22–27.
Piontek, M., Hengels, K.J., Porschen, R., Strohmeyer, G. (1993) *Journal of Cancer Pharmacology and Clinical Oncology* **119**, 697–699.
Poirot, M., Garnier, M., Bayard, F., Riviere, I., Traore, M., Wilson, M., Fargin, A., Faye, J.C.H. (1990) *Biochemical Pharmacology* **40**, 425–429.
Purohit, A., Reed, M.J. (1992) *International Journal of Cancer* **50**, 901–905.
Reidy, G.F., Murray, M. (1989) *Biochemical Pharmacology* **38**, 195–199.
Rowlands, M.G., Parr, I.B., McCague, R., Jarman, M., Goddard, P.M. (1990) *Biochemical Pharmacology* **40**, 283–289.
Santer, S.J., Santen, R.J. (1993) *Journal of Steroid Biochemistry and Molecular Biology* **45**, 383–390.
Sartor, P., Vacher, P., Mollard, P., Duffy, B. (1988) *Endocrinology* **123**, 534–540.
Spatz, M., Waisman, A., Kaye, A.M. (1992) *Journal of Steroid Biochemistry and Molecular Biology* **41**, 711–714.
Speirs, V., Adams, E.R., White, M.C. (1993) *Journal of Steroid Biochemistry and Molecular Biology* **46**, 605–613.
Teo, C.C., Kon, O.L, Sim, K.Y., Ng, S.C. (1992) *Journal of Medicinal Chemistry* **35**, 1330–1339.
Van den Koedijk, C.D.M.A., Vis van Heemst, C., Elsendoorn, G.M., Thijssen, J.H.H., Blankenstein, M.A. (1992) *Biochemical Pharmacology* **43**, 2511–2518.
Vasconcelles, M.J., Weitzman, S.A., Lee, S.A., Prachard, S., Gordon, L.I. (1990) *Free Radical Research Communications* **8**, 185–193.
Viano, I., Silvestro, L., Giubertoni, M., Diazani, C., Genazzani, E., DiCarlo, F. (1989) *Journal of Biological Regulators and Homeostatic Agents* **3**, 167–174.
Zimmermann, A., Keller, H. (1993) *Anticancer Research* **13**, 347–354.

8

Antioxidant Action of Tamoxifen and Related Compounds in Membranes and Lipoprotein Particles: Role in the Anticancer, Anti-multidrug Resistance and Cardioprotective Actions of Tamoxifen

A BRIEF INTRODUCTION TO MEMBRANES, LIPOPROTEINS AND LIPID PEROXIDATION

Outline of membrane structure, composition and function

Membranes are of fundamental importance to cell structure and function. In eukaryotic cells (both yeast and mammalian) membranes surround the cell (plasma membrane), form a continuous intracellular surface (endoplasmic reticulum) and form the structural basis of intracellular organelles such as mitochondria. In animal cells the dominant lipids in plasma membranes and intracellular organelles are various phospholipids based on glycerol; for example, phosphatidylserine, phosphatidylethanolamine, phosphatidylinositol and phosphatidylcholine, with the latter being the most common. The fatty acid side-chains of these phospholipids are also variable. In addition, sphingolipids, glycosphingolipids and gangliosides frequently occur in plasma membranes, whereas cardiolipin (diphosphatidylglycerol) is found predominantly in mitochondrial membranes. Cholesterol is found in large amounts in plasma membranes (often equimolar with the phospholipid). In contrast, endoplasmic reticulum and mitochondrial and nuclear membranes have a low cholesterol content. The cholesterol content of intracellular membranes such as the Golgi and secretory vesicle membranes is intermediate between those of the plasma membrane and the major intracellular organelles, and this may reflect their relationship with the plasma membrane in the process of endocytosis and exocytosis. In mammalian cells, membrane phospholipids contain large amounts of polyunsaturated fatty acid side-chains (Halliwell and Gutteridge, 1989), in contrast to yeast (see Chapter 9), where the phospholipid fatty acid side-chains are mostly saturated and monounsaturated; this is of importance because lipid peroxidation is broadly defined as the oxidative deterioration of polyunsaturated lipids (Halliwell and Gutteridge, 1989) (see below).

Lipids and proteins are the major constituents of biological membranes. The basis of the lipid bilayer structure reflects the amphipathic nature of membrane phospholipids. Phospholipids spontaneously associate to form bilayers such that the hydrophobic acyl regions are removed from contact with water while the hydrophilic polar head groups remain in contact with it (Kinsella, 1990; Lipowsky, 1991; Devaux, 1991). Studies on the lipid domains in biological membranes (Glaser, 1993) and lipid transmembrane asymmetry (Devaux, 1993) have been reported. The interaction and fusion of bilayers formed from unsaturated lipids has been investigated (Wolfe *et al.*, 1991) and the lipid arrangement in fluid model membranes has been analysed by the cross-linking of the phospholipid, phosphatidylethanolamine (Roth and Welt, 1991). In the contemporary basic model for membrane structure, extrinsic proteins are loosely adsorbed to the lipid bilayer, while the intrinsic proteins are imbedded in the bilayer and sometimes traverse the whole bilayer. Furthermore, both the protein and lipid components are capable of rapid lateral mobility.

In each half of the lipid bilayer, lipid and protein molecules can rapidly diffuse laterally, whereas migration from one bilayer to another (flip-flop) is rare and very slow, and this preserves the asymmetry of natural membranes (Devaux, 1991, 1993). This membrane fluidity (lateral diffusion possibility) is due to the presence of unsaturated and polyunsaturated fatty acid side-chains in many membrane lipids, which lowers the melting or phase transition temperature of the system. Membrane fluidity denotes the lateral diffusion of the lipid molecules (some authors include molecular rotation in this fluidity concept; see below): the fluidity of the bilayer in plasma membranes is determined by the composition of the acyl groups, the presence of cholesterol and the polar group of the phospholipid. Increasing the cholesterol and the saturated fatty acid content of a membrane both have the effect of increasing the order (in the thermodynamic sense) of the hydrocarbon matrix, and this increase in order is generally referred to as the determinant and definition of decreased membrane fluidity (Gurr and Harwood, 1991; New, 1992a). The introduction of cholesterol has a condensing effect on the acyl chains of the polar lipid, which are usually in a fluid state, and makes the membrane more rigid by restricting molecular motion. Cholesterol abolishes the sharp temperature-induced phase transition and prevents the formation of crystalline gel areas, whilst inhibiting the overall flexing motion of the hydrocarbon chains (New, 1992a). In addition, cholesterol has been reported to induce fluid-phase immiscibility in membranes (Sankarano and Thompson, 1991). The intracellular transport of cholesterol has also been studied (Liscum and Dahl, 1992). Cholesterol is a known modulator of membrane function (Yeagle, 1991) and it is of interest that the membrane interaction of calcium channel antagonists can be modulated by cholesterol (Mason, 1993), which has important implications for the activity of membrane-modulating anticancer drugs such as tamoxifen. The structure of lipoprotein particles is also of interest: the low-density lipoprotein (LDL) particle is composed of a large central core of cholesteryl ester and triglycerides surrounded by a monolayer of phospholipid molecules and free cholesterol, with the apoprotein B embedded in this outer layer (see review by Rice-Evans and Bruckdorfer, 1992).

Membrane fluidity can be measured by nuclear magnetic resonance (NMR) or electron spin resonance (ESR) order parameters, and by fluorescence polarisation (anisotropy). The effects of cholesterol on the lipid membrane-disordering actions of ethanol have been studied using deuterium NMR and steady-state fluorescence anisotropy techniques (Johnson *et al.*, 1992). Membrane probes such as 1,6-diphenyl-1,3,5-hexatriene (DPH) are used to study membrane fluidity in both bilayer models such as liposomes (Jones and Cossins, 1992; Wiseman *et al.*, 1993d) and intact cells (Clarke *et al.*, 1990a). It has been found using fluorescence anisotropy (an increase in the fluorescence anisotropy ratio is indicative of a decrease in membrane fluidity) that the introduction of both cholesterol and α-tocopherol separately into dipalmitoly-phosphatidylcholine (DPPC) lipid bilayers had a rigidifying effect on the bilayer (Bisby, 1990).

Membrane fluidity has a strong influence on the activity of membrane enzymes and receptors. Indeed within the membrane the flexing of acyl chains and local disorder of the lipids may be required for the changes in protein conformation associated with membrane protein function. It is of considerable interest that the activity of hormonally activated adenylate cyclase, which catalyses the formation of cAMP, is very sensitive to membrane fluidity: increasing the cholesterol content of isolated plasma membranes caused a progressive decline in adenylate cyclase activity as membrane fluidity decreased (Houslay, 1985). Furthermore, essential fatty acid deficiency in rats caused an increase in membrane saturation and a decrease in both membrane fluidity and adenylate cyclase activity (Houslay, 1985), and the membrane phospholipid environment has been reported to be important in receptor interaction with the adenylate cyclase complex in intact cells (Jansson *et al.*, 1993).

Lipid peroxidation in membranes, lipoproteins and cancer cells, and its measurement

FREE RADICALS AND LIPID PEROXIDATION IN CANCER AND CARDIOVASCULAR DISEASE: AN OUTLINE

Superoxide, hydrogen peroxide and the hydroxyl radical are all mutagens generated by radiation and are also produced as by-products of normal human metabolism. Oxidants are an important group of agents that stimulate cell division, which is a critical factor in mutagenesis, and this may be related to the stimulation of cell division that is associated with the inflammatory process involved in wound healing (Ames *et al.*, 1993). Redox cycling of compounds (via reductases such as cytochrome P-450 reductase, which can catalyse one-electron reductions) results in the production of oxygen radicals, which can also be formed during metabolism by cytochromes P-450 (see Chapters 3 and 9) and peroxidases (Aust *et al.*, 1993). The cellular damage caused by cytochromes P-450 (see Chapters 3 and 9) under conditions of oxidative stress has been considered (see review by Serbinova *et al.*, 1992) and the chemistry of oxidative stress has been discussed (Spiteller, 1993). In some cases redox cycling of compounds can reduce molecular oxygen by one electron to generate superoxide, which in the presence of transition metals such as iron can generate the highly reactive hydroxyl radical, resulting in oxidative damage to lipids (see below), proteins and DNA bases (e.g., formation of 8-hydroxyguanine). This DNA damage is thought to be involved in the carcinogenic action of synthetic oestrogens, including diethylstilboestrol (Zhu *et al.*, 1993; Gutteridge, 1993).

The role of free radicals in human disease is widely recognised: free radical-mediated oxidative damage appears to be important in the development of cancer and cardiovascular disease (Halliwell *et al.*, 1992; Gutteridge, 1993; Ames *et al.*, 1993; Gey, 1993; Guyton and Kensler, 1993; McCord, 1993; Blankson *et al.*, 1993), although it should be noted that free radicals can arise in the disease state as a result of the underlying pathology rather than being the primary cause (Halliwell *et al.*, 1992; Gutteridge, 1993). Lipid peroxidation results in the production of mutagenic lipid epoxides, lipid hydroperoxides, lipid alkoxyl and peroxyl radicals and enals (α, β-unsaturated aldehydes) and these are thought to be involved in carcinogenesis, in addition to general cell damage (Goldstein and Witz, 1990; Cheeseman, 1993; Ames *et al.*, 1993): the lipid peroxidation product 2,3-epoxy-4-hydroxynonanal has been reported to be a tumour-initiating agent (Chung *et al.*, 1993). In addition, singlet oxygen, which is a mutagenic and high-energy form of oxygen, can be produced by lipid peroxidation, the respiratory burst from neutrophils or the transfer of energy from light. Furthermore, the intercellular messenger nitric oxide (identified as endothelium relaxing factor), which is also produced by the phagocytic respiratory burst (in addition to hydrogen peroxide, hypochlorous acid and superoxide) in response to infection (chronic infection leads to chronic phagocytic activity and chronic inflammation, which is a recognised risk factor for cancer), is likely to be a human endogenous and exogenous (nitric oxide and related oxides are present also in cigarette smoke and car exhaust emissions) carcinogen (Arroyo *et al.*, 1992; Routledge *et al.*, 1993; Ames *et al.*, 1993). Nitric oxide is also a possible initiator of lipid peroxidation as a result of its reaction with superoxide to form the hydroxyl radical (via peroxynitrite) (see below). The pathological consequences of the interaction of free radicals with lipids have been discussed (Rice-Evans and Burdon, 1993). Tumour cells show differences in susceptibility to lipid peroxidation compared to normal cells, and this is reflected in the membrane fluidity of these cells (Galeotti *et al.*, 1984; Cheeseman, 1993). Phospholipid metabolism in human breast cancer cells has been studied using ^{31}P magnetic resonance spectroscopy (Kalra *et al.*, 1993) and cell and membrane lipid analysis, by proton magnetic resonance spectroscopy, in five breast cancer cell lines has been reported (Lemoyec *et al.*, 1992).

Lipid peroxidation, associated with the oxidative deterioration of polyunsaturated lipids—saturated fatty acids and monounsaturated fatty acids are more resistant to oxidative attack than polyunsaturated fatty acids—can be divided into two main stages: initiation and propagation (see Figure 8.1) (Halliwell and Gutteridge, 1989). The first chain-initiation step can be defined as the initial abstraction of a hydrogen atom (e.g., by a hydroxyl radical) in a peroxide-free lipid system. Following abstraction of the first hydrogen atom from a methylene group of a polyunsaturated fatty acid, molecular rearrangement occurs to stabilise the carbon radical formed, and this results in the formation of a conjugated diene. This conjugated diene often reacts with oxygen to give a peroxyl radical: peroxyl radicals are capable of abstracting a hydrogen atom from another adjacent fatty acid side-chain and this is the propagation stage of lipid peroxidation. The peroxyl radical combines with the hydrogen atom that it abstracts to form a lipid hydroperoxide. The carbon radical formed can react with oxygen to form another peroxyl radical, thus enabling the chain reaction of lipid peroxidation to continue. Abstraction of hydrogen atoms by the peroxyl radicals during the propagation stage of lipid peroxidation is an additional

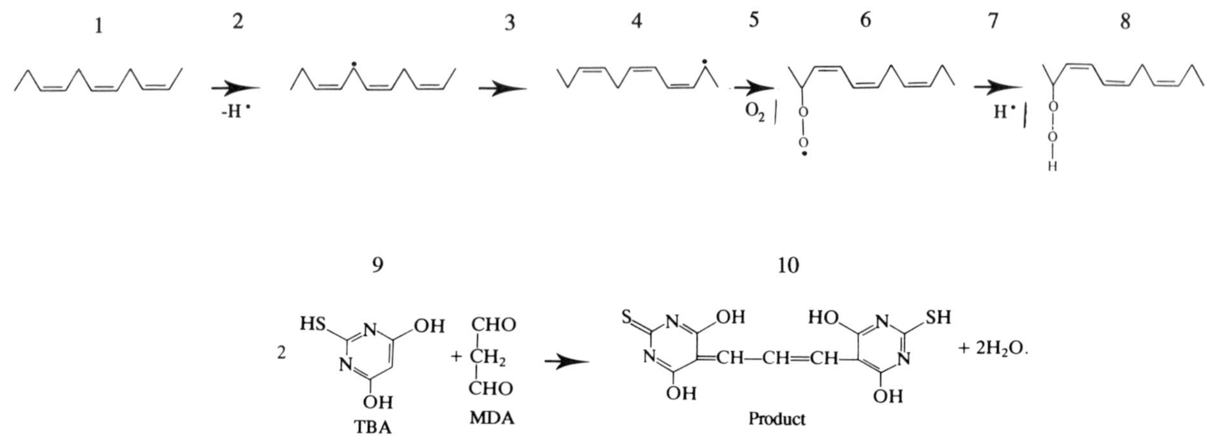

Figure 8.1. A schematic idealized model for the peroxidation of a fatty acid with three double bonds and also the TBA test

(1) A fatty acid with three double bonds
(2) Initiation of lipid peroxidation by abstraction of a hydrogen
(3) Rearrangement of the molecular structure follows
(4) A conjugated diene is formed that absorbs in the UV at 234 nm
(5) Uptake of oxygen occurs
(6) A peroxyl radical is formed
(7) The peroxyl radical abstracts a hydrogen from another fatty acid side-chain, causing a chain reaction (propagation of lipid peroxidation)
(8) The lipid hydroperoxide formed can be fragmented to malondialdehyde (MDA) and other products
(9) In the TBA test, MDA and related compounds react with TBA to generate a coloured product
(10) The product of the TBA reaction is a chromophore that absorbs at 532 nm and fluoresces as 553 nm

form of initiation, but this should really be referred to as stimulation of lipid peroxidation (Halliwell and Gutteridge, 1989). The formation of peroxides in amino acids and proteins exposed to oxygen free radicals has also been reported (Gebicki and Gebicki, 1993). It is of associated interest that the programmed lipid peroxidation of membranes resulting in the generation of the kinked phospholipids that permit local molecular mobility has been reported and a peroxidative theory of membrane fluidity control suggested (Jain *et al.*, 1993). There is also evidence for a concerted reaction between lipid hydroperoxides and polypeptides (Fruebis *et al.*, 1992).

Lipid peroxidation can be divided into two classes: 'enzymic' and 'non-enzymic' (Halliwell and Gutteridge, 1989). Peroxidation stimulated by adding Fe(II), Fe(III)/ascorbate, 'azo initiators' or synthetic hydroperoxides to lipid is usually referred to as 'non-enzymic'. The sources and role of iron in lipid peroxidation have been considered (see review by Minotti, 1993), and destruction of vitamin E and protein thiol oxidation associated with iron-initiated lipid peroxidation have been reported (Linseman *et al.*, 1993). When the antioxidant ascorbate is added with Fe(III) at low concentrations it can be considered to be acting as a pro-oxidant by reducing Fe(III) to Fe(II), which then decomposes lipid peroxides to generate peroxyl and alkoxyl radicals. Lipid peroxides are present in trace amounts in all commercially available lipids and membrane fractions isolated from disrupted cells. Alkoxyl and peroxyl radicals can abstract a hydrogen atom and stimulate lipid peroxidation (see above): here, therefore, there is no requirement for hydroxyl radical formation and first chain initiation. In addition, the equilibrium between polyunsaturated fatty acid alkoxyl radicals and the carbon-centred epoxyallylic radicals appears to be predominantly towards the epoxyallylic radical and this cyclization may, therefore, be a key step in the amplification of lipid peroxidation by polyunsaturated fatty acid hydroperoxides (Wilcox and Marnett, 1993).

'Enzymic' lipid peroxidation refers to the action of enzymes — cyclooxygenase and lipoxygenase — which catalyse the controlled peroxidation of their fatty acid substrates; and also to the increase in the rate of lipid peroxidation of membrane lipids caused by the addition of Fe(III) complexes with xanthine and xanthine oxidase, which generates the superoxide radical. This radical in turn reduces Fe(III) to Fe(II) and the latter stimulates lipid peroxidation as described above. The term 'enzymic' is also used to describe microsomal lipid peroxidation, which can be stimulated by the presence of NADPH (reduced form of nicotinamide adenine dinucleotide phosphate) and Fe(III) salts (added as complexes with ADP, pryophosphate or ethylenediaminetetraacetic acid (EDTA)). The reduced form of the cytochrome P-450 reductase enzyme, and the reduced cytochrome P-450, can donate electrons to some Fe(III) complexes, thus generating Fe(II), which stimulates peroxidation. In these examples, where reduced iron complexes are being used to stimulate lipid peroxidation, the systems are not really enzymic because the enzyme system is acting only to reduce the iron complexes (Halliwell and Gutteridge, 1989).

LIPID PEROXIDATION IN MICROSOMES, LIPOSOMES, LIPOPROTEIN PARTICLES AND CANCER CELLS

Microsomes

Microsomes are a heterogeneous mixture of vesicles derived from both endoplasmic reticulum and plasma membrane. The role of endogenous non-haem iron in microsomal redox reactions has been studied (Minotti, 1992). Furthermore, studies using rat liver microsomes have shown that both Fe(II) and Fe(III) are required for lipid peroxidation to occur (with maximal rates observed at a ratio of 1 : 1), and that ascorbate stimulated iron-catalysed lipid peroxidation acts by reducing the Fe(III) to Fe(II) (Miller and Aust, 1989). However, when the ascorbate concentration was sufficient to reduce all the Fe(III) to Fe(II) the ascorbate inhibited lipid peroxidation. In addition, simultaneous addition of ascorbate and organic hydroperoxides resulted in enhanced lipid peroxidation, indicating a synergistic pro-oxidant effect of ascorbate on hydroperoxide-dependent lipid peroxidation (Laudicina and Marnett, 1990). Furthermore, incubation with NADPH resulted in enzyme-catalysed microsomal lipid peroxidation mediated by endogenous iron (with mainly hydroperoxides as the primary products), which was increased in rate by the addition of low concentrations of either Fe(II) or Fe(III) ions (Morini *et al.*, 1990). It is possible that a higher peroxidation rate was observed because the low iron concentrations enhanced the breakdown of the formed hydroperoxides, thus further promoting the peroxidation process by the propagation step. Radicals produced by the reaction of hydroperoxides with rat liver microsomal fractions have been detected (Greenlay and Davies, 1992). The disadvantages of using rat liver microsomes as a test system for the antioxidant ability of drugs including tamoxifen and its metabolites include the presence of endogenous antioxidants (e.g., vitamin E), and the probability that their amounts can be variable with different preparations (Halliwell and Gutteridge, 1989).

Liposomes

Liposomes are used extensively as a model membrane system in the study of lipid peroxidation. The use of liposomes has many distinct advantages and has provided new information concerning the reaction mechanism of lipid peroxidation and consequent membrane damage, in addition to the mode of action of antioxidant compounds and drugs. Liposomes are artificial lipid structures, and are made by the shaking or sonicating of phospholipids in aqueous suspension; whereupon they first form micelles, but as more phospholipids are added liposomes are formed as either multilamellar vesicles, small unilamellar vesicles or indeed large unilamellar vesicles, depending upon the method of preparation used (New, 1992b). The role of enzymes, NADPH–cytochrome P-450 reductase and cytochrome P-450 in Fe(III)-ADP/NADPH-dependent lipid peroxidation, has been investigated in liposomes prepared from rat liver microsomal phospholipids, and with the addition of the purified enzymes (Sevanian *et al.*, 1990). It was found that the coupled role of these enzymes in lipid peroxidation was to provide overall the two electrons required for oxygen reduction and formation of lipid hydroperoxide (Sevanian *et al.*, 1990). Site-specific mechanisms of initiation of lipid peroxidation by chelated iron have been reported, using charged micelles as an alternative to liposomes (Fujii *et al.*, 1991). It is of interest that Mn(II) is an antioxidant, and the mechanism of its inhibition of phospholipid peroxidation has been investigated (Tampo and Yonaha, 1992).

Lipoprotein particles

The oxidative modification of low-density lipoproteins (LDL), in particular peroxidation-induced alterations in surface charge (aldehydic breakdown products of lipid peroxidation such as malodialdehyde and 4-hydroxynonenal alter the surface charge of LPD via modification of the ε-amino groups of the lysine residues), is thought to be a precondition for uptake by the non-down-regulating scavenger receptor of macrophages (see review by Krieger, 1992) during foam cell formation and, therefore, is important in the pathogenesis of in atherosclerosis (see Steinberg *et al.*, 1989; Rice-Evans and Bruckdorfer, 1992; Esterbauer *et al.*, 1992; Ross, 1993; Aviram, 1993; Leake, 1993; Schwartz *et al.*, 1993; Wiseman *et al.*, 1993c). However, the mechanism of the initiation of LDL oxidation is uncertain (Halliwell, 1993). The hydroxyl radical is a species capable of initiating the peroxidation of LDL and is formed by the reaction of transition metal ions (such as Fe(III) and Cu(II)) with hydrogen peroxide and of the superoxide radical with nitric oxide (via the intermediate peroxynitrite); although the role of the nitric oxide radical in macrophage-mediated oxidation of LDL has not yet been fully ascertained (Halliwell, 1993). It should be noted that in most *in vitro* experiments, reactions involving preformed peroxides in the LDL are being observed and not initiation: peroxides could be generated by lipoxygenases (15-lipoxygenases but probably not 5-lipoxygenase could be of importance) or be formed from endogenous peroxidation or even originate from dietary fats. Indeed, the 15-lipoxygenase-induced oxidative modification of LDL has been reported (Belkner *et al.*, 1993). Transition metal ions (present in advanced human arteriosclerotic lesions) and superoxide can decompose peroxides and so propagate the oxidation of LDL. The dynamics of the oxidation of LDL by free radicals has been monitored (Noguchi *et al.*, 1993). Furthermore, the simultaneous generation of superoxide and nitric oxide can initiate lipid peroxidation in human LDL (Darley-Usmar *et al.*, 1992).

Cancer cells

In cancer cells, increasing the polyunsaturated fatty acid content of the plasma membrane, which can be achieved by diet (see Chapter 4), can enhance their susceptibility to undergo lipid peroxidation, thus inhibiting their growth (Burdon and Rice-Evans, 1989). Such modification of the fatty acid content of tumour cells could thus increase their sensitivity to lipid peroxidation and cell death in the presence of pro-oxidant antitumour drugs. The antitumour drug adriamycin when complexed with Fe(II) *in vitro* is a powerful stimulator of lipid peroxidation, probably because it efficiently decomposes traces of lipid hydroperoxides. It has been suggested that damage to cancer cell lines by adriamycin may be caused by oxygen radical generation. Furthermore, enrichment of leukaemic lymphoblast (L1210) cells with polyunsaturated fatty acids was found to increase their sensitivity to lipid peroxidation induced by adriamycin, resulting in growth inhibition and cell death. The biochemical effects of lipids on cancer therapy have been discussed (Burns and Spector, 1994). The role of pro-oxidants and mitochondrial calcium in apoptosis and oncogenesis has been considered (Richter, 1993), However, the action of antioxidant anticancer drugs such as tamoxifen should also be considered (Wiseman, 1994a, 1994b); see below.

MEASUREMENT OF LIPID PEROXIDATION

Lipid peroxidation can be detected and measured by a number of different methods. In outline, these include the oxygen electrode (to measure uptake of oxygen during peroxide decomposition reactions); analysis of fatty acids by gas–liquid chromatography (GLC) or high-performance liquid chromatography (HPLC) to measure loss of unsaturated fatty acids; fluorescence (to measure aldehydes); light emission (to measure excited carbonyls and singlet oxygen); diene conjugation (to measure diene-conjugated structures from ultraviolet (UV) absorbance increase at 230–235 nm); hydrocarbon gases (measurement of pentane and ethane); GLC/mass spectrometry (to measure the formation of lipid peroxides); and the thiobarbituric acid (TBA) test (to mesure TBA-reactive substances TBARS) (Halliwell and Gutteridge, 1989; Gutteridge and Halliwell, 1990; Halliwell and Chirico, 1993; Draper *et al.*, 1993).

In the TBA test the test material is heated with TBA under acid conditions and the formation of a pink chromogen is measured at 532 nm (see below and Figure 8.1). Decomposition of the lipid peroxides formed during lipid peroxidation results in the formation of carbonyl compounds, including malondialdehyde (MDA), and these are TBA reactive substances (TBARS). The MDA–TBA adduct is a pink-coloured compound, which in acid solution absorbs light at 532 nm and fluoresces at 553 nm. However, little free MDA is produced by most peroxidising systems and in fact most of the MDA that reacts in the TBA test is formed by the accelerated decomposition of lipid peroxides that occurs during heating under the acid conditions of the TBA test (Halliwell and Gutteridge, 1989; Gutteridge and Halliwell, 1990; Halliwell and Chirico, 1993). A comparative evaluation of the TBA methods for the determination of MDA in biological materials has been made (Draper *et al.*, 1993).

OVERVIEW OF MEMBRANE ANTIOXIDANTS

Tocopherols, ascorbate and cholesterol

Dietary antioxidants such as tocopherol, ascorbate and β-carotene are recognised to be protective against a wide range of human cancers (tocopherol and carotenoids protect against the oxidative DNA damage and cell division associated with carcinogenesis), and cardiovascular disease is associated with low plasma concentrations of these dietary antioxidants (they protect LDL against oxidative modification) (Ames *et al.*, 1993; Gey, 1993; Rice-Evans and Diplock, 1993). Indeed, tocopherols (e.g., α-tocopherol, vitamin E) can inhibit free radical-mediated lipid peroxidation in biomembranes and lipoprotein particles (see Aust *et al.*, 1993) and this is likely to be of importance in the prevention of both cancer and heart disease, respectively. A study of vitamin E and the risk of coronary heart disease in women has shown that among middle-aged women the use of vitamin E supplementation was associated with a reduced risk of coronary heart disease (Stampfer *et al.*, 1993), and this is of relevance to the prevention of both breast cancer and heart disease in this group by means of drug therapy and dietary supplementation (see Chapter 4). Vitamin E inhibits lipid peroxidation by donating a hydrogen atom (from the phenolic hydroxyl group present in the 6-hydroxychromane rings) to the chain-propagating lipid peroxyl and alkoxyl radicals, thus terminating the chain reaction and generating tocopheroxyl (tocopheryl) radicals of the tocopherol antioxidant. In addition, the role of cellular metabolism in the antioxidant function of vitamin E has been considered: metabolism of α-tocopheryl esters, which are inactive as antioxidants releases α-tocopherol, whereas reductive metabolism of α-tocopherolquinone (an oxidation product of α-tocopherol) produces α-tocopherylhydroquinone, which may also provide antioxidant protection (Liebler, 1993).

The antioxidant action of ascorbate (vitamin C), by regenerating α-tocopherol from the tocopheroxyl radical, has been found to be 10-fold greater than that of glutathione in α-tocopherol-enriched microsomes (Hiramatsu *et al.*, 1990). However, the intracellular concentration of glutathione is higher than that of ascorbate, thus glutathione could be the more effective antioxidant when expressed in terms of maintaining the level of intracellular vitamin E (Hiramatsu *et al.*, 1990). Although vitamin E is located in membranes and vitamin C in the aqueous phase, vitamin C is able to recycle vitamin E by regenerating the tocopheroxyl (chromanoxyl) radical of vitamin E such that the function of vitamin E as a free radical chain-breaking antioxidant is restored (Buettner, 1993). The interaction of vitamins C and E during free radical stress in plasma has been studied using ESR to make serial measurements of the ascorbate and tocopheroxyl free radicals (Sharma and Buettner, 1993). The tocopheroxyl radical only appeared after the virtual disappearance of the ascorbate radical, and this supports the experimental observations that suggest that vitamin E—the primary lipid-soluble small molecule antioxidant—and ascorbate—the terminal water-soluble small molecule antioxidant in biological systems—cooperate to protect lipids and lipid structures against peroxidation (Buettner, 1993). It is of interest that activated human neutrophils can accumulate ascorbate (concentrations as high as 14 mM can be achieved) and also recycle it (Washko *et al.*, 1993). The oxidation products of ascorbic acid have been reported to protect human LDL against atherogenic modifications, and this is an example of an antioxidant rather than the pro-oxidant activity of vitamin C that is observed in the presence of transition metal ions (Retsky *et al.*, 1993).

It has been shown that α-tocopherol homologues of differing hydrocarbon chain lengths exhibited different antioxidant potencies in rat liver microsomal membranes. The short-chain homologues have the highest efficiency of regeneration from their chromanoxyl radicals by ascorbate, or by NADPH-dependent electron transport, and therefore display the highest antioxidant potency (Kagan *et al.*, 1990a). Similarly, several synthetic vitamin E derivatives have been shown to be potent inhibitors of microsomal lipid peroxidation, and their relative potencies were found to be consistent with their intrinsic antioxidant properties as peroxyl radical scavengers (Battioni *et al.*, 1993).

Dietary tocotrienols have been reported to be antioxidants: they become incorporated into human LDL where they react with peroxyl radicals as efficiently as the corresponding tocopherol isomers (Suarna *et al.*, 1993). Reactions of the vitamin E model compound 2,2,5,7,8-pentamethylchromnan-6-ol with peroxyl radicals showed that the reaction medium controlled the balance between competing reactions of the chromanoxyl radical 2b, and the results were consistent with the formation of epoxides and 8a-substituted tocopherones as the predominant products of

α-tocopherol oxidation in biological membranes (Liebler *et al.*, 1993). The ability of vitamin E to protect membranes has been shown to be dependant on the nature of the pro-oxidant used. The relative importance of vitamin E as an antioxidant was diminished when peroxidation was initiated by complexes containing Fe(II), and enhanced when peroxidation involved peroxyl radicals (Scheschonka *et al.*, 1990). The role of α-tocopherol as an antioxidant and peroxyl radical scavenger (Smith *et al.*, 1993) in human LDL has been investigated and the recycling of vitamin E in human LDL has been reported (Kagan *et al.*, 1992). Furthermore, conditions under which the antioxidant vitamin E can act as a pro-oxidant have been reported: lipid peroxidation can be propagated within LDL by rection of the α-tocopheroxyl radical with polyunsaturated fatty acid side-chains in the lipid and, therefore, vitamin C and ubiquinol 10 (see below), which can reduce the α-tocopheroxyl radical and inhibit the peroxidation of vitamin E-containing LDL (Bowry *et al.*, 1992). *In vitro*, vitamin C and β-carotene also prevent LDL oxidation and may be protective against atherosclerosis (Maxwell, 1993). Furthermore, cardiovascular disease is associated with low levels of ascorbate, α-tocopherol and β-carotene (Ames *et al.*, 1993).

Oxidation of α-tocopherol to α-tocopheroquinone in human LDL resulted from the simultaneous generation of superoxide and nitric oxide; these radicals react to form peroxynitrite, which decomposes to form the hydroxyl radical and nitrogen dioxide (Hogg *et al.*, 1993). Furthermore, exposure of microsomes to nitric oxide or the sydnonimine SIN-1, which spontaneously decomposes to yield nitric oxide and the superoxide radical (see above), resulted in the loss of α-tocopherol and again the quinone derivative was the main oxidation product (De Groot *et al.*, 1993).

Protection by vitamin E, selenium and β-carotene against oxidative damage in rat liver slices and homogenates has been reported: the diet with a combination of all three antioxidants provided the most effective protection against oxidative damage to haem proteins, which correlated with the inhibitory effects of these compounds on lipid peroxidation (Chen *et al.*, 1993). In addition, α-tocopherol has been reported to abolish the lipid peroxidation caused by oxidative stress in transformed and nontransformed baby hamster kidney cells (Goldring *et al.*, 1993). Carotinoids have also been shown to inhibit lipid peroxidation and this is likely to be important to their cancer chemopreventive action (Zhang *et al.*, 1991).

A structural antioxidant action in the membrane is displayed by a number of compounds, such as α-tocopherol (Lucy, 1972; Bisby, 1990), cholesterol (Gutteridge, 1978; Kinsella, 1990; Wiseman *et al.*, 1990a, 1992a; Wiseman, 1994a, 1994b) and ubiquinones (Cabrini *et al.*, 1986). In the case of α-tocopherol this is in addition to the donation of a phenolic hydrogen atom to scavenge lipid peroxyl and alkoxyl radicals, which is referred to as a chain-breaking antioxidant action. This is observed as a characteristic time course: the test curves reach the same level as the control curve as the chain-breaking antioxidant is consumed (Halliwell, 1990; Halliwell and Gutteridge, 1990). When cholesterol is introduced into membranes, or membrane models such as liposomes, it has been reported to inhibit lipid peroxidation (Gutteridge, 1978). The structural antioxidant action of cholesterol in membranes is thought to occur by interaction between the hydrophobic sterol rings of cholesterol and the saturated, mono-unsaturated and polyunsaturated fatty acid side-chains of the membrane phospholipids. This interaction may partially immobilise the hydrocarbon chains particularly in the region close to the polar head of the phospholipid.

Cholesterol when introduced into phospholipid liposomes during their preparation inhibits membrane lipid peroxidation, because of a membrane stabilisation effect (Gutteridge, 1978; Wiseman *et al.*, 1990b; Wiseman, 1994a, 1994b). Although cholesterol can undergo oxidation, no cholesterol hydroperoxides were detected when cholesterol was introduced into liposomes that were subsequently peroxidised (Gutteridge, 1978): this suggests that cholesterol does not have a free radical scavenging anti-oxidant action. It appears, therefore, that both α-tocopherol and cholesterol have structural antioxidant roles in the membrane, whereas only α-tocopherol has an additional free radical scavenging activity. It is also of interest that 6-ketocholestanol, a naturally occurring oxygenated sterol (and derivative of cholesterol), has been reported to inhibit human neutrophil respiratory burst activity, probably by modification of the membrane structure (Vasconcelles *et al.*, 1990). The α-tocopherol molecule is usually localised in the hydrophobic zone of the lipid bilayer due to various interactions, which then enable it to stabilise microsomal and liposomal membranes against lipid peroxidation (Kagan *et al.*, 1990b; Serbinova *et al.*, 1991): fluorescence anisotropy (polarisation) measurements have shown that both cholesterol and α-tocopherol have a rigidifying effect on liposomal membranes (Bisby, 1990).

Ubiquinols

Ubiquinol is the only known lipid-soluble antioxidant that can be synthesised *de novo* in animal cells and for which an enzymic mechanism (the mitochondrial electron transport chain) exists that can regenerate the antioxidant from its oxidised form, which results from its inhibitory effect on lipid peroxidation. In addition, the high degree of hydrophobicity of ubiquinol and its presence in both membranes and LDL particles indicate its likely important role in protection against oxidative damage. Ubiquinol 10 (coenzyme Q_{10}), when introduced into liposomes during their preparation, efficiently scavenges free radicals and, therefore, is a chain-breaking antioxidant (Frei *et al.*, 1990). Ubiquinol 10 was found to be about as effective in preventing peroxidative damage to membranes as α-tocopherol, which is considered to be the most effective lipid-soluble antioxidant in humans. Ubiquinol 10 can subsequently be regenerated by electron carriers present in various biomembranes although not by ascorbate, in contrast to α-tocopherol. In addition, ubiquinol has been shown to be effective as an inhibitor of ascorbate and Fe(III)-ADP-induced lipid peroxidation in beef heart submitochondrial particles in the absence of vitamin E, but is likely to amplify the antioxidant effect of vitamin E. Studies have shown that ubiquinol 10 was consumed preferentially to α-tocopherol when both were introduced into liposomes that were then peroxidised (Frei *et al.*, 1990; Hiramatsu *et al.*, 1991). Furthermore, ubiquinol 10 has been reported to protect human LDL particles against lipid peroxidation more effectively than α-tocopherol (Stocker *et al.*, 1991). Dietary supplementation with coenzyme Q_{10} resulted in increased levels of ubiquinol 10 within circulating lipoproteins and increased resistance of human LDL to the initiation of lipid peroxidation (Mohr *et al.*, 1992). Ubiquinol 3 has also been reported to have an antioxidant activity (Landi *et al.*, 1992) and a comparison of ubiquinol 3 and ubiquinol 7 has shown that the two homologues behave as chain-breaking antioxidants with a similar effectiveness that was slightly lower than that of α-tocopherol (Fiorentini *et al.*, 1993).

Ubiquinones, which unlike ubiquinols and α-tocopherol cannot donate a phenolic hydrogen atom to scavenge lipid free radicals, can stabilise membranes against lipid peroxidation (Cabrini *et al.*, 1986), in addition to their role as electron carriers. This antioxidant action may be by a similar mechanism to that proposed for the structural antioxidant action of α-tocopherol (Lucy, 1972). Furthermore, ubiquinones synergistically enhance NADH and NADPH-dependent regeneration of α-tocopherol during electron flow in mitochondria and microsomes (Kagan *et al.*, 1990c). Ubiquinone 3 has been reported to have antioxidant activity in human LDL (Merati *et al.*, 1992).

Oestrogens and vitamin D

Inhibition of liposomal and microsomal lipid peroxidation by 17β-oestradiol has been reported (Sugioka *et al.*, 1987; Wiseman *et al.*, 1990a, 1990b; 1992b; Wiseman and Halliwell, 1993). Tamoxifen and 4-hydroxytamoxifen also inhibit lipid peroxidation in these systems (Wiseman *et al.*, 1990a, 1990b; 1992b; Wiseman and Halliwell, 1993; see below). 17β-Oestradiol has also been found to stabilise LDL particles against lipid peroxidation (Huber *et al.*, 1990) and this has now been shown for tamoxifen and 4-hydroxytamoxifen (Wiseman *et al.*, 1993c; see below). It is of related interest that oestrogen regulates LDL receptors at the post-transcriptional level in the rat and the mouse *in vivo* (Ajit *et al.*, 1993). In addition, the antioxidant properties of a range of steroids has been studied: 17β-oestradiol, 17α-oestradiol and oestriol were all found to have antioxidant properties, whereas testosterone, oestrone, progesterone, androstenedione, dehydroepiandrosterone, cortisol, tetrahydrocortisone, deoxycorticosterone and aldosterone had no significant antioxidant properties, and cortisone and corticosterone had slight pro-oxidant properties (Mooradian, 1993). It is of associated interest that the radioprotective effect of oestrogens and in particular the catecholoestrogen 2-hydroxyoestradiol is thought to be due to their antioxidant ability (Tomatsu *et al.*, 1993). Furthermore the carcinogenic oestrogens, diethylstilboestrol, hexoestrol and 17α-ethynyloestradiol (see Figure 8.2), which are likely to exert their carcinogenic action through DNA damage by the free radicals generated by the metabolism and redox cycling of these compounds (Zhu *et al.*, 1993), are all potent antioxidants (Wiseman and Halliwell, 1993). Compounds acting as antioxidants towards lipids may also exert pro-oxidant effects towards other molecules such as DNA and cannot be assumed to be safe for human use (Wiseman and Halliwell, 1993). Vitamin D is another membrane antioxidant of interest (Wiseman 1993; see Figure 8.3). Furthermore, vitamin D, its active metabolite and also synthetic analogues have been reported to have anticancer activity (Colston *et al.*, 1992a, 1992b). The clinical applications of vitamin D analogues have been discussed (Pols *et al.*, 1994).

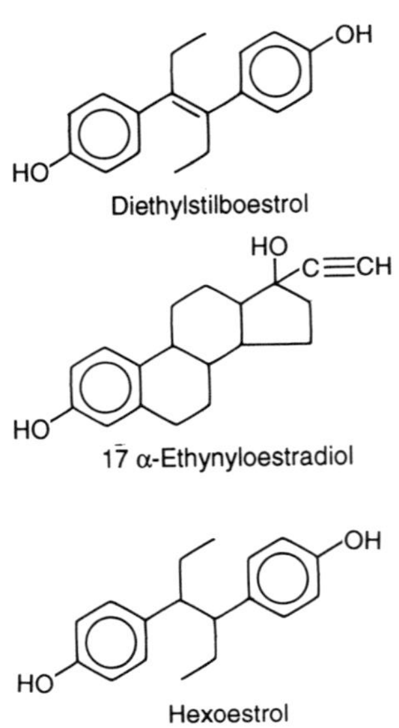

Figure 8.2. Synthetic oestrogens

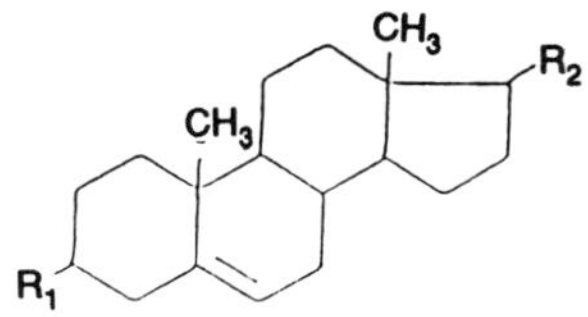

Cholesterol
$R_1 = OH, R_2 = CH(CH_3)(CH_2)_3CH(CH_3)_2$

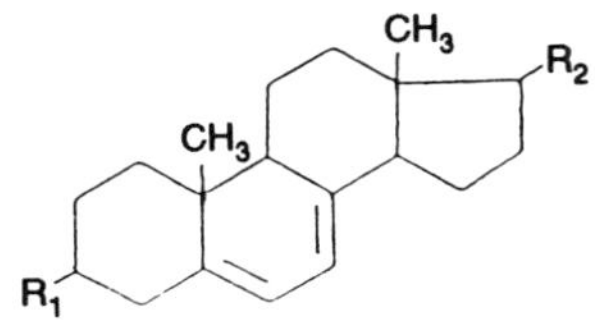

7-Dehydrocholesterol
$R_1 = OH, R_2 = CH(CH_3)(CH_2)_3CH(CH_3)_2$

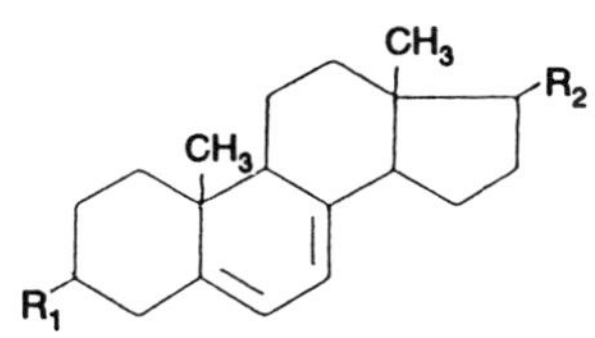

Ergosterol
$R_1 = OH, R_2 = CH(CH_3)CH{:}CHCH(CH_3)CH(CH_3)_2$

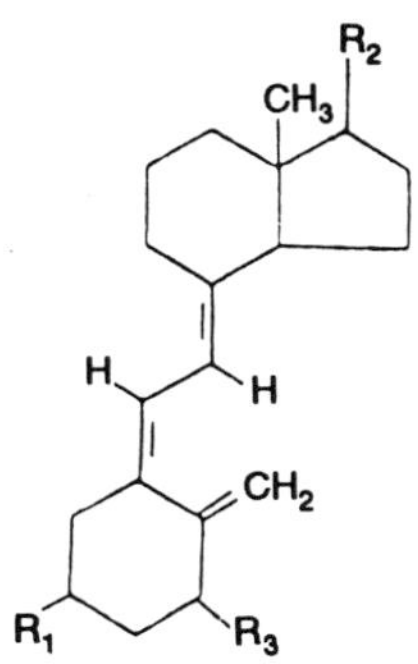

Ergocalciferol $R_1 = OH, R_2 = CH(CH_3)CH{:}CHCH(CH_3)CH(CH_3)_2, R_3 = H$ (Vitamin D_2)
Cholecalciferol $R_1 = OH, R_2 = CH(CH_3)(CH_2)_3CH(CH_3)_2, R_3 = H$ (Vitamin D_3)
1,25 Dihydroxycholecalciferol $R_1 = OH, R_2 = CH(CH_3)(CH_2)_3C(OH)(CH)_2, R_3 = OH$ (Active form of vitamin D)

Figure 8.3. Membrane antioxidants

Melatonin and dihydrolipoic acid

Studies both *in vivo* and *in vitro* have shown that melatonin (see Chapter 6) is an antioxidant (Pierrefiche *et al.*, 1993) and this is likely to be because of the indole structure of the molecule. Antioxidant activity has been reported for dihydrolipoic acid (DHLA) and its structural homologues both in membranes (scavenging of peroxyl radicals) and in aqueous phase (quenching of superoxide radicals and scavenging of peroxyl radicals); differences between the DHLA homologues in their antioxidant abilities in polar and apolar environments generally agreed with differences in their partition coefficients (Suzuki *et al.*, 1993).

THE ANTIOXIDANT ACTION OF TAMOXIFEN AND RELATED COMPOUNDS

Inhibition of microsomal and liposomal lipid peroxidation by tamoxifen and related compounds

Tamoxifen, its derivatives and 17β-oestradiol (see Figure 8.4) all inhibited lipid peroxidation in both microsomal and pre-formed liposomal systems (Wiseman *et al.*, 1990b, 1992b, 1993b; Wiseman and Halliwell, 1993; Wiseman, 1994a, 1994b). The IC_{50} values of these compounds (see Table 8.1) indicated that 4-hydroxytamoxifen was a better inhibitor of microsomal lipid peroxidation in both the Fe(III)-ascorbate and Fe(III)-ADP/NADPH systems, and of liposomal peroxidation, than tamoxifen, 3-hydroxytamoxifen or 17β-oestradiol. The similar effects of the compounds observed in the two microsomal systems also suggests that free radical intermediates are not being formed from the drugs because this finding eliminates the possibility that ascorbate might have re-reduced such intermediates, thus lowering the IC_{50} values observed in this system compared to the Fe(III)-ADP/NADPH system. Cholesterol and ergosterol had no inhibitory effect on either microsomal or liposomal peroxidation.

Tamoxifen and related compounds and 17β-oestradiol (all at their IC_{50} concentrations) inhibited microsomal and liposomal lipid peroxidation by an approximately constant percentage over the time course investigated. Furthermore, there was no evidence for a 'lag period' followed by an acceleration of peroxidation to the control rate that is often observed when chain-breaking antioxidants are added to a peroxidising lipid substrate. Compounds were added dissolved in ethanol, and ethanol itself was demonstrated to have no effect on peroxidation at this concentration (0.5% v/v): none of the compounds tested interfered with the TBA test and no inhibition was observed when the compounds were added to peroxidising microsomes or liposomes at the same time as the TBA reagents

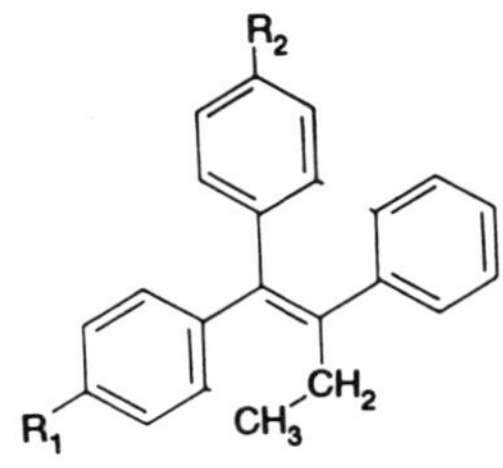

Tamoxifen $R_1 = H$, $R_2 = OCH_2CH_2N(CH_3)_2$
4-Hydroxytamoxifen $R_1 = OH$, $R_2 = OCH_2CH_2N(CH_3)_2$

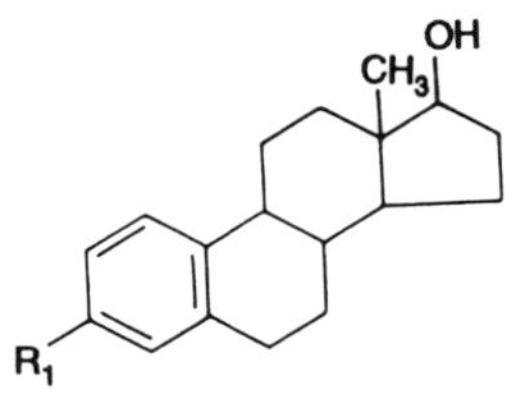

17 β-Oestradiol $R_1 = OH$

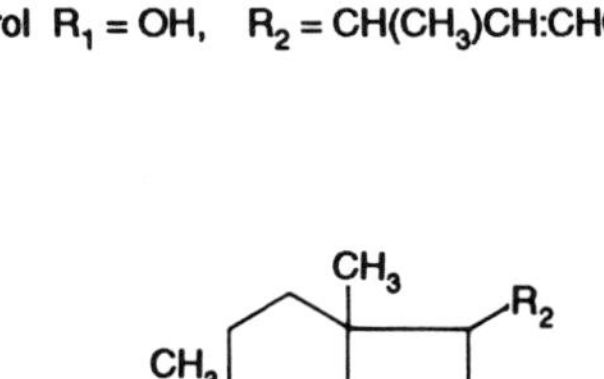

Ergosterol $R_1 = OH$, $R_2 = CH(CH_3)CH{:}CHCH(CH_3)CH(CH_3)_2$

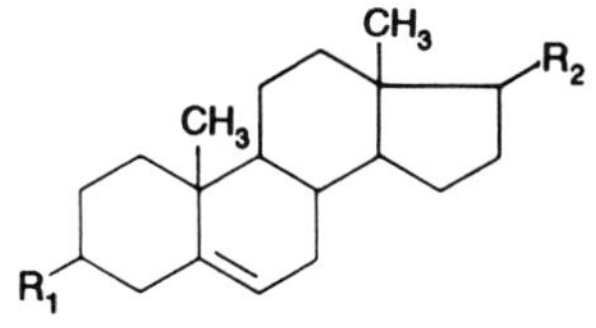

Cholesterol $R_1 = OH$, $R_2 = CH(CH_3)(CH_2)_3CH(CH_3)_2$

Figure 8.4. Inhibitors of lipid peroxidation

Table 8.1. IC_{50} values for the inhibition of microsomal and liposomal lipid peroxidation by tamoxifen and related compounds

	System		
		Liposomal	
Compound/drug	Microsomal (μM)	Pre-formed (μM)	Introduced into liposome (mM)
Tamoxifen	8	7	0.05
4-Hydroxytamoxifen	2	2	0.0036
3-Hydroxytamoxifen	13	—	—
cis-Tamoxifen	11	9	—
N-Desmethyltamoxifen	14	11	—
Cholesterol	NR	NR	0.72
Ergosterol	NR	NR	0.053
17β-Oestradiol	5	4	0.004

The lipid peroxidation was induced by Fe(III)-ascorbate in these systems.
NR = not reached. Data quoted from Wiseman, 1994b, and Wiseman *et al.*, 1993d.

instead of at the beginning of the incubation. Similar or enhanced inhibitory effects of these compounds on lipid peroxidation were obtained when butylated hydroxytoluene (BHT) was added at the end of the incubations to suppress peroxidation during the TBA test itself.

In the 'introduced into liposome' system tamoxifen inhibited lipid peroxidation to approximately the same extent as ergosterol (Wiseman *et al.*, 1990a). Cholesterol was a much less effective inhibitor than tamoxifen, whereas 4-hydroxytamoxifen and 17β-oestradiol were approximately equipotent: the latter two compounds were both more effective inhibitors of peroxidation than tamoxifen (see Table 8.1). These studies showed that the concentration of tamoxifen or ergosterol that had to be introduced into the membrane to achieve 50% inhibition of lipid peroxidation was approximately 15-fold less than for cholesterol. Moreover these IC_{50} values of 4-hydroxytamoxifen and 17β-oestradiol were approximately 200-fold less than for cholesterol, indicating the superiority of many compounds and drugs over the natural mammalian membrane component, cholesterol.

The likely physiological importance of these results is reflected in the finding that tamoxifen decreased plasma lipid peroxide levels and favourably altered the concentrations of antioxidant enzymes, including superoxide, catalase and glutathione peroxidase in post-menopausal but not pre-menopausal women with breast cancer (Thangaraju *et al.*, 1993). The lack of effect in pre-menopausal women may be because the dosage (10 mg twice a day) was inadequate and clearly further studies are required.

Computer-aided molecular modelling and calculation of the cholesterol coefficients of structural antioxidants in liposomes

Tamoxifen and 4-hydroxytamoxifen display a structural similarity to cholesterol, and this similarity has been shown by computer molecular modelling studies and by calculation of cholesterol coefficients (C_c) (see Table 8.2) from the slopes of the linear graphical plots (i.e., at the low compound/phospholipid ratios) derived from the ratio of percentage inhibition of lipid peroxidation by compound to percentage inhibition of lipid peroxidation by cholesterol, plotted against compound/phospholipid ratio in ox brain phospholipid liposomes (see Figure 8.5) (Wiseman *et al.*, 1992a; Wiseman, 1994a, 1994b). At high compound/phospholipid ratios tamoxifen, 4-hydroxytamoxifen and ergosterol were similar to cholesterol, whereas at low compound/phospholipid ratios tamoxifen and ergosterol and especially 4-hydroxytamoxifen and 17β-oestradiol displayed graphical plots that were highly divergent from cholesterol. The calculated cholesterol coefficients, therefore, indicate that both tamoxifen and ergosterol are superior to cholesterol as inhibitors of lipid peroxidation, and that this superiority is increased by approximately five-fold with 4-hydroxytamoxifen and 17β-oestradiol (Wiseman *et al.*, 1992a; Wiseman, 1994a, 1994b).

The computer molecular modelling system Chemmod (chemical modelling: White *et al.*, 1986) was used to quantify in terms of a root mean square (RMS) fit value the proposed structural similarity of tamoxifen (and more importantly 4-hydroxytamoxifen) to the membrane sterols cholesterol and ergosterol, and also to 17β-oestradiol (see Figure 8.6) (Wiseman *et al.*, 1992a). The relative binding affinity (RBA) for the oestrogen receptor of 4-hydroxytamoxifen is similar to that of 17β-oestradiol and is 100-fold higher than that of tamoxifen, while that of 3-hydroxytamoxifen (droloxifene: Wiseman *et al.*, 1992b) is 10-fold higher

Table 8.2. Cholesterol coefficient values for triphenylethylene drugs and sterol compounds. The cholesterol coefficient values were calculated from the slopes of the linear portions of the graphs plotted in Figure 8.5

Drug/compound	Cholesterol coefficient (C_c)
4-Hydroxytamoxifen	147
Tamoxifen	29
17β-Oestradiol	127
Cholesterol	0
Ergosterol	32

From Wiseman *et al.*, 1992a, with permission.

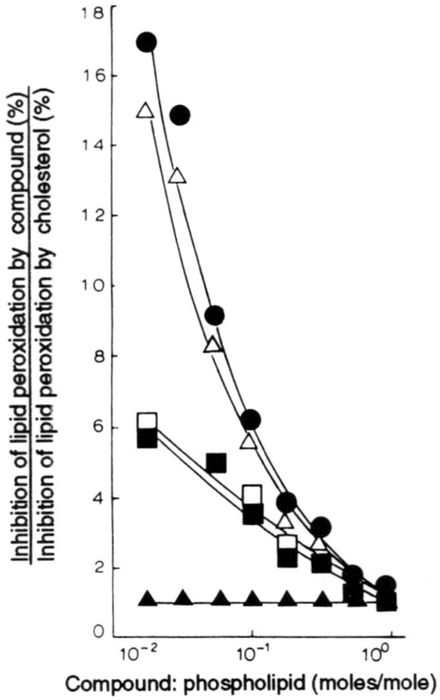

Figure 8.5. Inhibition of lipid peroxidation by 4-hydroxytamoxifen (•), tamoxifen (□), ergosterol (■) and 17β-oestradiol (△). Inhibition of lipid peroxidation by each of the compounds was compared to that observed for cholesterol (▲) and the ratios obtained were plotted against the compound: phospholipid molar ratio in ox brain phospholipid liposomes. The compounds were each introduced into liposomes during their preparation. From Wiseman *et al.*, 1992a, with permission

than that of tamoxifen. This is indicative of the importance of the ring position of the hydroxyl group on the tamoxifen molecule in relation to the structural mimicry of cholesterol and 17β-oestradiol that has been examined using computer molecular modelling techniques. These differences in binding affinity are reflected in the chemical structures; thus although tamoxifen, 4-hydroxytamoxifen and 3-hydroxytamoxifen mimic the steroid nucleus of 17β-oestradiol, only 4-hydroxytamoxifen has a hydroxyl group in the same ring position as 17β-oestradiol. The greater binding affinity reported for 4-hydroxytamoxifen, 3-hydroxytamoxifen and 17β-oestradiol compared to tamoxifen is reflected in their ability to inhibit lipid peroxidation more effectively than tamoxifen and is reflected in the cholesterol coefficients of tamoxifen, 4-hydroxytamoxifen and 17β-oestradiol.

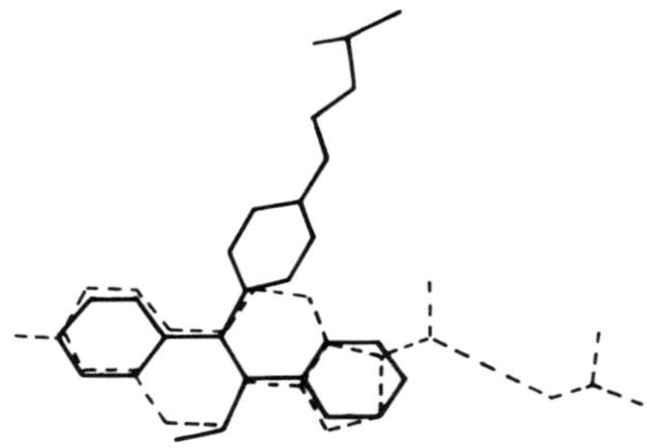

Tamoxifen-ergosterol

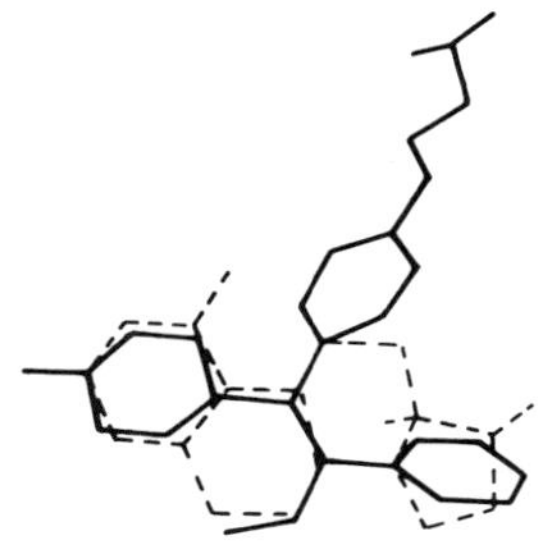

Tamoxifen-17β-oestradiol

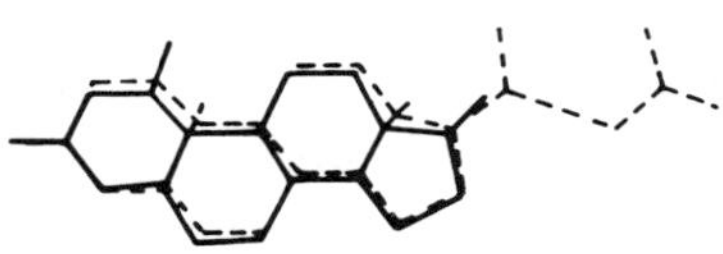

17β-oestradiol-cholesterol

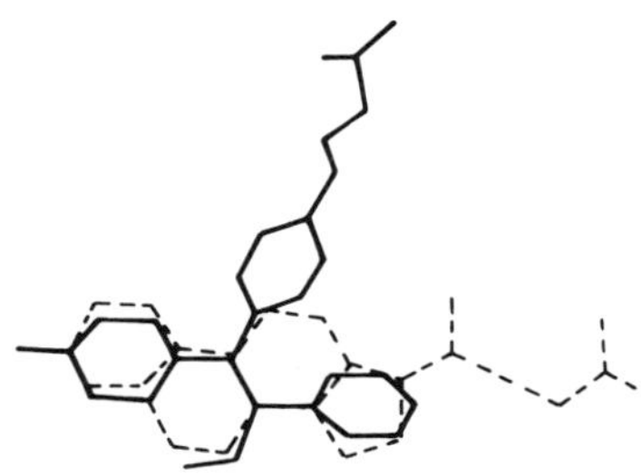

Tamoxifen-cholesterol

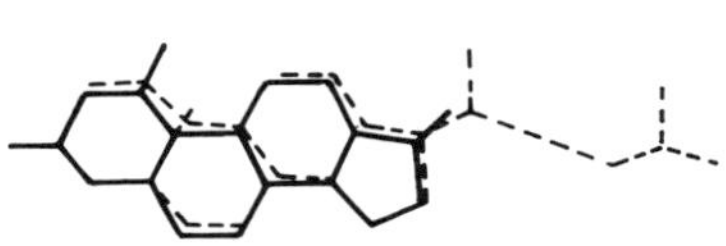

17β-oestradiol-ergosterol

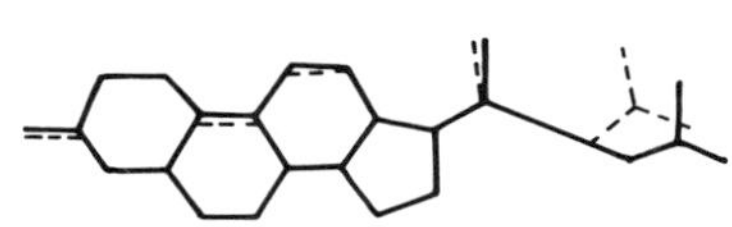

Ergosterol-cholesterol

Figure 8.6. Computer-graphic overlays of triphenylethylene drugs with sterol compounds. The data were generated using the Chemmod program. From Wiseman *et al.*, 1992a, with permission

Membrane-mediated mechanism of the antioxidant action of tamoxifen and its derivatives

The chemical structure of tamoxifen indicates that it is unlikely to act as a chain-breaking antioxidant because it does not possess easily donatable hydrogen atoms. Furthermore, chain-breaking antioxidants usually introduce a lag period into the peroxidation time course. However, this behaviour was not observed for tamoxifen or for 4-hydroxytamoxifen, 3-hydroxytamoxifen or 17β-oestradiol in either the microsomal or liposomal systems, even though 4-hydroxytamoxifen, 3-hydroxytamoxifen and 17β-oestradiol each possess a potentially donatable hydrogen atom (Wiseman *et al.*, 1990b, 1992b; Wiseman and Halliwell, 1993). Tamoxifen and 17β-oestradiol are highly lipophilic and would be expected to partition mostly into the membrane, with the cyclopentano, moiety of 17β-oestradiol (and the portion of tamoxifen that mimics this) being inserted into the lipid. These hydrophobic groups will be associated with the phospholipid fatty acid side-chains whilst the hydrophilic hydroxyl group of 17β-oestradiol (and 4-hydroxytamoxifen) will be orientated towards the aqueous phase.

The demonstration that tamoxifen and 17β-oestradiol structurally mimic cholesterol, as indicated by the computer molecular modelling results and by the cholesterol coefficient values (Wiseman *et al.*, 1992a) suggests that these molecules might mimic also the natural membrane-stabilising actions of cholesterol itself, observed as inhibition of lipid peroxidation (Wiseman *et al.*, 1990a). Cholesterol is proposed to act in this way via interaction between its hydrophobic rings and the saturated, monosaturated and polyunsaturated residues of phospholipid fatty acids. Additional evidence that the tamoxifen molecule is potentially able to adopt the C-ring configuration of the steroid nucleus has been provided by identification of products of UV irradiation of tamoxifen: the formation of a phenanthrene derivative of tamoxifen possessing this C-ring has been reported (Wilson and Reunitz, 1993).

Direct evidence exists for the ability of tamoxifen and also 17β-oestradiol to decrease membrane fluidity in human breast cancer cells (Clarke *et al.*, 1990a). Pharmacologically relevant concentrations of 17β-oestradiol, which has a similar efficacy as a structural antioxidant in membranes to that of 4-hydroxytamoxifen, decreased the membrane fluidity and also inhibited the growth of both the oestrogen receptor-positive MCF-7 breast cancer cell line and also the oestrogen receptor-negative cell line MDA-MB-436 (Clarke *et al.*, 1990a). Furthermore, tamoxifen, *cis*-tamoxifen, 4-hydroxytamoxifen, 17β-oestradiol and cholesterol have been found to decrease membrane fluidity in ox brain phospholipid liposomes, and a good positive correlation was demonstrated between decreased membrane fluidity and antioxidant ability (Wiseman *et al.*, 1993d; Wiseman, 1994a, 1994b, 1994c). The mechanism of the antioxidant action of tamoxifen and related compounds that share a structural similarity with cholesterol may, therefore, be by stabilisation of the membrane against lipid peroxidation through a decrease in membrane fluidity. The membrane antioxidant action of vitamin D may also be through this mechanism (Wiseman, 1993). It is also of interest that tamoxifen and cholesterol have been reported to decrease membrane permeability in ox brain phospholipid liposomes to a similar extent (Kayyali *et al.*, 1994) and this action may also arise from a decrease in membrane fluidity in the presence of these compounds.

MEMBRANE-MODULATING ACTION: ROLE IN ANTICANCER ACTION

Tamoxifen can decrease membrane fluidity in human breast cancer cells (Clarke *et al.*, 1990a) and membrane models (Wiseman *et al.*, 1993d), and this membrane-modulating ability may play an important role in its anticancer action. Plasma membranes from Morris hepatoma cells have a higher cholesterol/phospholipid ratio (Galeotti *et al.*, 1984), and microsomal membranes of Novikoff and Yoshida hepatoma cells have low levels of polyunsaturated fatty acids (Cheeseman, 1993) compared with normal cells, which causes a decrease in membrane fluidity. These membrane changes, if associated with cancer cells in general, compared with normal cells could be fortuitous in making their growth more readily inhibited by the membrane-modifying action of tamoxifen than that of normal cells (Wiseman *et al.*, 1993a, 1994a, 1994b). Furthermore, leukaemic cells and metastatic tumour cells have a higher plasma membrane fluidity than non-metastatic cells (Tarboletti *et al.*, 1989); therefore, decreasing the membrane fluidity with tamoxifen may restore contact inhibition between such cells by increasing the rigidity of the cells at cell junction contacts and thus oppose the metastasis of invasive epithelial malignancies of the breast that is aided by the generation of stromelysin 3 in the surrounding stromal cells (Basset *et al.*, 1990; Wolf *et al.*, 1993). Stromelysin 3 belongs to a subgroup of proteinases expressed in breast carcinoma fibroblastic cells and is implicated in tumour progression (Wolf *et al.*, 1993).

The ability of a tumour to grow beyond a certain size (usually a few millimetres in diameter, consisting of about 10^6 cells) requires induction of new capillary blood vessels (angiogenesis) and this has been found for breast cancer to correlate with metastasis and thus invasive breast carcinoma (Weidner *et al.*, 1991). Tamoxifen may, therefore, inhibit both the metastasis of tumour cells into the newly formed circulatory vessels by decreasing the fluidity of their highly fluid membranes, which is required for squeezing through capillaries and, via altered membrane structure, prevent the release of specific angiogenic molecules such as vascular endothelial growth factor from the tumour, which are required for angiogenesis (Weidner *et al.*, 1991; Kim K.J. *et al.*, 1993). This would hinder the process of malignant progression (previously detailed for human breast cancer by Clarke *et al.*, 1990b). In addition, the formation of metastases that could be caused by transfection with membrane-packaged genetic material following death by the apoptosis (programmed cell death) of cancer cells (Benson and Baum, 1993) could be decreased by tamoxifen through its ability to decrease plasma membrane fluidity. The anti-fluidity effect of tamoxifen could also contribute to its anticancer action by inhibiting the action of membrane enzymes, receptors and channels (see below).

MODULATION OF CELL SIGNALLING AND SECOND MESSENGER PATHWAYS: ROLE IN MEMBRANE-MEDIATED ANTICANCER ACTION?

The proposed ability of tamoxifen to inhibit breast cancer cell growth and division through decreased membrane fluidity (Clarke *et al.*, 1990a; Wiseman *et al.*, 1993d; Wiseman, 1994a, 1994b, 1994c) is likely to involve a second messenger system. This conclusion requires detailed consideration to be given to known mechanisms that have been reported to be affected by tamoxifen and other related systems. Adenylate cyclase catalyses the formation of cyclic AMP (cAMP) from ATP in response to hormone and growth regulator binding to cell surface receptors. These ligands send a stimulatory signal to adenylate cyclase via G-proteins (Neer and Clapham, 1988; Hardie, 1991). The activity of adenylate cyclase is known to be very sensitive to membrane fluidity. The activity of mammalian adenylate cyclase activity decreased as membrane fluidity decreased, probably because of restricted mobility of the components of the enzyme complex (Houslay, 1985), and effects of the membrane phospholipid environment on receptor interaction with the adenylate cyclase complex in intact cells have been reported (Jansson *et al.*, 1993). The decreased membrane fluidity, reported in the presence of tamoxifen, is likely to be inhibitory to the action of adenylate cyclase, decreasing cellular cAMP levels, which is inhibitory to the growth of some tumour cells (Dumont *et al.*, 1989). In addition, there is a known inhibition by tamoxifen of calcium calmodulin-dependent cAMP phosphodiesterase (see Chapter 7), which may be as a result of the membrane-modulating action of tamoxifen, and could result in high cAMP levels; this may be inhibitory to growth in certain cancer cells (Dumont *et al.*, 1989), in contrast to the effect discussed above.

It is possible that tamoxifen inhibits the formation of the second messengers of the phosphoinositide system. In mammalian tumour cells decreased membrane fluidity in the presence of tamoxifen could prevent the receptor-mediated hydrolysis of membrane-bound PIP_2 by polyphosphoinositide phosphodiesterase (a phospholipase C) to yield the intracellular signals inositol 1,4,5-triphosphate (IP_3) and diacylglycerol (DAG). Indeed this could contribute to the previously proposed inhibitory effects of tamoxifen on protein kinase C (see Chapter 7), which is activated directly by DAG as well as by tumour-promoting phorbol esters (DAG mimics) such as 12-*O*-tetradecanoylphorbol 13-acetate (TPA). This suggestion could also apply to other calcium effector systems such as calcium calmodulin-dependent cAMP phosphodiesterase (see above), because IP_3 releases calcium ions from endoplasmic reticulum that activate this enzyme, in addition to activating the protein kinase C.

Phosphomonoester (PME) is associated with proliferation in human breast cancer; in a ^{31}P magnetic resonance spectroscopy study tamoxifen caused changes in the PME/ATP ratio in two breast cancer tumours where tamoxifen had stabilised the disease, and the PME peak consisted predominantly of phosphoethanolamine, with a smaller contribution from phosphocholine (Kalra *et al.*, 1993). The regulation of phospholipid turnover by tamoxifen has been studied in human breast cancer cells: tamoxifen (10^{-6} M) treatment led to an increase of ^{32}P incorporation into phosphoinositides and a decrease of ^{32}P incorporation into phosphatidylcholine (Krasil'nikov *et al.*, 1993). Addition of TPA weakened the inhibitory effect of tamoxifen on phosphatidylcholine turnover and this suggests that the action of tamoxifen can be mediated through an alteration of the growth signal-transducing system (Krasil'nikov *et al.*, 1993). Protein kinase C is a calcium- and phospholipid-dependent enzyme that mediates the transmembrane signalling of a wide range of extracellular stimuli, including growth factors, hormones and other biologically active substances, resulting in the phosphorylation of various cellular proteins believed to be involved in proliferative control (see Chapter 7).

It is of interest, therefore, that membrane-modulation by oxysterols may modify the activity of protein kinase C (Moos *et al.*, 1991). Inhibition of protein kinase C may also be by mechanisms relating to decreased membrane fluidity in the presence of tamoxifen and conformational change in membrane proteins, discussed above for calcium calmodulin-dependent cAMP phosphodiesterase. This is confirmed in part by a proposed model for DAG and TPA binding to protein kinase C, which illustrates the importance of this enzyme being able to undergo conformational change. In outline, each activator is hydrogen-bonded to sulphydryl groups of cysteine residues, and to the carbonyl of an asparagine within the cysteine-rich regions of protein kinase C, thereby inducing a conformational change leading to the disruption of the association between the inhibitory pseudosubstrate sequence and the active centre of protein kinase C (Gschwendt *et al.*, 1991).

Lipid peroxidation in rat liver microsomes has been reported to be inhibited by the tumour promoter phorbol-12-myristate-13-acetate (PMA) and it has been proposed that protein kinase C, when activated by PMA (or other activators) could stimulate cell proliferation (as it is known to in most but not all cell types) by preventing the accumulation of the products of lipid peroxidation (Baldenkov *et al.*, 1988), which can be toxic to dividing cells (Burdon *et al.*, 1989, 1990; Burton and Rice-Evans, 1989). In contrast,

PMA, increased lipid peroxidation and cell damage in cultured hepatocytes (Von Ruecker *et al.*, 1989) and indeed TPA have also been reported to induce oxidative stress (Duran and Dereny, 1991). It is of interest, therefore, that TPA can also act as an inducer for the NAD(P)H:quinone reductase gene through the antioxidant responsive element (ARE) in the 5′-flanking region of this gene: this element is responsible for the basal level of expression of the gene in addition to transcriptional activation by phenolic antioxidants and metabolisable planar aromatic compounds (Favreau and Pickett, 1993). The oxidants hydrogen peroxide and linoleic acid hydroperoxide modulated protein kinase C activity and increased DAG levels in endothelial cells: hydrogen peroxide caused an increase in membrane-associated protein kinase C activity but also caused partial loss of cytosolic protein kinase C activity (Taher *et al.*, 1993).

It is of related interest that oxygen radicals have been suggested to be second messengers in systems such as the expression of the monocyte chemoattractant protein JE/MCP-1 and the monocyte colony-stimulating factor CSF-1 in response to tumour necrosis factor α, and the enzyme NADPH-dependent oxidase may be involved (Satriano *et al.*, 1993). Furthermore, the effect of oxidative stress on receptors and signal transmission has been considered (Vandervliet and Bass, 1992); for example, oxidative stress has been reported to induce a human gene encoding a protein tyrosine phosphatase: the level of protein tyrosine phosphorylation is involved in cell cycle control and regulation of cellular proliferation (Keyse and Emslie, 1992). This gene may therefore play an important role in regulating the human cellular response to environmental stress.

ANTIOXIDANT-MEDIATED ANTICARCINOGENIC POTENTIAL

DNA damage mediated by the hydroxyl radical has been reported in the DNA of invasive ductal carcinoma (IDC) of the female breast and is likely to be involved in malignant transformation (Malins and Haimanot, 1991; Malins *et al.*, 1993). In one study DNA from IDC showed a nine-fold increase in the altered DNA bases 8-hydroxyguanine, 8-hydroxyadenine and 2,6-diamino-4-hydroxy-5-formamidopyrimidine compared to the control value (Malins and Haimanot, 1991), and a large increase in the carcinogenic hydroxy adducts (e.g., 8-hydroxyguanine) was also observed in another study on DNA from IDC (Malins *et al.*, 1993). Free radical-mediated damage is also implicated in inflammatory breast cancer (Jaiyesimi *et al.*, 1992) and the role of macrophages in human breast cancer has also been considered (Vanetten *et al.*, 1992). Tamoxifen has been reported to suppress the production of hydrogen peroxide by human neutrophils (Lim *et al.*, 1992; Wei and Frenkel, 1993; Troll *et al.*, 1994): hydrogen peroxide is capable of malignant transformation of cells and tumour promotion, and it can also react with transition metal ions that are in close proximity with nuclear DNA to produce the hydroxyl radical. Tamoxifen could, therefore, act as an anticarcinogenic agent by suppressing hydrogen peroxide production by neutrophils, thus preventing hydroxyl radical-mediated DNA damage. It is of related interest that hydrogen peroxide and superoxide at low concentrations are important growth regulators in addition to the established cell growth signal transduction pathways (see above) in HeLa cancer cells (Burdon and Gill, 1993). Furthermore, dose-dependent induction of DNA single-strand breaks by hydrogen peroxide paralleled growth inhibition of the MCF-7 breast cancer cell line (see Chapter 5) and the MCF-10A line of immortalised but not transformed human breast epithelial cells (Djuric *et al.*, 1993).

Lipid peroxidation has been suggested to have a role in breast cancer risk: urinary excretion of the mutagen malonaldehyde was found to be approximately double in women with mammographic dysplasia (high risk) than in women without these radiological changes (Boyd and McGuire, 1991). Furthermore, the likely contribution of genotoxic carcinogens to human breast cancer has been discussed (Biggs *et al.*, 1993) and a currently favoured model for the carcinogenic action of both the oxygen free radicals and the lipid hydroperoxides arising from lipid peroxidation involves alterations in membrane processes and cellular signals, which lead to DNA damage by an oxidative genotoxic mechanism (Vaca *et al.*, 1988; Goldstein and Witz, 1990; Cheeseman, 1993; Ames *et al.*, 1993). Tamoxifen may also play an an anticarcinogenic role by inhibiting the formation of the reactive intermediates and products arising from lipid peroxidation in the nuclear membrane (Wiseman and Halliwell, 1994) that could damage nuclear DNA. Indeed, tamoxifen has been reported to decrease plasma lipid peroxide levels in breast cancer patients (Thangaraju *et al.*, 1993) and this action of tamoxifen should be investigated further in women treated prophylactically with tamoxifen (see Chapter 4). This anticarcinogenic action of tamoxifen could therefore contribute to its ability to prevent breast cancer (Wiseman *et al.*, 1994).

REVERSAL OF MULTIDRUG RESISTANCE

The failure of chemotherapy is a significant problem in cancer treatment with cytotoxic chemotherapeutic drugs. It has been observed that some tumours that initially show sensitivity to a particular chemotherapeutic regime become resistant to the same or different anticancer drugs. This resistance not only to a particular cytotoxic drug but also to a wide range of other drugs used in cancer chemotherapy is referred to as multidrug resistance (MDR; Pasman and Schouten, 1993). Tumours that are insensitive to initial therapy are considered to be intrinsically resistant. An MDR phenotype can result from the over-production in resistant cells of a transmembrane P-170 glycoprotein. This protein appears to cause MDR through an ATP-dependent drug efflux mechanism, which enables it to pump out of the cell molecules such as the cytotoxic anthracyclines (e.g., Adriamycin, which is also referred to as doxorubicin) and the vinca alkaloids (e.g. vinblastine). This prevents the accumulation of drugs to an effective cytotoxic concentration. In humans the *mdr-1* gene encodes the p-170 glycoprotein, and determining the extent of expression of this gene has important implications for the use of resistance modifiers in clinical trials (Twentyman, 1992). A study of the presence of P-170 glycoprotein in haematological malignancies showed that at diagnosis 14–62% of all patients showed P-170 glycoprotein expression, whereas 29–62% of previously treated patients were positive for P-170 glycoprotein: this slight increase in the frequency of P-170 glycoprotein in previously treated patients may be as a result of early mutation and selection by the cytotoxic drug, and chemotherapy itself could induce expression of the P-170 glycoprotein pump, (Pasman and Schouten, 1993). The reversal of P-170 glycoprotein-associated MDR is therefore a challenge that has attracted considerable interest (see reviews by Lehnert, 1993, and Pearson and Cunningham, 1993). However, MDR is likely to be due to other factors in addition to P-170 glycoprotein-mediated resistance and indeed P-170 glycoprotein is expressed by a wide range of normal non-cancerous cells (Pearson and Cunningham, 1993).

Pharmacological agents including tamoxifen, have been identified that antagonise the action of the P-170 glycoprotein pump. Reversal by tamoxifen of P-170 glycoprotein induced MDR in human and murine leukaemic cells (Berman *et al.*, 1991) and P-170 glycoprotein-expressing cell lines (Stuart *et al.*, 1992); also vinblastine resistance in multidrug-resistant cell lines (Kirk *et al.*, 1993) may be related to the reported ability of tamoxifen to decrease membrane fluidity in human cancer cells (Clarke *et al.*, 1990a) and model membranes (Wiseman *et al.*, 1993d). Decreased membrane fluidity in the presence of tamoxifen could directly inhibit P-170 glycoprotein function possibly by altering its conformation (Wiseman 1994a, 1994b, 1994c; Leonessa *et al.*, 1994). Furthermore, tamoxifen has been reported to decrease drug efflux from liposomes, and inhibition of a similar basal mechanism for drug removal in cancer cells may contribute to its anti-MDR action (Kayyali *et al.*, 1994). Membrane-mediated anti-MDR activity is another mechanism of action in addition to antioxidant ability displayed by both tamoxifen and antifungal azoles, as itraconazole, which is used in the prevention of fungal infections in immunocompromised cancer patients has been shown to reverse daunorubicin resistance in murine leukaemic cells (Gupta *et al.*, 1991), and ketoconazole has been found to have a similar membrane antioxidant ability to tamoxifen (see Chapter 9). Another anti-MDR drug, verapamil, is thought to compete with cytotoxic drugs as a P-170 glycoprotein substrate, while cyclosporin A has been suggested to interact with calmodulin and/or cause perturbations of the cell membrane (Pearson and Cunningham, 1993).

Clinical effects of tamoxifen as an enhancer of etoposide cytotoxicity have been reported (Stuart *et al.*, 1992; Millward *et al.*, 1994). Tamoxifen has also been used in combination with vinblastine as a MDR reversal agent in phase I clinical trials (Trump *et al.*, 1992). Furthermore, tamoxifen increased the cytotoxic effects of Adriamycin and vinblastine, and increased vinblastine accumulation in MCF-7 human breast cancer cells (Leonessa *et al.*, 1994). Tamoxifen in combination with recombinant human interferon-α (see Chapter 6) has been reported to modulate doxorubicin resistance (Kang and Perry, 1993), and differential effects of tamoxifen and the pure oestrogen antagonist ICI 182 780 (see Chapter 10) in human drug-resistant leukaemia cell lines have been reported (Zalebergy *et al.*, 1993). Combinations of epirubicin with verapamil and/or tamoxifen have also been investigated in cell cultures (Czejka *et al.*, 1993). In addition, increased chemosensitivity to doxorubicin in intrinsically multidrug-resistant human colon carcinoma cells has been achieved by prolonged exposure to verapamil (Toffoli *et al.*, 1993). Furthermore, tamoxifen or verapamil has been shown to enhance the growth inhibition by doxorubicin of an ovarian cell line that expresses the P-glycoprotein (Wasserman *et al.*, 1992). It is of interest that tamoxifen is starting to be used in the treatment of human hepatocellular carcinoma (HCC; see Chapter 4), because HCC does not respond to chemotherapy: one of the main mechanisms for the drug resistance in HCC is an elevated expression of the *mdr-1* gene, and the combined use of tamoxifen and cyclosporin A (but not verapamil) showed significant synergism on the sensitivity of both high and low *mdr-1* expressor HCC cell lines to doxorubicin (Kim J.H. *et al.*, 1993).

IMPORTANCE OF ANTIOXIDANT ACTION OF TAMOXIFEN TO ITS CARDIOPROTECTIVE ACTION

Cardiovascular benefits have been reported in clinical studies on the treatment of breast cancer with tamoxifen: the incidence of fatal myocardial infarction was significantly less in the tamoxifen-treated group (McDonald and Stewart, 1991; see Chapter 4). Furthermore, tamoxifen lowers serum cholesterol levels significantly and favourably affects lipid and lipoprotein profiles (Love, 1992; Thangaraju, *et al.*, 1994). Some of the beneficial cardiovascular effects of tamoxifen may be related to its antioxidant ability, as tamoxifen protects rat cardiac membranes against the damage caused by lipid peroxidation (Wiseman *et al.*, 1993b; Wiseman, 1994a): the role of lipid peroxidation in cardiovascular injury (Kukreja and Hess, 1992) and the development of atherosclerosis (Regenstrom *et al.*, 1992) is well

Table 8.3. IC_{50} values for inhibition of copper-dependent LDL lipid peroxidation by tamoxifen, 4-hydroxytamoxifen and 17β-oestradiol. Values are deduced from the graphs shown in Figure 8.7 which show the inhibition of copper-dependent LDL peroxidation, measured as TBARS, by the compounds and in which each point represents the mean ±S.D. of three separate assays.

Compound	IC_{50} (μM)
Tamoxifen	29.3
4-Hydroxytamoxifen	1.9
17β-Oestradiol	3.1

From Wiseman *et al.*, 1993c, with permission.

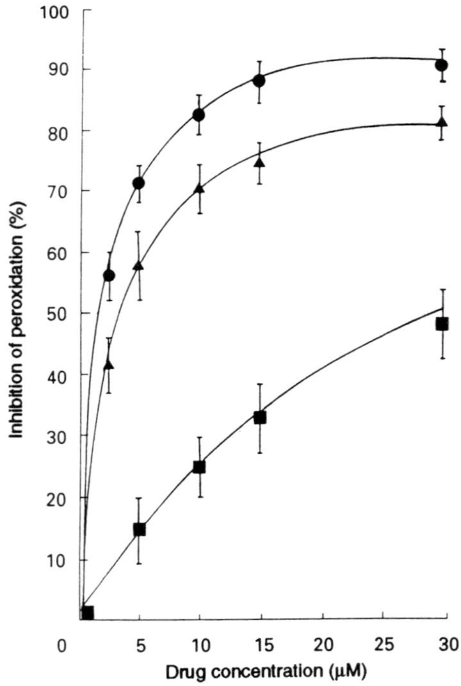

Figure 8.7. Concentration-dependent inhibition of $CuCl_2$-dependent LDL peroxidation (measured as TBARS). LDL (0.2 mg/ml) at pH 7.4 was incubated at 37°C with 15 μM $CuCl_2$ for 2 h and peroxidation was measured using the TBA assay. The results are expressed as percentage inhibition of peroxidation in the presence of tamoxifen (■), 4-hydroxytamoxifen (•) or 17β-oestradiol (▲) all in the range 0–30 μM. Results are means ±SD, $n = 3$. From Wiseman *et al.*, 1993c, with permission

documented. It is of related interest that the antioxidant antifungal agent ketoconazole (see Chapter 9) has been reported to have an effect on cholesterol precursors and LDL kinetics in hypercholesetrolaemia (Gyling *et al.*, 1993). Oxidative damage to LDL plays an important role in the development of atherosclerosis (see above) and it is of some interest that fragmentation of DNA in macrophages exposed to oxidised LDL has been observed (Reid *et al.*, 1993). Tamoxifen can protect human LDL against copper ion-dependent lipid peroxidation (4-hydroxytamoxifen was even more effective; see Table 8.3) and these highly lipophilic compounds are likely to accumulate in the atheromal plaques in damaged arterial wall to achieve the protective concentrations reported (see Figures 8.7 and 8.8) (Wiseman *et al.*, 1993c). Therefore, some of the cardiovascular benefits of tamoxifen therapy may be associated with this antioxidant protection of LDL. Furthermore, the prophylactic use of tamoxifen to prevent breast cancer might thus additionally provide long-term cardiovascular benefits (Wiseman *et al.*, 1994; Wiseman, 1994d). It is known that 17β-oestradiol also protects LDL against oxidative damage (Huber *et al.*, 1990; Rifici and Khachadurian, 1992) and is superior to the antiatherogenic antioxidant

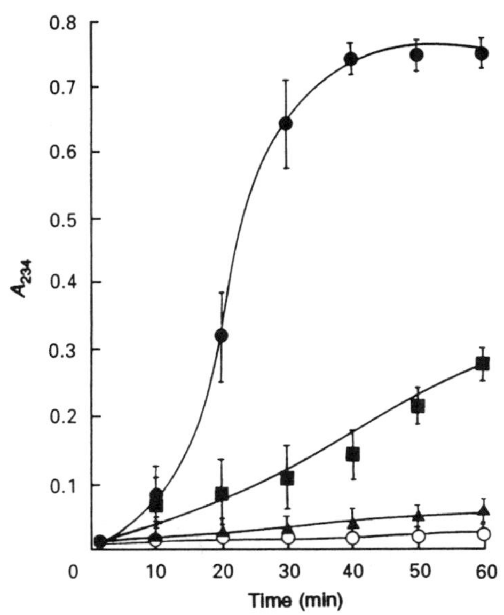

Figure 8.8. Time course of $CuCl_2$-induced conjugated-diene formation. Conjugated-diene formation in LDL (0.1 mg/ml) at pH 7.4, incubated at 37°C with 15 μM $CuCl_2$ for 1 h, was measured by difference spectroscopy and is expressed as A_{234} in the control (containing 0.5% (v/v) ethanol) (•) or in the presence of tamoxifen (■), 4-hydroxytamoxifen (○) or 17β-oestradiol (▲), all at a concentration of 15 μM. Results are means ±SD, $n = 3$. From Wiseman *et al.*, 1993c, with permission

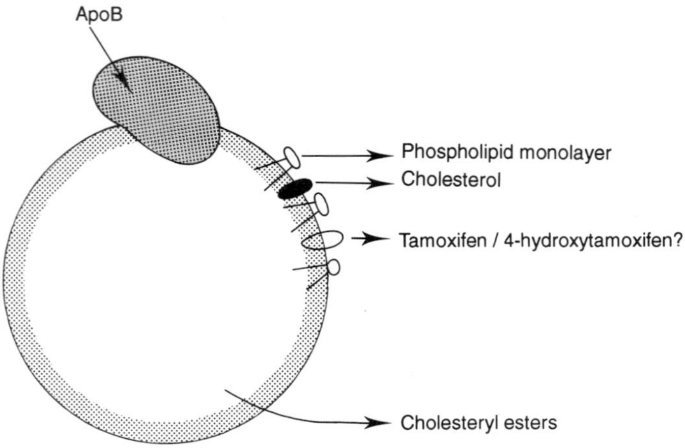

Figure 8.9. A simplified representation of the structure of LDL and the interaction of tamoxifen with LDL

probucol as an antioxidant in LDL (Huber *et al.*, 1990), but less effective than 4-hydroxytamoxifen: the cardiovascular benefits of hormone replacement therapy in post-menopausal women are well recognised (Stampfer *et al.*, 1991; see Chapter 4). Tamoxifen (and 4-hydroxytamoxifen) may act in a similar way to 17β-oestradiol to stabilise LDL against lipid peroxidation, by interaction between their hydrophobic rings and the polyunsaturated residues of the phospholipid layer of LDL (see Figure 8.9) (Wiseman *et al.*, 1993c; Wiseman, 1994a); this suggestion is supported by the decrease in membrane fluidity, and thus lipid peroxidation, arising from similar interactions in liposomal membranes (Wiseman *et al.*, 1993d).

REFERENCES

Ajit, R., Srivastava, K., Baumann, D., Schonfeld, G. (1993) *European Journal of Biochemistry* **216**, 527–578.

Ames, B.N., Shigenaga, M.K., Hagen, T.M. (1993) *Proceedings of the National Academy of Sciences USA* **90**, 7915–7922.

Arroyo, P.L., Hatch-Pigott, V., Mower, H.F., Cooney, R.V. (1992) *Mutation Research* **281**, 193–202.

Aust, S.D., Chignell, C.F., Bray, T.M., Kalyanaraman, B., Mason, R.P. (1993) *Toxicology and Applied Pharmacology* **120**, 168–178.

Aviram, M. (1993) *Atherosclerosis* **98**, 1–10.

Baldenkov, G.N., Serbinova, R.A., Balkalova, R.A., Tkachuk, V.A., Kagan, V.E., Stoytchem, T.S.S. (1988) *Free Radical Research Communications* **4**, 277–281.

Basset, P., Bellcoq, J.P., Wolf, C., Stoll, I., Hutin, P., Limacher, J.M., Podhajer, O.L., Chenard, M.P., Rio, M.C., Chambon, P. (1990) *Nature* **348**, 699–704.

Battioni, J.P., Fontecave, M., Jaouen, M., Mansuy, D. (1991) *Biochemical and Biophysical Research Communications* **174**, 1103–1108.
Belkner, J., Wiesner, R., Rathman, J., Barnett, J., Sigal, E., Kuhn, H. (1993) *European Journal of Biochemistry* **213** 251–261.
Benson, J.R., Baum, M. (1993) *Lancet* **341**, 1288.
Berman, E., Adams, A., Duigou-Osterndorf, R., Godfrey, L., Clarkson, B., Andreeff, M. (1991) *Blood* **77**, 818–825.
Biggs, P.J., Warren, W., Venitt, S., Stratton, M.R. (1993) *Mutagenesis* **8**, 275–283.
Bisby, R.H. (1990) *Free Radical Research Communications* **8**, 299–306.
Blankson, D.D., Kestin, M., Rifai, N. (1993) *Clinics in Laboratory Medicine* **13**, 463–480.
Bowry, V.W., Ingold, K.U., Stocker, R. (1992) *Biochemical Journal* **288**, 341–344.
Boyd, N.F., McGuire, V. (1991) *Free Radical Biology and Medicine* **10**, 185–190.
Buettner, G.R. (1993) *Archives of Biochemistry and Biophysics* **300**, 535–755.
Burdon, R.H., Gill, V. (1993) *Free Radical Research Communications* **19**, 203–213.
Burdon, R.H., Rice-Evans C. (1989) *Free Radical Research Communications* **6**, 345–358.
Burdon, R.H., Gill, V., Rice-Evans C. (1989) *Free Radical Research Communications* **7**, 149–159.
Burdon, R.H., Gill, V., Rice-Evans C. (1990) *Free Radical Research Communications* **11**, 65–76.
Burns, C.P., Spector, A.A. (1994) *Journal of Nutritional Biochemistry* **5**, 114–123.
Cabrini, L., Pasquali, P., Tadolini, B., Sechi, A.M., Landi, L. (1986) *Free Radical Research Communications* **2**, 85–92.
Cheeseman, K.H. (1993) In *DNA and Free Radicals* (eds B. Halliwell, O.I. Aruoma), Ellis Horwood, Chichester, pp. 109–144.
Chen, H., Pellet, L.J., Andersen, H.J., Tappel, A.L. (1993) *Free Radical Biology and Medicine* **14**, 473–482.
Chung, F.L., Chen, H.J.C., Guttenplan, J.B., Nishikawa, A., Hard, G.C. (1993) *Carcinogenesis* **14**, 2073–2078.
Clarke, R., Vanden Berg, H.W., Murphy, R.F. (1990a) *Journal of the National Cancer Institute* **82**, 1702–1705.
Clarke, R., Dickson, R.B., Brunner, N. (1990b) *Annals of Oncology* **1**, 401–407.
Colston, K.W., Chander, S.K., Mackay, A.G., Coombes, R.C. (1992a) *Biochemical Pharmacology* **44**, 693–702.
Colston, K.W. Mackay, A.G., James, S.Y., Binderup, L., Chander, S.K., Coombes, R.C. (1992b) *Biochemical Pharmacology* **44**, 2273–2280.
Czejka, M.J., Schenk, T., Scheithauer, W. (1993) *Pharmazie* **48**, 124–129.
Darley-Usmar, V.M., Hogg, N., O'Leary, V.J., Wilson, M.T., Moncada, S. (1992) *Free Radical Research Communications* **17**, 9–20.
De Groot, H., Hegi, U., Sies, H. (1993) *Federation of European Biochemical Societies Letters* **315**, 139–142.
Devaux, P.F. (1991) *Biochemistry* **30**, 1163–1172.
Devaux, P.F. (1993) *Current Opinions in Structural Biology* **3**, 489–494.
Djuric, Z., Everett, C.K., Luongo, D.A. (1993) *Free Radical Biology and Medicine* **14**, 541–547.
Draper, H.H., Squires, E.J., Mahmoodi, H., Wu, J., Agarwal, S., Hadley, M. (1993) *Free Radical Biology and Medicine* **15**, 353–364.
Dumont, J.E, Jauniaux, J.C., Roger P.P. (1989) *Trends in Biochemical Sciences* **14**, 61–71.
Duran, H.A., Dereny, B.M. (1991) *Carcinogenesis* **12**, 2047–2052.
Esterbauer, H., Gebicki, J., Puhl, H., Jurgens, G. (1992) *Free Radical Biology and Medicine* **13**, 341–390.

Favreau, L.V., Pickett, C.B. (1993) *Journal of Biological Chemistry* **268**, 19875–19881.
Fiorentini, D., Cabrini, L., Landi, L. (1993) *Free Radical Research Communications* **18**, 201–219.
Frei, B., Kim, M.C., Ames, B.N. (1990) *Proceedings of the National Academy of Sciences USA* **87**, 4879–4883.
Fruebis, J., Parthasarathy, S., Steinberg, D. (1992) *Proceedings of the National Academy of Sciences USA* **89**, 10588–10622.
Fujii, T., Hiramoto, Y., Terao, J., Fukuzawa, K. (1991) *Archives of Biochemistry and Biophysics* **284**, 120–126.
Galeotti, T. Borrello, S., Palombini, G., Masotti, L., Ferrari, M.B., Cavatorta, P., Arcioni, A., Stremmenos, C., Zannoni, C. (1984) *Federation of European Biochemical Societies Letters* **164**, 169–173.
Gebicki, S., Gebicki, J.M. (1993) *Biochemical Journal* **289**, 743–766.
Gey, K.F. (1993) *British Medical Bulletin* **49**, 679–699.
Glaser, M. (1993) *Current Opinions in Structural Biology* **3**, 475–481.
Goldring, C.E.P., Rice-Evans, C.A., Burdon, R.H., Rao, R., Haq, I., Diplock, A.T. (1993) *Archives of Biochemistry and Biophysics* **303**, 429–435.
Goldstein, B.D., Witz, G. (1990) *Free Radical Research Communications* **11**, 3–10.
Greenlay, T.L., Davies, M.J. (1992) *Biochimica et Biophysica Acta* **1116**, 192–203.
Gschwent, M., Kittstein, W., Marks, F. (1991) *Trends in Biochemical Sciences* **16**, 167–169.
Gupta, S., Kim, J., Gollapudi, S. (1991) *Journal of Clinical Investigation* **87**, 1467–1469.
Gurr, M.I., Harwood, J.L. (1991) *Lipid Biochemistry* 4th edn, Chapman & Hall, London.
Gutteridge, J.M.C. (1978) *Research Communications in Chemical Pathology and Pharmacology* **22**, 563–572.
Gutteridge, J.M.C. (1993) *Free Radical Research Communications* **19**, 141–158.
Gutteridge, J.M.C., Halliwell, B. (1990) *Trends in Biochemical Sciences* **15**, 129–135.
Guyton, K.Z., Kensler, T.W. (1993) *British Medical Bulletin* **49**, 523–544.
Gyling, H., VanHanen, H., Miettnen, T.A. (1993) *Journal of Lipid Research* **34**, 59–68.
Halliwell, B. (1990) *Free Radical Research Communications* **9**, 1–32.
Halliwell, B., (1993) *Current Opinion in Lipidology* **4**, 382–384.
Halliwell, B., Chirico, S. (1993) *American Journal of Clinical Nutrition* **57**, 15S–25S.
Halliwell, B., Gutteridge, J.M.C. (1989) *Free Radicals in Biology and Medicine* 2nd edn, Oxford University Press, Oxford.
Halliwell, B., Gutteridge, J.M.C. (1990) *Archives of Biochemistry and Biophysics* **280**, 1–8.
Halliwell, B., Gutteridge, J.M.C., Cross, C.E. (1992) *Journal of Laboratory and Clinical Medicine* **119**, 598–620.
Hardie, D.G. (1991) *Biochemical Messengers, Hormones Neurotransmitters, and Growth Factors,* Chapman & Hall, London.
Hiramatsu, M., Velaso, R.D., Packer, L. (1990) *Free Radical Biology and Medicine* **9**, 459–464.
Hiramatsu, M., Velaso, R.D., Wilson, D.S., Packer, L. (1991) *Research Communications in Chemical Pathology and Pharmacology* **72**, 231–242.
Hogg, N., Darley-Usmar, V.M., Wilson, M.T., Moncada, S. (1993) *Federation of European Biochemical Societies Letters* **326**, 199–203.
Houslay, M.D. (1985) *Proceedings of the Nutrition Society* **44**, 157–165.
Huber, L.A., Scheffler, E., Poll, T., Ziegler, R., Dressel, H.A. (1990) *Free Radical Research Communications* **8**, 167–173.

Jain, S., Thomas, M., Kumar, G.P., Laloraya, M. (1993) *Biochemical and Biophysical Research Communications* **195**, 574–580.

Jaiyesimi, I.A., Buzdar, A.U., Hortobagyi, G. (1992) *Journal of Clinical Oncology* **10**, 1014–1024.

Jansson, C., Harmala, A.S., Torvola, D.M., Slotte, J.P. (1993) *Biochimica et Biophysica Acta* **1145**, 311–319.

Johnson, D.A., Valenzuela, C.F., Zidovetzki, R. (1992) *Biochemical Pharmacology* **44**, 769–774.

Jones, G.R., Cossins, A.R. (1992) In *Liposomes: A Practical Approach* (ed. R.R.C. New), IRL Press, Oxford, pp. 183–220.

Kagan, V.E., Serbinova, E.A., Packer, L. (1990a) *Archives of Biochemistry and Biophysics* **282**, 221–225.

Kagan, V.E., Serbinova, E.A., Bakalova, R.A., Stoytchev, T.S., Ernin, A.N., Priliko, L.L., Evstigneeva, R.P. (1990b) *Biochemical Pharmacology* **40**, 2403–2413.

Kagan, V., Serbinova, E., Packer, L. (1990c) *Biochemical and Biophysical Research Communications* **3**, 851–857.

Kagan, V.E., Serbinova, E.A., Forte, T., Scita, G., Packer, L. (1992) *Journal of Lipid Research* **33**, 385–398.

Kalra, R., Wade, K.E., Hands, L., Styles, P., Camplejohn, R., Greenall, M., Adans, G.E., Harris, A.L., Radda, G.K. (1993) *British Journal of Cancer* **67**, 1145–1153.

Kang, Y., Perry, R.R. (1993) *Cancer Research* **53**, 3040–3045.

Kayyali, R., Marriott, C., Wiseman. H. (1994) *Federation of European Biochemical Societies Letters* **344**, 221–224.

Keyse, S.M., Emslie, E.A. (1992) *Nature* **359**, 644–647.

Kim, J.H., Chung, J.B., Park, I.S., Kim, B.S., Yoo, N.C. Choi, J.H., Roh, J.K., Kim, H.S., Kwon, O.H., Lee, K.S. (1993) *Yonsei Medical Journal* **34**, 35–44.

Kim, K.J., Bing, L., Winer, J., Armanin, M., Gillett, N., Phillips, H.S., Ferrara, N. (1993) *Nature* **362**, 841–844.

Kinsella, J.E. (1990) *Journal of Parenteral and Enteral Nutrition* **14**, 200–217.

Kirk, J., Houlbrook, S., Stuart, N.S.A., Stratford, I.J., Harris, A.L., Carmichael, J. (1993) *European Journal of Cancer* **29A**, 1152–1156.

Krasil'nikov, M.A., Shatskaya, V.A., Kuzmina, Z.V., Barinov, V.V., Letyagin, V.P., Bassalyk, L.S. (1993) *Acta Endocrinologica* **128**, 543–548.

Krieger, M. (1992) *Trends in Biochemical Sciences* **17**, 141–146.

Kukreja, R.C., Hess, M.L. (1992) *Cardiovascular Research* **26**, 641–655.

Landi, L., Cabrini, L., Fiorentini, D., Stefanelli, C., Pedulli, G.F. (1992) *Chemistry and Physics of Lipids* **61**, 121–130.

Laudicina, D.C., Marnett, L.J. (1990) *Archives of Biochemistry and Biophysics* **278**, 73–80.

Leake, D.S. (1993) *British Heart Journal* **69**, 476–478.

Lehnert, M. (1993) *European Journal of Cancer* **29A**, 636–637.

Lemoyec, L., Tatoud, R., Eugene,, M., Grauville, C., Primot, I., Charlemagne, D., Calvo, F. (1992) *British Journal of Cancer* **66**, 623–628.

Leonessa, F., Jacobson, M., Boyle, B., Lippman, J., McGarvey, M., Clarke, R. (1994) *Cancer Research* **54**, 441–447.

Liebler, D.C. (1993) *Critical Reviews in Toxicology* **23**, 147–169.

Liebler, D.C., Burr, J.A., Matsumoto, S., Matsuo, M. (1993) *Chemical Research in Toxicology* **6**, 351–355.

Lim, J.S., Frenkel, K., Troll, W. (1992) *Cancer Research* **52**, 4969–4972.

Linseman, K.L., Lason, P., Braughler, J.M., McCall, J.M. (1993) *Biochemical Pharmacology* **45**, 1477–1482.

Liscum, L., Dahl, N.K. (1992) *Journal of Lipid Research* **33**, 1239–1254.
Lipowsky, R. (1991) *Nature* **349**, 475–481.
Love, R.R. (1992) In *Introducing New Treatments for Cancer* (ed. C.J. Williams), John Wiley & Sons, Chichester, pp. 341–358.
Lucy, J.L. (1972) *Annals of the New York Academy of Sciences* **203**, 4–11.
Malins, D.C., Haimanot, R. (1991) *Cancer Research* **51**, 5430–5432.
Malins, D.C., Holmes, E.H., Polissar, N.' Gunselman, S.J. (1993) *Cancer*, **71**, 3036–3043.
Mason, R.P. (1993) *Biochemical Pharmacology* **45**, 2173–2184.
Maxwell, S.R. (1993) *Journal of Clinical Pharmacy and Therapeutics* **18**, 85–95.
McCord, J.E. (1993) *Clinical Biochemistry* **26**, 351–357.
McDonald C.C., Stewart, H.J. (1991) *British Medical Journal* **303**, 435–437.
Merati, G., Pasquali, P., Vergani, C., Landi, L. (1992) *Free Radical Research Communication* **15**, 11–18.
Miller, D.M., Aust, S.D. (1989) *Archives of Biochemistry and Biophysics* **271**, 113–119.
Millward, M.J., Lien, E.A., Robinson, A., Cantwell, B.M.J. (1994) *Oncology* **51**, 79–83.
Minotti, G. (1992) *Archives of Biochemistry and Biophysics* **297**, 189–382.
Minotti, G. (1993) *Chemical Research in Toxicology* **6**, 134–146.
Mohr, D., Bowry, V.W., Stocker, R. (1992) *Biochimica et Biophysica Acta* **1126**, 247–254.
Mooradian, A.D. (1993) *Journal of Steroid Biochemistry and Molecular Biology* **45**, 509–511.
Moos, C., Deloulne, J.C., Baudier, J., Revel, M.O., Bischoff, P., Hieth, H., Luu, B. (1991) *Biochemie* **73**, 1321–1326.
Morini, P., Casalino, E., Marcotrigiano, G.O., Landriscina, C. (1990) *Biochimica and Biophysica Acta* **1046**, 207–213.
Neer, E.J., Clapham, D.E. (1988) *Nature* **333**, 129–134.
New, R.R.C. (1992a) In *Liposomes: A Practical Approach* (ed. R.R.C. New), IRL Press, Oxford, pp. 1–32.
New, R.R.C. (1992b) In *Liposomes: A Practical Approach* (ed. R.R.C. New), IRL Press, Oxford, pp. 33–161.
Noguchi, N., Gotoh, N., Niki, E. (1993) *Biochimica et Biophysica Acta* **1168**, 348–357.
Pasman, P.C., Schouten, H.C. (1993) *Netherlands Journal of Medicine* **42**, 218–231.
Pearson, C.K., Cunningham, C. (1993) *Trends in Biotechnology* **11**, 511–516.
Pierrefiche, G., Topall, G., Courboin, G., Henriet, I., Laborit, H. (1993) *Research Communications in Chemical Pathology and Pharmacology* **80**, 211–223.
Pols, H.A.P., Birkenhager, J.C., Van Leewen, J.P.T.M. (1994) *Clinical Endocrinology* **40**, 285–292.
Regenstrom, J., Nilsson, J., Tornvall, P., Landou, C., Hamsten, A. (1992) *Lancet* **339**, 1183–1186.
Reid, V.C., Hardwick, S.J., Mitchinson, M.J. (1993) *Federation of European Biochemical Societies Letters* **332**, 218–220.
Retsky, K.L., Freeman, M.W., Frei, B. (1993) *Journal of Biological Chemistry* **268**, 1304–1309.
Rice-Evans, C., Bruckdorfer, K.R. (1992) *Molecular Aspects of Medicine* **13**, 1–111.
Rice-Evans, C., Burdon, R. (1993) *Progress in Lipid Research* **32**, 71–110.
Rice-Evans, C.A., Diplock, A.T. (1993) *Free Radical Biology and Medicine* **15**, 77–96.
Richter, C. (1993) *Federation of European Biochemical Societies Letters* **325**, 104–107.
Rifici, V.A., Khachadurian, A.K. (1992) *Metabolism* **41**, 1110–1114.
Ross, R. (1993) *Nature* **362**, 801–809.
Roth, M.R., Welt, W. (1991) *Biochimica et Biophysica Acta* **1063**, 242–246.

Routledge, M.N., Wink, D.A., Keefer, L.K., Dipple, A. (1993) *Carcinogenesis* **14**, 1251–1254.
Sankarano, M.B., Thompson, T.E. (1991) *Proceedings of the National Academy of Sciences USA* **88**, 8686–8696.
Satriano, J.A., Shuldiner, M., Hora, K., Xing, Y., Sham, Z., Schlondroff, D. (1993) *Journal of Clinical Investigation* **92**, 1564–1571.
Scheschonka, A., Murphy, M.E., Sies, H. (1990) *Chemico-Biological Interactions* **74**, 233–252.
Schwartz, C.J., Valente, A.J., Sprague, E.A. (1993) *American Journal of Cardiology* **71**, 9B–14B.
Serbinova, E., Kagan, V., Backer, D.H.L. (1991) *Free Radical Biology and Medicine* **10**, 263–276.
Serbinova, E., Ivanova, S., Kirova, A., Kitanova, S., Packer, L., Kagan, V. (1992) *Advances in Experimental Medicine and Biology* **316**, 223–230.
Sevanian, A., Nordenbrand, K., Kim, E., Ernster, L., Hochstein, P. (1990) *Free Radical Biology and Medicine* **8**, 145–152.
Sharma, M.K., Buettner, G.R. (1993) *Free Radical Biology and Medicine* **14**, 649–653.
Smith, D., O'Leary, V.J., Darley-Usmar, V.M. (1993) *Biochemical Pharmacology* **45**, 2195–2202.
Spiteller, G. (1993) *Journal of Lipid Mediators* **7**, 199–222.
Stampfer, M.J., Colditz, G.A., Willett, W.C., Manson, J.E., Rosner, B., Speizer, F.E., Hennekens, C.H. (1991) *New England Journal of Medicine* **325**, 756–762.
Stampfer, M.J., Hennekens, C.H., Manson, J.E., Colditz, G.A., Rosner, B., Willett, W.C. (1993) *New England Journal of Medicine* **328**, 1444–1449.
Steinberg, D., Parthasarathy, S., Carew, T.E., Khoo, J.C., Witzum, J.L. (1989) *New England Journal of Medicine* **320**, 915–924.
Stocker, R., Bowry, V.W., Frei, B. (1991) *Proceedings of the National Academy of Sciences USA* **88**, 1646–1650.
Stuart, N.S.A., Philip, P., Harris, A.L., Tonkin, K., Houlbrook, S., Kirk, J., Lien, E.A., Carmichael, J. (1992) *British Journal of Cancer* **66**, 833–839.
Suarna, C., Hood, R.L., Dean, R.T., Stocker, R. (1993) *Biochimica et Biophysica Acta* **1166**, 163–170.
Sugioka, K., Shimosegawa, Y., Nakano, M. (1987) *Federation of European Biochemical Societies Letters* **210**, 37–39.
Suzuki, Y.J., Tsuchiya, M., Packer, L. (1993) *Free Radical Research Communications* **18**, 115–122.
Taher, M.M., Garcia, J.G., Natarajan, V. (1993) *Archives of Biochemistry and Biophysics* **303**, 260–266.
Tampo, Y., Yonaha, M. (1992) *Free Radical Biology and Medicine* **13**, 115–120.
Tarboletti, G., Perin, L., Bottazzi, B. (1989) *International Journal of Cancer* **44**, 707–713.
Thangaraju, M., Ilanchezian, S., Ezhilarasi, R., Sachdanandam, P. (1993) *Medical Science Research* **21**, 721–723.
Thangaraju, M., Kumar, K., Gandhirajan, R., Sachdanandam, P. (1994) *Cancer* **73**, 659–663.
Toffoli, G., Tumiotto, L., Gigante, M., Dallarche, M.G., Perin, T., Bolocchi, M. (1993) *European Journal of Cancer* **29A**, 1776–1777.
Tomatsu, A., Komura, S., Ohishi, N., Nakanishi, M., Yagi, K. (1993) *Journal of Clinical Biochemistry and Nutrition* **15**, 43–49.
Troll, W., Lim, J.S. Frenkel, K. (1994) In ACS Symposium Series 547, *Food Phytochemicals for Cancer Prevention II, Teas, Spices and Herbs* (eds C.T. Ho, T. Osawa, M.T. Huang, R.T. Rosen) American Chemical Society, Washington D.C., pp. 116–121.

Trump, D.L., Smith, D.C., Ellis, P.G., Rogers, M.P., Schold, S.C., Winer, E.P., Panella, T.J., Jordan, V.C., Fine, R.L. (1992) *Journal of the National Cancer Institute* **84**, 1811–1815.
Twentyman, P.R. (1992) *Journal of the National Cancer Institute* **84**, 1458–1461.
Vaca, C.E., Wilhelm, J., Harms-Ringdahl, M. (1988) *Mutation Research* **195**, 137–149.
Vandervliet, A., Bass, A. (1992) *Chemico-Biological Interactions* **85**, 95–116.
Vanetten, J.P., Ashmead, B.J., Cavers, D., Fletcher, R., Thornton, I.G., Antonsen, B.L., Coy, P., Brigden, M.L. (1992) *British Journal of Cancer* **66**, 220–221.
Vasconcelles, M.J., Weitzman, S.A., Lee, S.A., Prachard, S., Gordon, L.I. (1990) *Free Radical Research Communications* **8**, 185–193.
Von Ruecker, A.A., Han-Jeon, B.E., Wild, M., Bidlingmier, F. (1989) *Biochemical and Biophysical Research Communications* **163**, 836–842.
Washko, P.W., Wang, Y., Levine, M. (1993) *Journal of Biological Chemistry* **268**, 15531–15535.
Wasserman, L., Aviram, R., Levavi, H., Ovadia, J., Shneyuor, Y., Frisch, A., Blau, O., Beery, E., Novogrosky, A., Nordenberg, J. (1992) *European Journal of Cancer* **28**, 22–27.
Wei, H., Frenkel, K. (1993) *Carcinogenesis* **14**, 1195–1201.
Weidner, N., Semple, J.P., Welch, W.R., Folkman, J. (1991) *The New England Journal of Medicine* **324**, 1–8.
White, D., Tyler, J., Lindley, M. (1986) *Computers in Chemistry* **10**, 193–199.
Wilcox, A.L., Marnett, L.J. (1993) *Chemical Research in Toxicology* **6**, 413–416.
Wilson, S., Reunitz, R.C. (1993) *Journal of Pharmaceutical Sciences* **82**, 571–574.
Wiseman, H. (1993) *Federation of European Biochemical Societies Letters* **326**, 285–288.
Wiseman, H. (1994a) *Trends in Pharmacological Sciences* **15**, 83–89.
Wiseman, H. (1994b) *Methods in Enzymology* Volume **234**, Chapter 61, 602–614.
Wiseman, H. (1994c) *Talking Medicine* **5**, 5–9.
Wiseman, H. (1994d) *Lancet* **343**, 598.
Wiseman, H., Halliwell, B. (1993) *Federation of European Biochemical Societies Letters* **332**, 159–163.
Wiseman, H., Halliwell, B. (1994) *Free Radical Biology and Medicine* (in press).
Wiseman, H., Cannon, M., Arnstein, H.R.V., Halliwell, B. (1990a) *Federation of European Biochemical Societies Letters* **274**, 107–110.
Wiseman, H., Laughton, M.J., Cannon, M., Arnstein, H.R.V., Halliwell, B. (1990b) *Federation of European Biochemical Societies Letters* **263**, 192–194.
Wiseman, H., Cannon, M., Arnstein, H.R.V., Barlow, D.J. (1992a) *Biochimica et Biophysica Acta* **1138**, 197–202.
Wiseman, H., Smith, C., Halliwell, B., Cannon, M., Arnstein, H.R.V., Lennard, M.S. (1992b) *Cancer Letters* **66**, 61–68.
Wiseman, H., Cannon, M., Arnstein, H.R.V., Halliwell, B. (1993a) *Biochimica et Biophysica Acta* **1181**, 201–206.
Wiseman, H., Cannon, M., Arnstein, H.R.V., Halliwell, B. (1993b) *Biochemical Pharmacology* **45**, 1851–1855.
Wiseman, H., Paganga, G., Rice-Evans, C., Halliwell, B. (1993c) *Biochemical Journal* **292**, 635–638.
Wiseman, H., Quinn, P., Halliwell, B. (1993d) *Federation of European Biochemical Societies Letters* **330**, 53–56.
Wiseman, H., Rice-Evans, C., Halliwell, B. (1994) *Breast Cancer Research and Treatment* **29**, 307.
Wolf, C., Rouger, N., Lutz, Y., Adida, C. Loriot, M., Bellocq, J.P., Chambon, P., Basset, P. (1993) *Proceedings of the National Academy of Sciences USA* **90**, 1843–1847.

Wolfe, J., Perez, E., Bonanno, M., Chapel, J.P. (1991) *European Biophysics Journal* **19**, 275–281.
Yeagle, P.L. (1991) *Biochemie* **73**, 1303–1310.
Zalebergy, J.R., Hu, X.F., Ching, M., Wakeling, A., Wall, D.M., Marschner, I.C., Deluiso, M. (1993) *Cancer Chemotherapy and Pharmacology* **33**, 123–129.
Zhang, L.X., Cooney, R.V., Bertram, J.S. (1991) *Carcinogenesis* **12**, 2109–2114.
Zhu, B.T., Roy, D., Liehr, J.G. (1993) *Endocrinology* **132**, 577–583.

9

Inhibitory Action of Tamoxifen in a Yeast Tumour Model and the Potential Anti-*Candida* and Antiviral Use of Tamoxifen

INHIBITION OF GROWTH IN THE YEAST TUMOUR MODEL

Control of yeast growth

Yeast systems have the advantage over bacterial systems of possessing virtually all the cellular components of higher eukaryotic cells and, therefore, the same target sites for drug action. Yeast cells also bear some resemblance to tumour cells within the body, because they are able to grow rapidly and semi-anaerobically, in contrast to cultured mammalian cells. The yeast species referred to throughout is *Saccharomyces cerevisiae*, unless stated otherwise. The important role of yeast in cancer research, especially in relation to cell growth has been reviewed (Hartwell, 1992); yeast has many features that make it useful in this connection, including the construction of recombinant forms that contain human genes on known chromosomes. Studies on yeast also have the benefit of enabling the identification of anti-yeast drugs, which may be of clinical use.

S. cerevisiae has spheroid or ovoid cells (diameter approximately 3 μm), which proliferate by forming a single bud-like appendage into which a full complement of daughter chromosomes moves during mitotic division. This bud is then pinched off to yield a smaller daughter cell (Robinow and Johnson, 1991; Herskowitz, 1992). *S. cerevisiae* cells bud at either axial or bipolar sites depending on their cell type, and bud site selection is controlled by at least five genes *bud-1/rsr-1*, *bud-2*, *bud-3*, *bud-4* and *bud-5*.

The Bud-1 protein has a similar sequence to Ras, a small GTP-binding protein; the Bud-2 protein is a GTPase-activating protein (GAP) for the Bud-1 protein and is necessary for proper bud site selection in *S. cerevisiae* (Park *et al.*, 1993). The Bud-2 protein has a similar sequence to the catalytic domain of Ras GAPs. In addition, the Bud-5 protein is similar to Cdc-25, a GDP–GTP exchange factor (see below).

Yeast growth is controlled by the nature and concentration of the carbon source, and the availability of oxygen. The lower rate of glycolysis that occurs in the presence of oxygen is known as the Pasteur effect; conversely, the absence at high glucose concentrations of the enzymes needed for respiration resulting from catabolite (glucose) repression of the synthesis of the respiratory enzymes is known as the Crabtree effect (Ratledge and Evans, 1989). However, in some strains of *S. cerevisiae* the Crabtree effect appears to be not solely mediated by glucose repression: the aerobic fermentation of galactose (a non-repressing carbon source) in galactose-limited continuous cultures gave identical results to that of glucose (Sierkstra *et al.*, 1993). The culture medium must contain all the essential elements for growth in proportions similar to those occurring in the yeast biomass (Ratledge and Evans, 1989). The glycolytic pathway in *S. cerevisiae* is activated by fermentable sugars at several steps, and mutants with deletions of genes coding for enzymes of the upper part of glycolysis have been used to investigate the triggering mechanisms (Boles *et al.*, 1993). The signalling process correlated with temporal changes in the glucose 6-phosphate concentration but not with its absolute levels, and this suggests an adaptational mechanism. Furthermore, effects of glucose concentration in the culture medium on the protein and phosphate concentration of *S. cerevisiae* cells have been reported (Pejin and Razmovski, 1993).

In yeast the GTP form of the Ras protein (see Chapter 6) can directly modulate adenylate cyclase (Manser *et al.*, 1994) and in *S. cerevisiae* addition of glucose to starved cells results in the transient rise in intracellular cAMP that induces a protein phosphorylation cascade: the glucose signal is mediated by the Cdc-25/Ras/adenylate cyclase pathway, where the role of Cdc-25 is to catalyse the GDP–GTP exchange on Ras, and the sequence of Ras–guanyl nucleotide exchange factors is highly conserved from yeasts to mammals (see Chapter 6). Phosphorylation of Cdc-25 in response to glucose results in its partial relocalisation to the cytoplasm, reducing its accessibility to membrane-bound Ras, and thus in its dissociation from Ras (Gross *et al.*, 1992). Furthermore, members of the Ras superfamily of GTP-binding proteins are involved in many cellular functions, including signal transduction and protein transport, and a GTPase-activating protein (GAP of Ypt-6 protein) has been found in *S. cerevisiae* that interacts specifically with the the Ypt-6 protein, a member of the Ypt(yeast)/Rab(mammalian) family of GTP-binding proteins (Strom *et al.*, 1993). Activation of the Ras–adenylate cyclase system *in vitro* by glucose in *S. cerevisiae* mutants lacking glucose-phosphorylating enzymes has been reported (Pardo *et al.*, 1993). These mutants, which are unable to produce the glucose-induced increase of cAMP levels *in vivo*, appear to have an active signal transduction mechanism, therefore, and their lack of response to glucose *in vivo* may arise from the absence of intracellular acidification. Ras is implicated in growth factor-stimulated signalling pathways involving both tyrosine and serine/threonine kinases, and it is of interest that a brain serine/threonine protein kinase, which has a sequence related to that of the yeast protein Ste-20 (implicated in pheromone response pathways) may be a target for the $p21^{ras}$-related proteins Cdc-42 and Rac-1 (Manser *et al.*, 1994).

S. cerevisiae has a limited reproductive capacity, which is measured by the number of times an individual cell divides, and there is evidence that it is the relative levels of a senescence factor and Ras that determines whether a cell ceases to divide and senesces (Jazwinski *et al.*, 1993). Controlled expression of the transforming gene of the Harvey murine sarcoma virus (*v-Ha-ras*) extended the lifespan of *S. cerevisiae* nearly two-fold. The normal homologues of this oncogene, *ras-1* and *ras-2*, are important in the control of cell growth and the cell cycle in yeast, and it appears that the expression of *v-Ha-ras* interferes with this control. It is of interest also that in yeast containing a single *ras* gene in which glycine 19 (equivalent to glycine 12 in mammalian *ras*, although Gs (GTP-binding stimulator of adenylate cylase) rather than Ras couples receptors to adenylate cyclase in mammals) is mutated, normal mitotic division is still possible in rich medium. In *S. cerevisiae* a high concentration of cAMP is an absolute requirement for normal mitotic division, and cAMP exerts its role as a second messenger in yeast by activation of a specific cAMP-sensitive protein kinase, which regulates cell metabolism by phosphorylation of individual proteins (Rose, 1989). In starved yeast, however, a 'yeast equivalent of cancer' occurs in that there is no decrease in cAMP and no cessation of growth, or indeed any switch to meiosis and spore formation (Hardie, 1991). It could be that use of such yeast mutants would be an interesting and informative adaptation of the yeast tumour model that has been used to investigate the action of tamoxifen.

Growth inhibition in yeast

S. cerevisiae has been used to investigate the action of tamoxifen (Wiseman *et al.*, 1994a, 1994b) and other antitumour drugs, such as Adriamycin (Wilkie and Collier, 1987) and methylglyoxal bis(guanylhydrazone) (MGBG: Cheng *et al.*, 1990). MGBG has been shown to possess clinical activity against acute myelocytic leukaemia and in the yeast test system it inhibits the growth of yeast, both on plates and in culture (Cheng *et al.*, 1990). The antiproliferative effects of MGBG on tumours are thus reflected

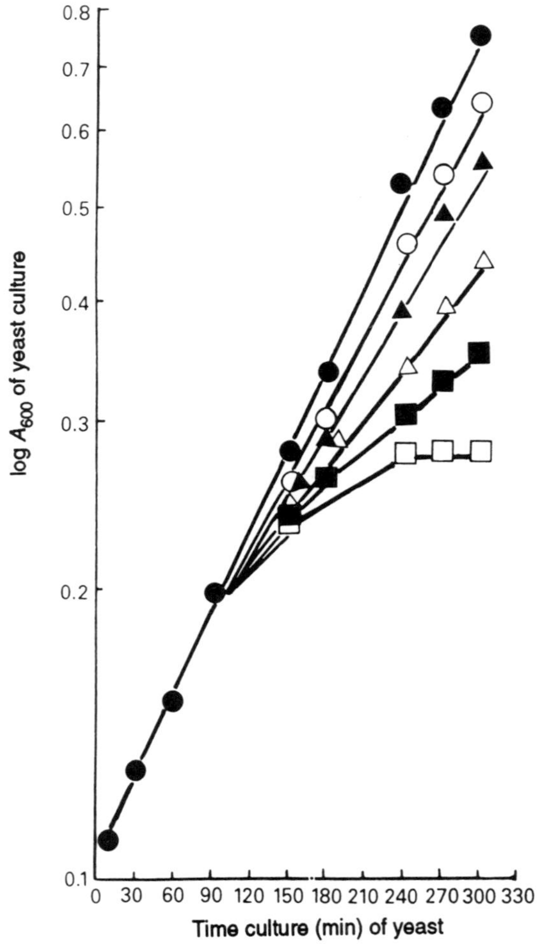

Figure 9.1. Dose dependency of inhibition of growth of Saccharomyces cerevisiae (A224A) by tamoxifen. A224A was grown in YEPD medium at 30°C, and at an A_{600} of 0.2 tamoxifen was added (with or without an equimolar amount of 17β-oestradiol) to give the final drug concentrations 3.75 μM (▲), 7.5 μM (△), 15 μM (■) and 30 μM (□), all with a final concentration of ethanol of 1% (v/v) (a control containing 1% (v/v) ethanol (○) was also included together with an untreated control (●)). The presence of the 17β-oestradiol did not significantly affect the growth inhibition levels due to tamoxifen (these superimposed points are not shown). From Wiseman *et al.*, 1989, with permission

in its inhibition of growth in the yeast system. Anthracyclines such as Adriamycin are widely used in the treatment of acute leukaemia, breast cancer, Hodgkin's disease and sarcomas, and Adriamycin has been shown to inhibit the growth of yeast (Wilkie and Collier, 1987).

Tamoxifen, *cis*-tamoxifen and *N*-desmethyltamoxifen were all found to be potent growth inhibitors of the growth of *S. cerevisiae* (A224A), grown in a glucose-containing medium (see Figure 9.1) (Wiseman *et al.*, 1989, 1990a, 1993a, 1994; Wiseman, 1994a, 1994b). 4-Hydroxytamoxifen, however, had no effect on yeast growth, probably because it is a polar compound and is unable to enter the yeast cell. *cis*-Tamoxifen was of similar effectiveness to tamoxifen, indicating that this effect was not stereospecific. 17β-Oestradiol had no effect on yeast growth or indeed on the inhibition of yeast growth by tamoxifen. This suggests that this yeast tumour model system was probably oestrogen independent. 17β-Oestradiol is, however, a polar compound and, as found for 4-hydroxytamoxifen, may not be able to enter the yeast cell. Nevertheless, it has been reported that 17β-oestradiol was able to reduce the normally extended generation time (due to the unbudded period) of old cells of *S. cerevisiae* back to nearer the normal generation time when grown in glucose-containing but not glycerol-containing media (Motizuki and Tsurugi, 1992). Furthermore, 17β-oestradiol equally elevated the cAMP level of the old cells in either medium up to the level of the young cells but elevated the ATP level of only those in the glucose-containing medium, and it is possible that 17β-oestradiol reduces the unbudded period of the old cells by stimulating energy metabolism through elevation of the cAMP level.

A decrease in the viability of the yeast cells, in addition to inhibition of growth, is a valuable indicator of the cellular toxicity of a drug. Tamoxifen treatment caused a rapid decrease in viability, which was fully established after 1 h (H. Wiseman, unpublished observations). This shows that tamoxifen is highly effective as an anti-yeast agent, and the observation that there was no lag phase prior to the decrease in viability suggests that metabolic activation of tamoxifen is not required (see Chapter 3). A lowered potency of tamoxifen on plates (high minimum inhibitory concentration value on plates) in comparison to liquid culture was observed, and this is a generally observed phenomenon for growth inhibitors, which may relate to differences in the uptake of both nutrients and drug.

Tamoxifen was as effective as the antifungal azoles miconazole and clotrimazole (see Figure 9.2) as an inhibitor of yeast growth (H. Wiseman, unpublished observations). Ketoconazole, however, was a poor inhibitor of yeast growth compared to tamoxifen. It has been reported that ketoconazole at a concentration of 200 μM completely inhibits the growth of *S. cerevisiae* (Kelly *et al.*, 1991), which is in contrast to the maximum concentration of ketoconazole of 30 μM used in the comparative study with tamoxifen (H. Wiseman, unpublished observations). It is of related interest

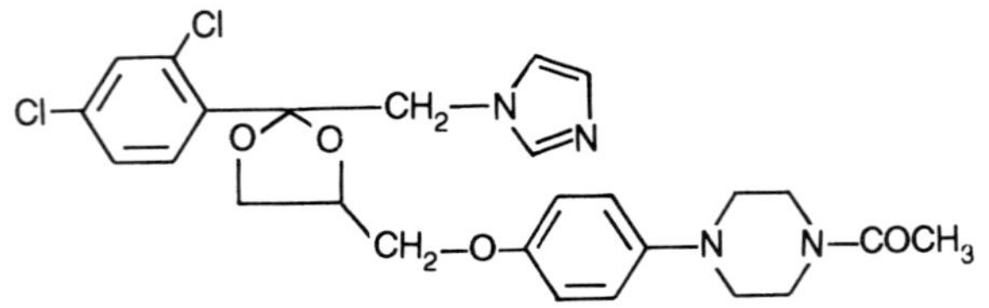

Ketoconazole

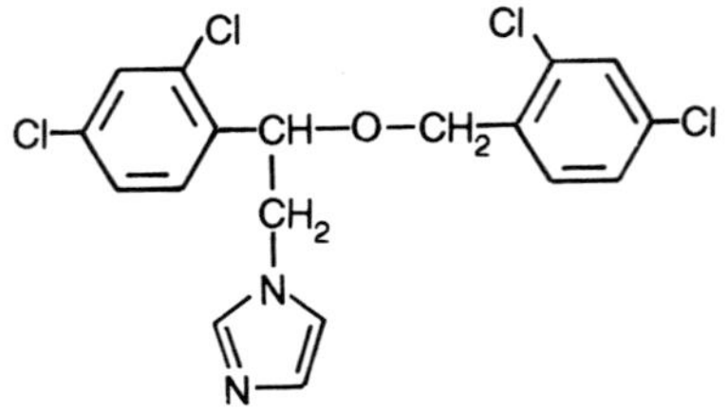

Miconazole

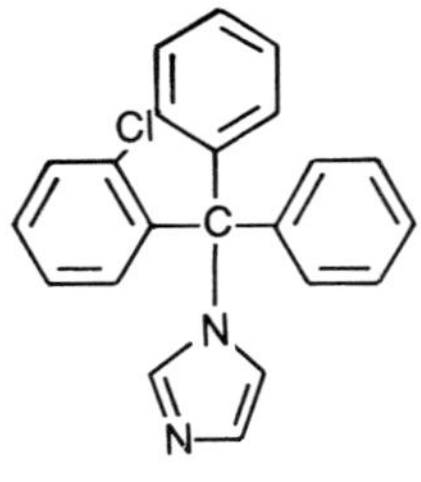

Clotrimazole

Figure 9.2. Structures of the azole antifungal drugs ketoconazole, miconazole and clotrimazole

that the ability of ketoconazole to inhibit the growth of human breast cancer cells in culture has been compared to that of tamoxifen (see Chapter 5); ketoconazole (1 nM to 1 μM) decreased MCF-7 cell proliferation in a time- and dose-dependent manner and also caused an accumulation of these cells in the G_0–G_1 phase of the cell cycle (Najid and Ratinaud, 1991).

ACTION ON YEAST SUBCELLULAR TARGET SITES

The yeast mitochondrial system

In mammalian model systems it is difficult to demonstrate the primary antimitochondrial activity of antitumour drugs. In contrast, yeast cells (and their mitochondria: Guerin, 1991) have been used to establish this for the cytotoxic anticancer drugs Adriamycin (Wilkie and Collie, 1987) and MGBG (Cheng *et al.*, 1990). A good indication of primary antimitochondrial activity is the inhibition of growth of yeast cells in non-fermentable medium (the carbon source used is usually glycerol) while growth continues in glucose medium, in the presence of the drug. This was found for both Adriamycin (Wilkie and Collier, 1987) and for MGBG (Cheng *et al.*, 1990). Primary antimitochondrial activity is, therefore, characterised by the ability of the cells to grow and divide only in the presence of a glycolysable sugar (e.g., glucose), because the glycolytic pathway is an alternative source of ATP, which is otherwise provided mainly by the mitochondria. However, inhibition of growth by tamoxifen was as high in the glycolytic medium as in the non-glycolytic (glycerol-containing) medium (Wiseman *et al.*, 1994b). This finding suggests that the mitochondrion is not a specific target site for tamoxifen in the yeast system and that tamoxifen is not an antimitochondrial agent in the strain of *S. cerevisiae* used.

In the yeast system, the *petite* mutant is a convenient tool for both the study of mitochondrial function and for screening drugs and chemicals for potential carcinogenicity. The *petite* mutation is an event of mainly unknown mechanism in which the mitochondrial genome is deleted so that only a fragment (usually not more than 5%) of the mitochondrial DNA survives transmission to daughter cells. Such daughter cells are respiratory defective and cannot grow in non-fermentable medium. The *petite* condition is a deletion mutation and thus is irreversible and stable. The mutation is very frequent—about 1% (10^{-2}) in most yeast strains. This makes diagnosis of mitochondrial change certain, because nuclear mutations are usually of the order of 10^{-6}. *Petite* colony formation can be induced by known mutagenic agents such as acriflavine and ethidium bromide, and thus the induction of the *petite* mutation is a useful criterion for testing drugs (including antitumour drugs) for mitochondrial genotoxicity and mutagenicity (Evans and McAthey, 1991; Cheng and Wilkie, 1991). It is of interest in this connection that induction of the *petite* mutation in *S. cerevisiae* by a series of trypanocidal drugs has been reported (Ferguson and Sunberg, 1991). Treatment of yeast with MGBG was found to produce a significantly higher frequency of *petite* colonies than in the control (Cheng *et al.*, 1990). Adriamycin was also found to induce the *petite* mutation (Wilkie and Collier, 1987). Tamoxifen, however, did not induce the mitochondrial mutant *petite* (H. Wiseman, unpublished observations) and thus was not mutagenic in mitochondrial DNA. Thus tamoxifen is unlikely to be generally genotoxic, at least in yeast.

Cytochrome P-450-dependent enzymes

Cytochrome P-450-enzymes are a family of haemoproteins (see Chapter 3).

Cytochrome P-450 enzymes have been shown to be present and active in *S. cerevisiae* (King and Wiseman, 1987). In the yeast system, adriamycin is metabolised by the cytochrome P-450 dependent mixed-function oxidase system, accepting electrons from the NADPH–cytochome P-450 reductase flavoprotein component of the cytochrome P-450 system. The major sterol in yeast membranes is ergosterol. The pathway of ergosterol biosynthesis in yeast has many similarities to the pathway of cholesterol biosynthesis in mammalian tissue, and indeed as far along the pathway as lanosterol the pathways of biosynthesis are identical. In both pathways lanosterol is a key intermediate, and the lanosterol 14α-demethylation reaction of the C32 methyl group is an essential and rate-limiting step. This step is thought to be catalysed by cytochrome P-450-dependent lanosterol 14α-demethylase, in both mammalian cells and yeast cells. This could be a target site for antitumour drugs in the yeast tumour model system as well as for antifungal drugs such as ketoconazole, miconazole and clotrimazole (Vanden Bossche *et al.*, 1988; Vanden Bossche, 1988).

The ability of miconazole to inhibit aromatase, the cytochrome P-450 enzyme that mediates the synthesis of oestrogens from androgen precursors (Covey, 1988), has led to its proposed use in the treatment of advanced breast cancer, as an inhibitor of peripheral oestrogen synthesis (Jones *et al.*, 1991). Furthermore, ketoconazole inhibits the 17–20 lyase activity of the cytochrome P-450 enzyme 17α-hydroxylase/17–20 lyase, thus inhibiting the synthesis of androgens such as testosterone but not the glucocorticoid cortisol (Vanden Bossche, 1988; Laughton *et al.*, 1990; Mainwaring, 1991). This has led to the use of ketoconazole in the treatment of prostatic cancer because most of these cancers are controlled by the level of androgens, especially testosterone (Laughton *et al.*, 1990). The ability of antitumour drugs to inhibit cytochrome P-450-dependent lanosterol 14α-demethylase, and other cytochrome P-450 dependent enzymes, could be studied, therefore, using the yeast tumour model. It is possible that if the synthesis of ergosterol is blocked by a drug such as tamoxifen that causes inhibition of growth in the yeast system, then growth could potentially be restored by the addition of exogenous ergosterol. Yeast, however, has been shown to take up ergosterol only under strict anaerobic conditions, when ergosterol cannot be synthesised (Cartwright *et al.*, 1989): addition of ergosterol to the culture medium at the same time as the tamoxifen had no effect on the inhibition of growth by tamoxifen (H. Wiseman, unpublished observations), even though inhibition of P-450-dependent lanosterol α-demethylase by tamoxifen can be postulated.

Protein kinase C

Tamoxifen has been reported to influence cellular signal transduction by its ability to bind calmodulin and to inhibit calcium calmodulin-dependent cAMP phosphodiesterase and protein kinase C from mammalian sources; this is discussed in Chapter 7. A protein kinase C has been identified in *S. cerevisiae* and this was activated by the simultaneous addition of calcium, diacylglycerol and phosphatidylserine (Ogita *et al.*, 1990). Tumour-promoting phorbol esters did not activate this enzyme, in contrast to mammalian protein kinase C. Furthermore, yeast protein kinase C had a distinctly different substrate specificity to the mammalian enzyme. The exact role of this yeast enzyme in cellular regulation and cell cycle control is not yet known. In yeast it has been reported that the essential functions of yeast calmodulin for cell proliferation can be carried out by half-calmodulins (molecules with drastic deletions at either the N- or C-terminal domains of the protein: Sun *et al.*, 1991). This is of interest because tamoxifen has been reported to bind to calmodulin and thus inhibit its action (see Chapter 7). Similarities between vertebrate and yeast calmodulins have been investigated, including a study of their calcium-binding and structural properties (Starovasnik *et al.*, 1993). It is of related interest that a calcium and calmodulin-dependent protein kinase has been partially purified from *S. cerevisiae* and it has been suggested that it may have a role in transduction by the mating pheromone α (Miyakawa *et al.*, 1989). The protein kinase activity of the yeast preparation was found to be stimulated at least eight-fold by the simultaneous presence of calmodulin and calcium. Furthermore, stimulation of the enzyme was found to be strongly inhibited by trifluoperazine, a calmodulin antagonist. In addition, the substrate specificities for yeast and mammalian cAMP-dependent protein kinases are similar though not identical (Denis *et al.*, 1991). Other protein kinases of interest in yeast include the Cdc-2/Cdc-28 protein kinases that control the cell cycle (see below). Protein kinase C-β_1 from the rat is functional in yeast: expression of its cDNA in *S. cerevisiae* introduced novel phorbol ester binding sites, which stimulated a specific calcium- and phospholipid-dependent catalytic activity *in vitro*, and this was consistent with a fully functional protein, which phosphorylates yeast proteins *in vivo* (Riedel *et al.*, 1993). In addition, phorbol ester activation of protein kinase C-β_1 *in vivo* leads to the stimulation of extracellular protein uptake, changes in cell morphology and an increase in the doubling time of *S. cerevisiae*. These findings suggest that there are compatible aspects of the signalling pathways in higher and lower eukaryotes and support the use of studies on yeast in determining the action of drugs such as tamoxifen. It is of interest also that a Ca^{2+} transport system that does not belong to the plasma membrane type Ca^{2+}-ATPase family but instead to the family of endomembrane type ATPases has been reported in *S. cerevisiae* (Okorokov *et al.*, 1993). These findings increase the potential usage of the yeast tumour model system in the investigation of the mode of action of an anticancer drug such as tamoxifen, although there is as yet no evidence for a direct interaction between tamoxifen and these enzymes in the yeast system.

Oestrogen-binding protein in yeast

The oestrogen receptor is an important target site for antitumour drugs which have an antioestrogen action, for example tamoxifen. Although this target site is found in oestrogen-responsive tumour models such as the human breast cancer cell line MCF-7 (see Chapter 5), it is not clear whether an analogous functional target site exists in the yeast system for the testing of antioestrogen antitumour drugs. *S. cerevisiae* has two mating types, *a* and α. Each mating type secretes one peptide hormone *a* and α factor respectively, which act on the opposite mating type to promote conjugation; this can be considered to be a hormonal system analogous to the mammalian one. It is also of interest that the human oestrogen receptor, when expressed in yeast, stimulates inhibition of transcription in a strictly hormone (oestradiol)-dependent manner, as in mammalian cells, indicating a striking conservation of the underlying regulatory mechanisms (Metzger *et al.*, 1988). In addition, a high level of expression of a biologically active oestrogen receptor has been reported in *S. cerevisiae* (McDonnell *et al.*, 1991). It was found in studies where *S. cerevisiae* cytosol was screened with a series of ^{3}H-labelled steroids that an oestrogen-binding protein could be identified, which had a high affinity for the vertebrate oestrogens (oestradiol, oestrone and oestriol), moderate affinity for progesterone, but negligible affinity for corticosterone and androgens. Tamoxifen, however, showed only a low affinity for the yeast oestrogen-binding protein (Burshell *et al.*, 1984). The binding specificity profile for the *S. cerevisiae* oestrogen-binding protein is unique and quite unlike that of the mammalian oestrogen receptor. Although the oestrogen-binding protein in the yeast tumour model system is probably analogous to the oestrogen receptor found in mammalian systems, the ability of the oestrogen-binding protein to act as a target site for antitumour drugs such as tamoxifen is not yet established. It is also of interest that the gene for a high-affinity corticosteroid-binding protein (CBP) from the pathogenic yeast *Candida albicans* has been cloned and expressed; when this protein was over-expressed in *S. cerevisiae* it displayed a steroid hormone-binding profile comparable with that of the native protein (Malloy *et al.*, 1993). Heat-shock proteins (HSP) 56 (also known as FK506 binding protein 59), 90 and 70 are known to associate with steroid receptors, including the glucocorticoid and progesterone receptors, and may maintain the receptors in an inactive state; another HSP, HSP-27, is thought to play an important role in the growth and progression of breast cancer cells and in their drug resistance (see Chapter 6). It is interesting, therefore, that an HSP-56 homologue complexed with HSP-90/HSP-70 has been detected in yeast (Tai *et al.*, 1993).

Biosynthesis of DNA, RNA and of protein in yeast

DNA BIOSYNTHESIS AND CELL CYCLE CONTROL

The nuclear DNA (14×10^3 kilobase pairs) of *S. cerevisiae* is distributed among 16 discrete chromosomes, each containing a single DNA molecule. DNA synthesis in yeast does not usually occur throughout the mitotic cycle, being restricted to the S phase. This phase is preceded by the G_1 phase (when separation of the bud from the parent cell occurs) and is followed by the G_2 and M phases, when growth of spindles, chromosomal segregation and the terminal cytokinesis events that bud off the daughter cell occur (Robinow and Johnson, 1991; Williamson, 1991; Herskowitz, 1992; Park *et al.*, 1993). The replication of chromosomes during the S phase and their segregation during mitosis is common to all eukaryotic cell cycles, including that of yeast. The sequence—S phase precedes mitosis and mitosis precedes the S phase of the succeeding cell cycle—is usually strictly adhered to, thus ensuring an orderly progression through the cell cycle (Newlon, 1989; Broek *et al.*, 1991). All of the DNA synthesis genes of *S. cerevisiae* are periodically expressed and hence are under cell cycle control. It has been reported that DSC1 (DNA synthesis control) is a transcription factor periodically active in the cell cycle and is likely to be a key protein controlling DNA synthesis; its regulation is thus of importance in understanding cell cycle control of the S phase (Lowndes *et al.*, 1991).

In *S. cerevisiae* the protein kinase product of the *cdc-28* gene has been found to be homologous to the Cdc-2+ gene product (i.e., protein kinase p34) of the fission yeast, *Schizosaccharomyces pombe* (Draetta, 1990; Freeman and Donoghue, 1991; Hartwell, 1992). Alterations in the state of this protein kinase (by tyrosine phosphorylation and dephosphorylation) can allow a cell to be reprogrammed from entering mitosis to undergoing S phase (Broek *et al.*, 1991). The Cdc-2+ gene product and its homologue are the central cell cycle regulators in species ranging from yeast to humans (Draetta, 1990; Hartwell, 1992). Furthermore, the *rum-1+* gene has been identified as a regulator of progression through the G_1 phase of the cell cycle in fission yeast: *rum-1+* influences determination of the length of G_1, dependence of S phase on the completion of mitosis and retardation of mitosis until G_1 is complete (Moreno and Nurse, 1994). In *S. pombe* the Swi6 protein is required for transcription of the periodically expressed genes required for DNA synthesis (Lowndes *et al.*, 1992). Furthermore, in *S. cerevisiae*, a transcription factor composed of the Swi6 and Swi4 proteins (called SBF) activates the transcription of the G_1-specific cyclins encoded by *cln-1* and *cln-2* (see above) and thus has a central role in modulating cell cycle start-specific transcription (Dirick *et al.*, 1992; Primig *et al.*, 1992; Moll *et al.*, 1993). The Cdc kinase also regulates the assembly of the mitotic spindle required for chromosomal assembly via a phosphorylation-induced activation of a chromosomal protein at the interphase/mitosis, transition and there is also a requirement for mitotic chromatin (Yeo *et al.*, 1994).

In yeast cell cycle progression requires the periodic activation of the genes that code for the cyclin proteins, which bind and activate the Cdc-2+/Cdc-28 protein kinase. This protein kinase associates with a succession of different cyclins (Clns and Clbs): the cell cycle events are initiated in G_1 phase by Cln-3, which promotes accumulation of Cln-1 and Cln-2, and this leads to the cell cycle commitment point start. In S phase, Clb-5 and Clb-6 replace Cln-1 and Cln-2 and at M phase this again changes and Cdc-28 binds Clb-1 and Clb-2 (Moll *et al.*, 1993; Nasmyth and Hunt, 1993). It is of associated interest that the p21 protein has been identified as a universal inhibitor of cyclin-dependent kinases (CDK): in normal human fibroblasts cyclin-dependent kinases exist in multiple quaternary units, each containing a CDK, cyclin, proliferating cell nuclear antigen and the p21 protein; however, in many transformed cells proliferating cell nuclear antigen and p21 are lost from these multiprotein enzymes (Xiong *et al.*, 1993; Nasmyth and Hunt, 1993).

In *S. cerevisiae* the *rad-9* gene-dependent G_1 arrest of the cell cycle occurs following DNA damage, for example by ultraviolet (UV) light or X-rays, to enable repair of lesions that could result in lethal or mutagenic damage during DNA synthesis, and the *rad-9* gene product may interact with cellular components common to the G_1/S and G_2/M transition points in the cell cycle of this yeast (Siede *et al.*, 1993; Nasmyth and Hunt, 1993). In addition, the *rad-3* gene of *S. cerevisiae* is required for excision repair of UV-damaged DNA and is essential for cell viability (Guzder *et al.*, 1994). The protein encoded by the *rad-3* gene has a high degree of homology with the human *ercc-2*(*xpd*) gene product: mutations in *xpd* cause the cancer-prone syndrome xeroderma pigmentosum. The mammalian transcription factor and tumour suppressor protein p53 protein (see Chapter 6) as found for *rad-9* is not required for normal cell growth or division but is required to shut down S phase after treatment with UV light, and it is the inappropriate DNA replication that occurs in p53 mutant cells that can generate the mutations that lead to cancer (Nasmyth and Hunt, 1993). It is possible that p53 normally controls the gene for the p21 protein that inhibits a wide range of cyclin-dependent kinases (Nasmyth and Hunt, 1993). Furthermore, p53 can function as a transcription factor in yeast (Scharer and Iggo, 1992). Replication protein A (RPA) has been identified as a binding protein for p53: RPA (a multisubunit complex containing three polypeptides) appears to be important for unwinding DNA origins, and p53 interacts with and prevents the ability of RPA to bind single-stranded DNA *in vitro* (Dutta *et al.*, 1993). All. three genes for the three subunits of RPA are essential for yeast viability (Pietenpol and Vogelstein, 1993).

RNA BIOSYNTHESIS

Yeast DNA is transcribed by three distinct and separable forms of RNA polymerase: this is true for eukaryotic cells in general, and each polymerase transcribes a different set of genes for each of messenger RNA (mRNA), ribosomal RNA (rRNA) and transfer RNA (tRNA). The yeast RNA polymerases all resemble the bacterial RNA polymerase, which transcribes all the genes of a bacterial genome, in that they are all large (M_r 4–6 $\times 10^5$) and composed of a number of different polypeptide chains (Oliver and Warmington, 1989). RNA polymerase I in *S. cerevisiae* transcribes the ribosomal genes into a precursor rRNA that is eventually processed to give the two large rRNAs (25S and 18S) and one of the two small RNAs (5.8S) found in ribosomes. The function of RNA polymerase II is to transcribe all the DNA coding for mRNA and some of the smaller-sized RNAs, such as the small nuclear RNAs. RNA polymerase III transcribes the genes coding for tRNA, 5S rRNA and a number of other small RNAs. RNA synthesis is regulated in yeast primarily at the level of transcriptional initiation. Yeast promoter elements can be considered to be either basic elements or regulatory elements, although the distinction between these two categories is not always clear (Oliver and Warmington, 1989; Hawkins, 1991). The basic elements determine the site(s) of initiation and the efficiency of transcriptional initiation at each site, following transcriptional activation or depression by the regulatory elements. The TATA box and CT block, which are present in many yeast genes, are both basic elements. The regulatory elements include positive regulatory sequences (upstream activation sites, UASs) and negative elements (upstream repression sites, URSs) (Oliver and Warmington, 1989; Hawkins, 1991).

In yeast the transcription factor TFIIIB (a transcription initiation factor) only is required for transcription by yeast RNA polymerise III (Kassavetic *et al.*, 1989; Paule, 1990). It has been reported that yeast transcriptional activators can be generated, which contain no yeast protein sequences. Thus it was found that approximately 1% of the short peptides encoded by *Escherichia coli* genomic DNA fragments act as transcriptional activating regions in yeast when fused to either the yeast transcriptional activator Gal-4 or to the bacterial repressor Lex-A (Ruden *et al.*, 1991). The structure $m^7G(5')ppp(5')Pu$ is the 'cap' found at the 5′ end of most mRNAs of *S. cerevisiae*. Transcriptional activation by Gal-4 requires an acidic region at its carboxyl terminus; however, when this domain is deleted Gal-4 can still function when this is accompanied by a mutation in the *Sug-1* gene (an essential gene in yeast). The predicted amino acid sequence of Sug-1 closely resembles that of the Tbp-1 and Mss-1 human proteins which modulate expression by the HIV *tat* gene (Swaffield *et al.*, 1992). A direct interaction of the HIV transactivator Tat protein with the human basal transcription factor TFIID has also been reported (Kashanchi *et al.*, 1994). Furthermore, the yeast Gal-11 protein has been identified as a transcription factor that enhances basal transcription *in vitro* and also enhances transcription activated by general regulatory factor 1, Gal-4–AH, or Gal-4–VP16 to the same extent as the basal transcription (Sakurai *et al.*, 1993). This suggests that the Gal-11 protein is a positive cofactor of basal and activator-induced transcription *in vitro*. It is of considerable interest that the *rad-3* gene of *S. cerevisiae* (see above) is essential for transcription by RNA polymerase II (Guzder *et al.*, 1994).

PROTEIN BIOSYNTHESIS

The mechanism of protein biosynthesis has been discussed in great detail (see Arnstein and Cox, 1992). The 5′ end of a yeast mRNA is thought to be the start point for transcription and also plays an important part in the initiation of translation. The 5′ cap may also protect mRNA *in vivo* against 5′-exonuclease digestion. The poly(A) tail (added post-transcriptionally to mRNA at the 3′ end) is about 50 nucleotides long in yeast and also protects mRNA against attack by nucleases. *S. cerevisiae* ribosomes comprise a 60S large subunit containing a 25S rRNA molecule (compared to the 28S rRNA molecule found in many other eukaryotes) and a 40S small subunit containing an 18S rRNA molecule. Additionally, 5S rRNA and 5.8S rRNA are both present in the 60S subunit (Lee, 1991). Yeast cells, in common with other eukaryotic cells, have ribosomes attached to the endoplasmic reticulum, which synthesise both integral membrane proteins and proteins for secretion (e.g., the peptide mating factor α); they also possess large numbers of free cytosolic polysomes. *S. cerevisiae* has been used extensively as a model system for studies of eukaryotic translation (Muller and Trachsel 1990). Translation initiation in *S. cerevisiae* closely resembles the cap-dependent initiation pathway in higher eukaryotes, whereby the ribosomes recognise and bind to the mRNA at the 5′ cap structure and scan the leader region to find the initiator codon AUG. Alternatively, there is evidence for internal initiation, whereby the ribosomes bind internally to mRNA. The elongation process is very similar in prokaryotes and lower and higher eukaryotes. The ribosome moves in relation to the mRNA in the 5′ to 3′ direction while incorporating amino acid residues into the growing polypeptide chain. The secondary structure, upstream AUG codons in the 5′ leader region, RNA sequences flanking the AUG initiation codon and the post-transcriptionally added 3′-poly(A) tail are all features known to affect the translational efficiency of mRNA in yeast. It is of interest that the elongation factor 1α determines the susceptibility of a mouse fibroblast variant (BALB/c 3T3) to malignant transformation (Tatsuka *et al.*, 1992). It is of related interest that in eukaryotic cells, including yeast, the accumulation of unfolded proteins in the endoplasmic reticulum triggers a signalling pathway from the endoplasmic reticulum to the nucleus. The *ern-1* gene in yeast codes for a 1115 amino acid protein (Ern-1 protein) whose glycosylated N-terminal is located inside the endoplasmic reticulum and whose cytoplasmic C-terminal carries a Cdc-2+/Cdc-28-related kinase activity (Mori *et al.*, 1993). It has been suggested that the Ern-1 protein is required for signalling from the endoplasmic reticulum to the nucleus: binding of a ligand to the Ern-1 protein results in transduction of a message across the endoplasmic reticulum membrane, resulting in the activation of a specific set of transcription factors.

ACTION ON THE BIOSYNTHESIS OF DNA, RNA AND OF PROTEIN

Antitumour drugs such as Adriamycin and actinomycin D have been shown to intercalate between DNA bases, interfering with DNA replication and the transcription of RNA. Actinomycin D inhibits the synthesis of RNA at concentrations much lower than those needed to inhibit the synthesis of DNA. The features of the DNA required for interaction with actinomycin D are guanine–cytosine pairs, a double-stranded helical structure, and the sugar moiety has to be deoxyribose (Franklin and Snow, 1989). Adriamycin inhibits DNA initiation and elongation, and RNA initiation, at adenine–thymine base pairs. Treatment with Adriamycin also results in DNA strand breakage, perhaps as a result of interaction and/or as a result of oxidant generation. In the yeast test system, Adriamycin has been found to intercalate with DNA and thus has been classified as one of the mutagens/carcinogens which block mitochondrial biogenesis and induce the *petite* mutation. Actinomycin D cannot enter yeast cells, and thus cannot be tested in this system.

Pre-treatment of rat fetal forelimb *in vitro* with tamoxifen (100 μM) for 16 h resulted in inhibition of both [^{3}H]thymidine incorporation into DNA (87% at $t = 120$ min) and [^{3}H]leucine incorporation into protein (75% at $t = 120$ min) (Stewart and Stern, 1986). In the yeast system, although inhibition of protein synthesis (incorporation of [^{3}H]leucine) was observed following the addition of tamoxifen to the culture, it occurred simultaneously with inhibition of RNA synthesis (incorporation of [^{3}H]uridine) (see Figure 9.3) (Wiseman *et al.*, 1990b, 1990c) and also DNA synthesis indicated by incorporation of [^{3}H]adenine (Wiseman *et al.*, 1994a). Similar results were observed in the human ovarian tumour SK-OV-3 cell line (Wiseman *et al.*, 1994a); inhibition of DNA, RNA and protein synthesis by tamoxifen was again simultaneous in the SK-OV-3 cell line. These results indicate, therefore, that tamoxifen is not a specific inhibitor of biosynthesis of DNA, RNA or of protein. The processes of biosynthesis of DNA, RNA and protein are thus unlikely to be primary target sites for the growth-inhibitory action of tamoxifen in both yeast and tumour cells. It is possible that the observed simultaneous inhibition of DNA, RNA and protein

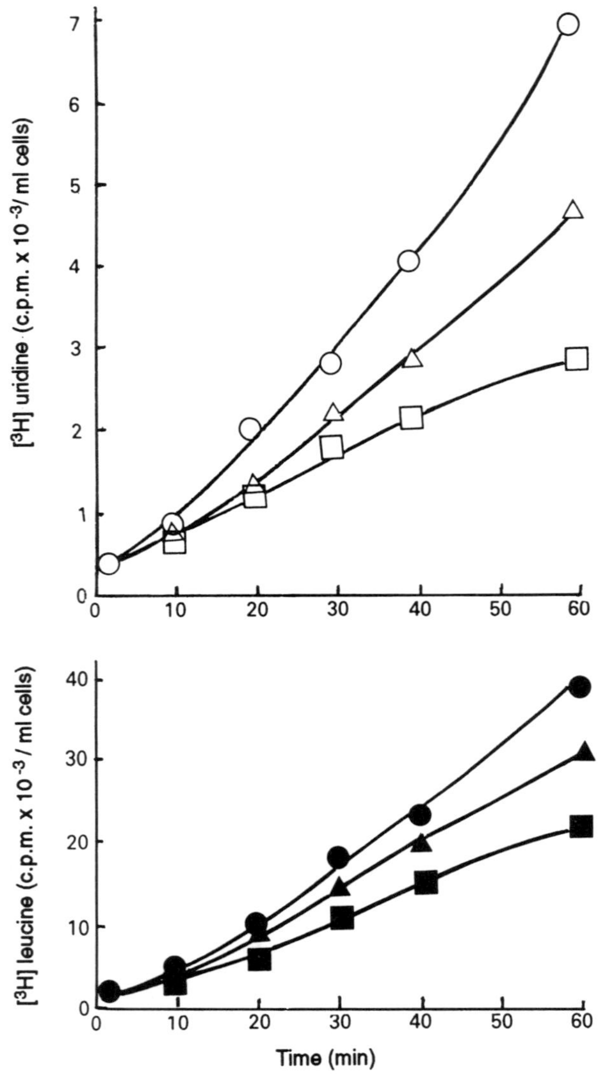

Figure 9.3. Inhibition by 30 μM tamoxifen of the incorporation of [^{3}H]uridine into RNA and [^{3}H]leucine into protein (in A224A) and partial protection by 20 mM ascorbate. Incorporation of [^{3}H]uridine into RNA and [^{3}H]leucine into protein (○) and (•), respectively, for the controls containing 0.5% (v/v) ethanol, is simultaneously inhibited by 30 μM tamoxifen (□) and (■), respectively, and partially protected by 20 mM ascorbate (△) and (▲), respectively. From Wiseman *et al.*, 1990b, with permission

synthesis (Wiseman *et al.*, 1994a) may be features of the reported tamoxifen-induced apoptosis (Couldwell *et al.*, 1994). Although it is probable that membrane lipid synthesis is inhibited at the same time as these other cellular processes, because normal membrane fluidity (decreased by tamoxifen) is a likely requirement for further membrane synthesis, this could not be demonstrated as incorporation of labelled acetate could not be achieved (H. Wiseman, unpublished observations). This is probably because of uptake problems, in contrast to positive results reported with *Candida* species (Vanden Bossche *et al.*, 1980); and indeed this may be one disadvantage of using *S. cerevisiae*. It is of related interest that the anti-*Candida* agent cispentacin has been found to inhibit the biosynthesis of RNA and protein in *C. albicans* (Capobianco *et al.*, 1993).

ACTION IN A BACTERIAL SYSTEM

In addition to the eukaryote yeast, prokaryotic microorganisms such as the bacterium *E. coli* have also played an important role in the discovery of anticancer drugs in complex mixtures of natural products and in determining the mode of action of known agents. The main advantages of the bacterial system are their rapid response, low cost and sensitivity. Their major limitations are that most baterial proteins are not recognised by drugs (ligands) active against eukaryotic proteins, and the bacterial cell wall may exclude some drugs. Tamoxifen was found not to be an inhibitor of either growth of *E. coli* or protein synthesis in a cell-free translation system derived from this bacterium (H. Wiseman, unpublished observations), indicating that tamoxifen is not an inhibitor of 70S ribosomal function and thus of prokaryotic protein synthesis. The inability of tamoxifen to inhibit bacterial growth suggests that the bacterial cell wall may, in association with the cell membranes, exclude tamoxifen, in contrast to eukaryotic cells, including yeast.

THE PRO-OXIDANT OR ANTIOXIDANT ACTION OF TAMOXIFEN AND OTHER ANTITUMOUR DRUGS IN YEAST

The ability of adriamycin to accept electrons from microsomal and nuclear flavoproteins resulting in the formation of a semiquinone free radical, and ultimately in the formation of superoxide and hydroxyl free radicals, has been demonstrated in animal cells and in isolated cardiac submitochondrial particles, and this mechanism may be involved in the cardiotoxicity of Adriamycin (Doroshow *et al.*, 1990; Kojima *et al.*, 1993; Gutteridge, 1993). In yeast the toxic effect of Adriamycin was mostly reversed by an exogenous supply of glutathione (Wilkie and Collier, 1987). Vitamin E, which was found to be an antioxidant in the yeast system and was only slightly less effective than glutathione in protecting against Adriamycin toxicity, may be more readily administered to patients than glutathione. Furthermore glutathione, vitamin E and vitamin C were all found to protect the yeast cells against the toxicity and antimitochondrial activity of MGBG, and this suggests that toxic free radical metabolites of this drug are of importance in its cellular activity (Cheng *et al.*, 1990). Adriamycin and MGBG are pro-oxidant antitumour drugs and this has important implications for both their mechanisms of action and therapeutic usefulness. In addition, the role of glutathione in the cytotoxicity of alkylating agents in human breast cancer cells has been reported (Chen and Waxman, 1994).

The pro-oxidant or antioxidant status of tamoxifen has been investigated both in the yeast system and in membrane systems *in vitro* (see below). The antioxidants ascorbate, glutathione and *N*-acetylcysteine all conferred partial protection against the inhibition of growth and biosynthesis of RNA and of protein caused by tamoxifen (see Table 9.1 and Figure 9.3) (Wiseman *et al.*, 1990a, 1990b, 1990c). Similar results were observed for *cis*-tamoxifen and *N*-desmethyltamoxifen, with the exception that the inhibition of RNA synthesis caused by *cis*-tamoxifen was virtually unprotectable by antioxidants (H. Wiseman, unpublished observations). The reason for this may be related to the increased potency of *cis*-tamoxifen, compared to tamoxifen, as an inhibitor of RNA synthesis (but not protein synthesis). Although glutathione can regenerate thiol groups from disulphide bridges in proteins, the main antioxidant role of ascorbate with respect to thiol group maintenance is thought to be in the regeneration of glutathione from oxidised glutathione (Halliwell and Gutteridge, 1989, 1990; Halliwell, 1990). In addition, ascorbate can regenerate

Table 9.1. Reduction in tamoxifen-mediated inhibition of yeast growth by protective agents. The percentage inhibition is calculated from the reduction in A_{600} at 1.5× generation time of the control containing 0.5% (v/v) ethanol and protection is calculated from the reduction in inhibition and is expressed as a percentage of the unprotected inhibition. All values are shown as mean ± SD where $n \geqslant 4$

		Tamoxifen (μM)			
Additions	Effect on growth	3.75	7.5	15	30
None	Inhibition (%)	20 ± 3.0	40 ± 4.3	65 ± 4.4	80 ± 1.7
	Protection (%)	—	—	—	—
10 mM Glutathione	Inhibition (%)	2.9 ± 1.3	8 ± 1.3	28 ± 3.7	46 ± 2.0
	Protection (%)	86 ± 4.3	77 ± 5.2	56 ± 4.6	40 ± 3.3
10 mM *N*-Acetylcysteine	Inhibition (%)	2.8 ± 0.3	11 ± 1.2	34 ± 1.2	56 ± 1.4
	Protection (%)	84 ± 2.3	72 ± 1.3	50 ± 1.7	30 ± 2.3
20 mM Ascorbate	Inhibition (%)	1.6 ± 1.4	7 ± 1.4	20 ± 2.2	35 ± 2.9
	Protection (%)	92 ± 6.3	82 ± 3.0	68 ± 2.5	53 ± 4.0

From Wiseman *et al.*, 1990a, with permission.

membrane α-tocopherol, which is also a potent antioxidant (Cohen, 1989; Buettner, 1993; Sharma and Buettner, 1993). The partial protective action of the antioxidants against the inhibition of growth and biosynthesis of RNA and of protein by tamoxifen and related compounds in the yeast system may be related to protection of membrane protein thiol groups against oxidation, by the antioxidants preventing deleterious changes in protein and glycoprotein conformation, or restoration of thiol groups perhaps followed by formation of the correct disulphide bridges. Such changes in protein conformation may, therefore, restore the activity of important membrane enzymes adversely affected by the ability of tamoxifen to decrease membrane fluidity (Clarke *et al.*, 1990; Wiseman *et al.*, 1993b). Decreased membrane fluidity in the presence of tamoxifen can inactivate membrane proteins such as adenylate cyclase by causing them to undergo inappropriate conformational changes (see Chapter 8). Restoration, therefore, of the correct disulphide bridges by the action of antioxidants such as glutathione or ascorbate could allow the active conformation to be regained and thus protect the growth ability of the yeast cell (when dependent on cAMP for proliferation). Protection by the antioxidants glutathione and ascorbate may also be via maintenance of the correct thiol groups not only in membrane proteins but additionally in other proteins, and in enzymes such as those involved in the biosynthesis of DNA, RNA and of protein, and in cytochrome P-450-dependent enzymes. Indeed it has been proposed that metabolism of triphenylethylenes such as tamoxifen (see Chapter 3) may produce a reactive intermediate (T^* may be an epoxide metabolite of tamoxifen; see Chapter 3) that binds non-covalently to protein thiol groups (including the oestrogen receptor), thus altering their structure and activity (Kupfer and Bulger, 1990; Mani and Kupfer, 1991). Antioxidants such as glutathione and ascorbate could also counteract the free radicals, such as the superoxide formed during the metabolism of tamoxifen by one form of cytochrome P-450 (Turner *et al.*, 1991).

In this connection it is of great interest that an antioxidant protein (27 kDa) has been identified in *S. cerevisiae* that is induced by the presence of oxygen, Fe(III) or 2-mercaptoethanol and specifically prevents the inactivation of various yeast enzymes caused by a non-enzymic Fe(III)/oxygen/thiol mixed-function oxidation system but not by other mixed-function systems, where the thiol component is replaced, for example, by ascorbate as the electron donor (Kim *et al.*, 1989). This *in vivo* induction of an antioxidant protein in yeast may represent an adaptive response that has evolved to protect cells against the oxidative stress caused by thiol-dependent mixed-function oxidation systems but did not appear to be an HSP; the stress response in yeast has been reviewed (Mager and Ferreira, 1993). Indeed this thiol-specific antioxidant protein may be conserved in mammalian systems. Similarly, a thiol-specific antioxidant protein from *S. cerevisiae* can remove hydrogen peroxide and the hydroxyl radical, but only in the presence of dithiothreitol as a reducing agent (Lim *et al.*, 1993). In addition, *N*-ethylmaleimide (binds to thiol groups) was able to inhibit the action of the thiol-specific antioxidant protein, suggesting that it is the sulphydryl group of the cysteine residues that is important to the antioxidant action of the protein. Furthermore, this antioxidant protein can also prevent the strand breaks in DNA caused by the Fe(III)/oxygen/thiol mixed-function oxidation system, but not by an ascorbate mixed-function oxidation system, suggesting that the yeast antioxidant protein is a sulphur radical scavenger (Kwoon *et al.*, 1993). The gene for the antioxidant protein from *S. cerevisiae* has been cloned and found to have no sequence homology in its predicted amino acid residue sequence to those of the main mammalian antioxidant enzymes, including catalases, peroxidases and superoxide dismutase (Chae *et al.*, 1993). Furthermore, the 195-amino acid sequence of the thiol-specific antioxidant protein contains two cysteine residues, and is likely to be encoded on chromosome 13 of yeast nuclear DNA.

In *S. cerevisiae* the intracellular concentration of the antioxidant enzyme catalase increased on aeration of the culture without substrates or with ethanol and was inhibited on aeration with glucose following cell permeabilisation (Gille *et al.*, 1993). The enhanced catalase activity was probably due to *de novo* protein synthesis, whereas the inhibitory effect of glucose was caused by succinate (a major metabolite of glucose metabolism). Export of catalase to the cell surface and the extracellular catalase activity increased on aeration (Gille *et al.*, 1993). Furthermore the fluidity of the yeast cell membrane also increased during aeration. Also, both yeast and mammalian metallothioneins have been reported to functionally substitute for yeast copper–zinc superoxide dismutase, and this suggests that metallothioneins may protect against oxidative stress by acting as antioxidant proteins (Tamai *et al.*, 1993).

ADVANTAGES OF THE YEAST TUMOUR MODEL SYSTEM

It is clear that this system can contribute to the toxicity testing and determination of the mode(s) of action of antitumour drugs by providing a rapid and inexpensive method for assessing toxicity, perhaps in relation to the production of free radical metabolites and their removal by appropriate antioxidants. Where the cytochrome P-450-dependent mixed-function oxidase system is present it can activate the drug and it provides a target site, therefore, for use of appropriate inhibitors of yeast cytochrome P-450. In addition, there is the oestrogen-binding protein, protein kinases (including protein kinase C), biosynthesis of DNA, RNA and of protein and other important target sites such as the plasma membranes, which are as yet not well characterised as targets for antitumour drug action. Furthermore, the membranes of *S. cerevisiae* contain saturated and monounsaturated fatty acids (Ratledge and Evans, 1989). This is of significance in relation to membrane stability against lipid peroxidation (see below and Chapter 8); the structural requirements of sterols for correct membrane function in this yeast have been investigated (Nes *et al.*, 1993). The yeast system also has the advantage of similar signal transduction systems to those found in mammalian cells (Rose, 1989). The cAMP second messenger system that operates in yeast is thought to be similar to the mammalian one, although there is evidence for only one cAMP-sensitive protein kinase, in contrast to the multitude in the mammalian system. Adenylate cyclase generates cAMP from ATP in response to hormone or growth regulator binding to cell surface receptors, which send a stimulatory signal to adenylate cyclase via G-proteins (Neer and Clapham, 1988). In yeast, cAMP activates a protein kinase, which regulates cellular metabolism by phosphorylation of particular proteins (Rose, 1989). A phosphoinositide second messenger system, first discovered in mammalian cells, has been found also in yeast (Rose, 1989; Henschke and Rose, 1991), and indeed phosphoinositol 4,5-bisphosphate has been shown to be a requirement for cell division in *S. cerevisiae* (Uno *et al.*, 1988).

ENHANCEMENT OF THE MEMBRANE ANTIOXIDANT ACTION OF YEAST ERGOSTEROL

Yeast plasma membranes have a high ergosterol content and this neutral lipid largely replaces the cholesterol found in mammalian plasma membranes (see Figure 9.4). Yeast membranes contain a typically eukaryotic mixture of phospholipids, including phosphatidylserine, phosphatidylcholine, phosphatidylethanolamine, phosphatidylinositol, cardiolipin and sphingolipids (Ratledge and Evans, 1989). The fatty acid side-chains of membrane lipids in animal cells have unbranched carbon chains (mostly in the range 14–24 carbon atoms) and the double bonds (0–6) display the *cis* configuration. Yeast synthesises mostly 16- and 18-carbon fatty acids, which are usually saturated or monounsaturated (Ratledge and Evans, 1989). Ergosterol is a more potent membrane antioxidant than cholesterol (see Chapter 8) and is also thought to stabilise membranes against lipid peroxidation (Wiseman *et al.*, 1990d, 1993a; Wiseman, 1994a, 1994b). Vitamin D is another recently characterised membrane antioxidant thought to act in this way (Wiseman, 1993). The membrane antioxidant action of ergosterol was demonstrated by its ability to inhibit lipid peroxidation when introduced into phospholipid liposomes and by the ability of the yeast lipid fraction (containing ergosterol) to inhibit lipid peroxidation when introduced into ox brain phospholipid liposomes. Ergosterol is thought to stabilise membranes against lipid peroxidation by an interaction between its hydrophobic rings and the fatty acid side-chains of phospholipids, as

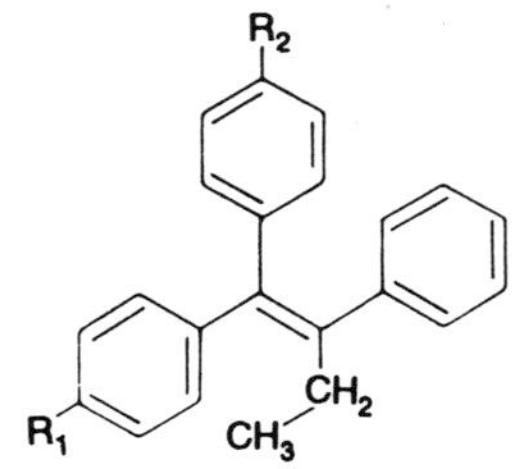

Tamoxifen $R_1 = H$, $R_2 = OCH_2CH_2N(CH_3)_2$

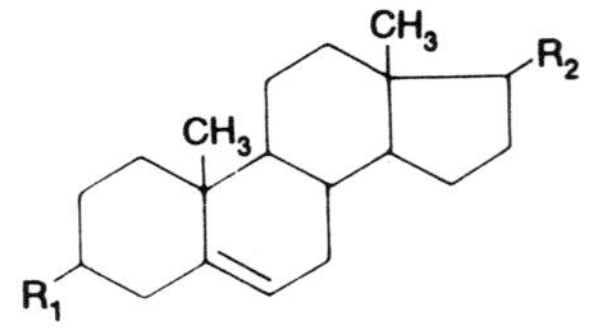

Cholesterol $R_1 = OH$, $R_2 = CH(CH_3)(CH_2)_3CH(CH_3)_2$

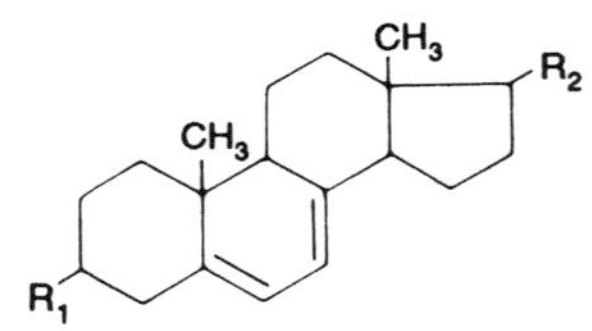

Ergosterol $R_1 = OH$, $R_2 = CH(CH_3)CH{:}CHCH(CH_3)CH(CH_3)_2$

Figure 9.4. Structural mimicry by tamoxifen of the mammalian membrane sterol cholesterol and the yeast membrane sterol ergosterol

proposed for the cholesterol that is present in mammalian cell membranes (see Chapter 8). The superior antioxidant action of ergosterol in comparison to cholesterol may indicate an evolutionary advantage of fungal cells over mammalian cells. It is only a disadvantage to the fungal cell to have membranes that are highly stabilised against lipid peroxidation when they are exposed to a drug (such as tamoxifen) that deleteriously stabilises the membrane beyond that achieved by ergosterol. The antioxidant action of ergosterol was shown also by the ability of yeast lipid fraction, or the ergosterol component of this fraction, when introduced into ox brain phospholipid liposomes to stabilise these membranes against lipid peroxidation (Wiseman *et al.*, 1993a). Furthermore, the phospholipid component of the yeast lipid fraction also stabilised the liposomes against lipid peroxidation, presumably by dilution of the polyunsaturated fatty acid side-chains of the ox brain phospholipids with the predominantly saturated and monounsaturated fatty acid side-chains in yeast phospholipids. Saturated and monounsaturated fatty acids are known to be highly resistant to peroxidative attack (Halliwell and Gutteridge, 1989). In addition, this explains also the inability of yeast microsomes, and also of liposomes prepared from yeast phospholipid (in which the inhibitory action of ergosterol has been eliminated), to peroxidise under the conditions successfully used for rat liver microsomes and ox brain phospholipid liposomes. Therefore a yeast-based test system for the antioxidant action of drugs such as tamoxifen has not been possible.

The lipid fraction extracted from yeast treated with tamoxifen was more effective at inhibiting lipid peroxidation, when introduced into ox brain phospholipid liposomes, than that from untreated yeast (see Figure 9.5 and Table 9.2) (Wiseman *et al.*, 1993a). This resulted from the additional action of tamoxifen above that of ergosterol and other membrane

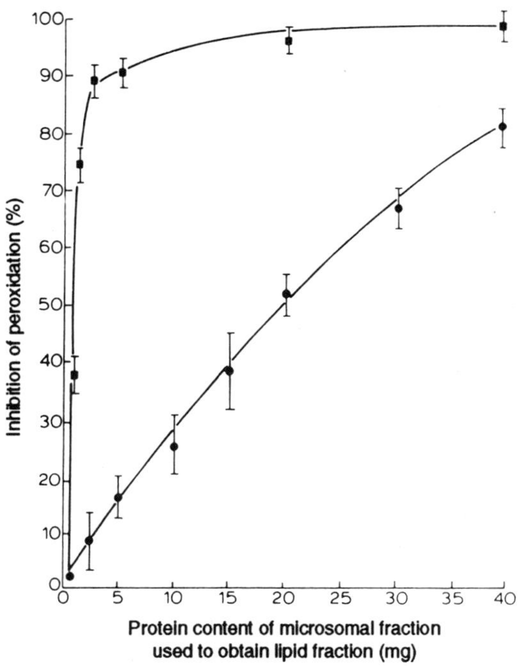

Figure 9.5. Inhibition of Fe(III)-dependent lipid peroxidation by yeast lipid fraction from microsomes obtained from (•) untreated and (■) tamoxifen-treated yeast introduced into liposomes. Results are shown as mean ± SD, $n = 3–9$ tests. From Wiseman *et al.*, 1993a, with permission

Table 9.2. IC_{50} values for the inhibition of liposomal lipid peroxidation by yeast lipid fraction obtained from microsomes from untreated and tamoxifen-treated yeast. Values are deduced from the graphs shown in Figure 9.5 in which each point represents the mean ± SD, $n = 3–9$ tests

Type of microsomal lipid fraction	IC_{50} value microsomal protein (mg)
Untreated	20
Tamoxifen-treated	1.2

From Wiseman *et al.*, 1993a, with permission

components, and indicates that tamoxifen accumulates also in the membranes of intact yeast treated with this drug: microsomal membranes prepared from untreated yeast were found to bind 0.3 mg of [^{3}H]tamoxifen per gram of microsomal protein. The lipid fraction from untreated yeast was found to inhibit iron-dependent liposomal lipid peroxidation in a concentration-dependent manner when introduced into ox brain phospholipid liposomes during their preparation. However, yeast lipid fraction from yeast that had been treated with tamoxifen again exerted a concentration-dependent inhibitory effect on lipid peroxidation but was more effective at inhibiting liposomal lipid peroxidation than that from untreated yeast. When ratios were calculated for inhibition of lipid peroxidation by tamoxifen-treated yeast lipid fraction to inhibition of lipid peroxidation by untreated yeast lipid fraction, and plotted against amounts of microsomal protein added (see Figure 9.6), the slope of the linear portion of the graph had a value of 2.0. This value was designated the tamoxifen enhancement coefficient (TEC). The TEC value of 2.0 thus quantifies the effectiveness of tamoxifen in enhancing the membrane antioxidant action of the ergosterol-containing yeast lipid fraction (Wiseman *et al.*, 1993a; Wiseman, 1994b).

In the yeast tumour model (using *S. cerevisiae* (A224A); (Wiseman *et al.*, 1989, 1990a; Wiseman, 1994b) a likely explanation of the potent inhibition of growth by tamoxifen, which has a potential application in the treatment of *Candida* species infections, may be in the deleterious further decrease in membrane fluidity beyond that achieved by ergosterol. The mechanism of the anti-yeast ability of tamoxifen, which has a potential clinical application in the treatment of *Candida* infections (Wiseman, 1994a; see below), may thus involve a further decrease in membrane fluidity that is harmful to the yeast cells. The decreased membrane fluidity reported for tamoxifen may be responsible for the growth-inhibitory action of tamoxifen in yeast because it could be inhibitory to the action of adenylate cyclase

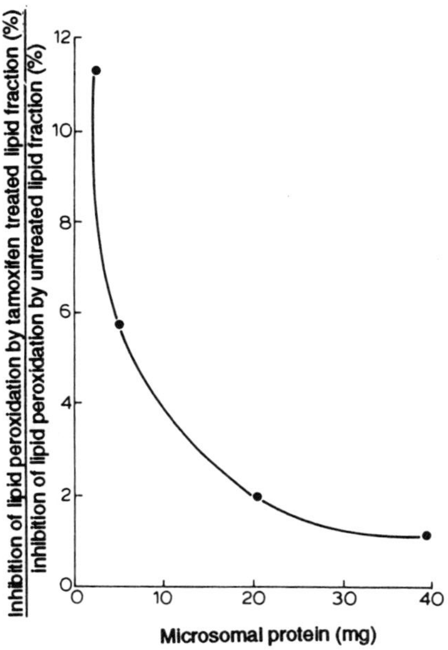

Figure 9.6. Enhanced inhibition of lipid peroxidation by yeast fraction obtained from microsomes from (•) tamoxifen-treated yeast introduced into liposomes. Inhibition of lipid peroxidation by yeast microsomal lipid fraction obtained from yeast treated with tamoxifen was compared to that observed from microsomal lipid fraction from untreated yeast and the ratios obtained were plotted against the protein content of the microsomes used to extract the lipid fraction. Results section and results were ± SD, $n = 3$–9 tests. From Wiseman *et al.*, 1993a, with permission

(see Chapter 8), thus decreasing cellular cAMP: yeast proliferation has an absolute requirement of cAMP.

MEMBRANE ANTIOXIDANT ACTION OF ANTIFUNGAL AZOLES: COMPARISON WITH CHOLESTEROL AND TAMOXIFEN

Tamoxifen and its metabolites have similar membrane antioxidant activities to the azole anti-*Candida* drugs, in particular ketoconazole (Wiseman *et al.*, 1991). The membrane-stabilising action of these drugs against lipid peroxidation in liposomal and microsomal membranes is thought to result from their structural similarity to the ergosterol, present in yeast cell membranes (see above). In addition to the well-established ability of ketoconazole to inhibit the action of the cytochrome P-450-dependent enzyme lanosterol 14α-demethylase (Vanden Bossche, 1988; Polak, 1990), thus preventing ergosterol synthesis and thus growth in fungal cells, it is possible that it might also have a structural antioxidant role in the membrane similar to that suggested for tamoxifen. Ketoconazole inhibits lipid peroxidation to about the same extent as 4-hydroxytamoxifen and to a greater extent than tamoxifen, and has a cholesterol coefficient (see Chapter 8) almost as high as 4-hydroxytamoxifen. In addition, ketoconazole does not disrupt membrane organisation, in contrast to miconazole and clotrimazole (Vanden Bossche, 1988; Polak, 1990), and has a closer structural similarity to lanosterol (and thus presumably cholesterol and ergosterol) than miconazole and clotrimazole (Lewis *et al.*, 1989). Indeed, the ability of miconazole to cause direct damage to the membrane has been related to its anti-yeast action (Beggs, 1992). It is likely that structural similarity to lanosterol is the basis of the ability of such azoles to bind to and thus inhibit the action of lanosterol 14α-demethylase. Further evidence for the structural similarity of these azoles, in particular ketoconazole, to sterols is provided by the report that they can mimic C_{21}-steroids in binding competitively to the active site of the 16-ene-C_{19}-steroid-synthesising enzyme in pig testicular microsomes (Nakajin *et al.*, 1991).

POTENTIAL CLINICAL USE AS AN ANTI-*CANDIDA* AND ANTIVIRAL AGENT

Anti-*Candida* action

Fungal infections occur frequently in cancer patients (Meunier, 1991), and itraconazole is used in the prophylactic treatment of fungal infections in immunocompromised cancer patients (Muhldorfer and Konig, 1990). Furthermore, *Candida albicans* (reviewed by Tuite, 1990) is a promoter of oral mucosal neoplasia (O'Grady and Reade, 1992), and the impact of the changing epidemiology of fungal infections in the 1990s has been reviewed (Pfaller and Wenzel, 1992). Fluconazole is used in the prevention of fungal infections in transplant patients (Goodman *et al.*, 1992; Quabeck *et al.*, 1992) and in AIDS patients (Nightingale *et al.*, 1992) and also to prevent the recurrence of bacterial meningitis (Saag *et al.*, 1992) in AIDS patients. Ketoconazole is used in the treatment of oral Candidosis in HIV-infected patients (Korting *et al.*, 1992). Opportunistic fungal infections are a considerable problem in AIDS patients (Viviani, 1992). Similar therapeutic uses may be found for tamoxifen in the future, particularly as pathogenic yeasts can develop resistance to azole derivative antifungal drugs (Odds, 1993). Tamoxifen has the further advantage for treatment of AIDS patients because it also has an anti-HIV action (see below). The possible therapeutic usage of tamoxifen for *Candida* infections is indicated by the ability of tamoxifen to inhibit the growth of *S. cerevisiae* (Wiseman *et al.*, 1989, 1993a,

1994a, 1994b; used initially as a model for *Candida*) and *C. albicans* ATCC 11651 grown *in vitro* (Beggs, 1993). Furthermore, use of tamoxifen or the azole ketoconazole inhibited *C. albicans* SC-9172, with similar effectiveness, in a rat vaginitis model (Mitchell *et al.*, 1988). A possible mechanism for the anti-yeast ability of tamoxifen is discussed above.

There is a clear case, therefore, for prospective and retrospective clinical evaluation of the incidence of the anti-*Candida* activity of tamoxifen in women taking this drug (Wiseman, 1994a, 1994b).

Antiviral action

Antiviral effects of tamoxifen have been reported, including the observation of regression and resolution of early herpetic lesions (Vennin *et al.*, 1992; Benson and Baum, 1993). Tamoxifen is also able to prevent the induction of viral replication by phorbol myristate acetate in promonocyte cells chronically infected with HIV-1 (Laurence *et al.*, 1990). In addition, associated clinical observations on HIV-infected people may be unreported at present (Wiseman, 1994a). Tamoxifen also inhibits the production of Moloney murine virions by fibroblastic A9 cells, which have no detectable oestrogen receptor (Chailleux *et al.*, 1993). Furthermore, tamoxifen and other protein kinase C inhibitors (see Chapter 7) inhibited the infectivity of the following enveloped viruses—vesicular stomatis virus, herpes simplex 1 virus, turkey herpes virus, vaccinia virus and Sindbis virus—but not the non-enveloped poliomyelitis virus on cultured human fibroblasts, and it has been suggested that protein kinase C is important in the infectivity of enveloped viruses, probably at the level of viral entry (Constantinescu *et al.*, 1991). The release of enveloped viruses from their host cells is associated with a perturbation of the cell plasma membrane. Stabilisation of the plasma membrane through the ability of tamoxifen to decrease membrane fluidity could prevent the lysis of viral-infected cells. It is possible, therefore, that the subcellular site of action of the viral inhibitory actions of tamoxifen is primarily the plasma membrane. This may be associated with initiation of transmembrane signalling events that lead to induction of viral inhibitory proteins such as interferon or the negative transforming growth factor, TGF-β (Benson and Baum, 1993).

Apoptosis and an increase in free radical levels are thought to be important in HIV activation, and the antioxidant *N*-acetylcysteine has been found to decrease viral particles in HIV chronically infected cells (Pani *et al.*, 1993; Malorni *et al.*, 1993). Furthermore, plant-derived antioxidants appear to have efficacy in inhibiting the activation of latent HIV in infected individuals by oxygen and free radicals (Greenspan, 1993). Antioxidants regulate the activation of the transcription factor NF-κ B (Adcock *et al.*, 1994) and the signal transduction pathways that lead to HIV expression. It has been reported that the glutathione precursor *N*-acetylcysteine inhibits NF-κ B activation and HIV expression under conditions where the main cellular antioxidant glutathione has been depleted and *N*-acetylcysteine cannot be converted to glutathione, and that glutathione depletion augments HIV production in a model of acute infection. This suggests that direct antioxidant action may be the mechanism for inhibition of HIV activation by the *N*-acetylcysteine and glutathione (Staal *et al.*, 1993). Studies on the antiviral action of tamoxifen and other antioxidants against constructed variants of the HIV virus may also be of interest in relation to the emergence of such variants during multiple-drug therapies (Emini *et al.*, 1993).

Designer antiviral agents could follow, because antiviral agents could be conveniently identified by membrane-modulating and antioxidant testing in model systems (Wiseman, 1994a).

REFERENCES

Adcock, I.M., Brown, C.R., Kwon, O., Barnes, P.J. (1994) *Biochemical Society Transactions* **22**, 186S.

Arnstein, H.R.V., Cox, R.A. (1992) *Protein Biosynthesis*, IRL Press/Oxford University Press, Oxford.

Beggs, W.H. (1992) *Research Communications in Chemical Pathology and Pharmacology* **77**, 249–252.

Beggs, W.H. (1993) *Research Communications in Chemical Pathology and Pharmacology* **80**, 125–128.

Benson, J.R., Baum, M. (1993) *Lancet* **341**, 1288.

Boles, E., Heinisch, J., Zimmermann, F.K. (1993) *Yeast* **9**, 761–770.

Broek, D., Bartlett, R., Crawford, K., Nurse P. (1991) *Nature* **349**, 388–393.

Buettner, G.R. (1993) *Archives of Biochemistry and Biophysics* **300**, 535–755.

Burshell, A., Stathis, P.A., Do, Y., Miller, S.C., Feldman, D. (1984) *Journal of Biological Chemistry* **259**, 3450–3456.

Capobianco, J.C., Zakula, D., Coen, M.L., Goldman, R.C. (1993) *Biochemical and Biophysical Research Communications* **190**, 1037–1044.

Cartwright, C.P., Rose, A.H., Calderbank, J., Keenan, M.H.J. (1989) In *The Yeasts*, Vol. 3, 2nd edn (eds A.H. Rose and J.S. Harrison), Academic Press, London, pp. 5–56.

Chae, H.Z., Kim, I.H., Kim, K., Rhee, S.G. (1993) *Journal of Biological Chemistry* **268**, 16815–16821.

Chailleux, C., Mesange, F., Bayard, F., Prats, A.C., Faye, J.C. (1993) *Molecular Pharmacology* **44**, 324–327.

Chen, L.H. (1989) *In Vivo* **3**, 199–210.

Chen, G., Waxman, D.J. (1994) *Biochemical Pharmacology* **47**, 1079–1088.

Cheng, L.L., Wilkie, D. (1991) *Biochemical Pharmacology* **42**, 1237–1240.

Cheng, L.L, Collier, D.C., Wilkie, D. (1990) *Cancer Letters* **51**, 213–220.

Clarke, R., van den Berg, H.W., Murphy, R.F. (1990) *Journal of the National Cancer Institute* **82**, 1702–1705.

Constantinescu, S.N., Cernescu, C.D., Popescu, L.M. (1991) *Federation of European Biochemical Societies Letters* **291**, 31–33.

Couldwell, W.T., Hinton, D.R., He, S., Chen, T.C., Sebat, I., Weiss, M.H., Law, R.E. (1994) *Federation of European Biochemical Societies Letters* **345**, 43–46.
Covey, D.F. (1988) In *Sterol Biosynthesis Inhibitors* (eds D. Berg and M. Plempel), Ellis Horwood, Chichester, pp. 534–571.
Denis, C.L., Kemp, B.E., Zoller, M.J. (1991) *Journal of Biological Chemistry* **266**, 17932–17935.
Dirick, L., Moll, T., Auer, H., Nasmyth, K. (1992) *Nature* **357**, 508–513.
Doroshow, J.H., Kaman, S.A., Chu, F.F., Esworthy, S. (1990) *Pharmacology and Therapeutics* **42**, 359–370.
Draetta, G. (1990) *Trends in Biochemical Sciences* **15**, 378–383.
Dutta, A., Ruppert, J.M., Aster, J.C., Winchester, E. (1993) *Nature* **365**, 79–82.
Emini, E.A., Graham, D.J., Gotlib, L., Condra, J.H., Byrnes, V.W., Schleif, W.A. (1993) *Nature* **364**, 679.
Evans I., McAthey, P. (1991) In *Genetically Engineered Proteins and Enzymes from Yeast: Production Control* (ed. A. Wiseman), Ellis Horwood, Chichester, pp. 11–74.
Ferguson, L.R., Sunberg, R.J. (1991) *Antimicrobial Agents and Chemotherapy* **35**, 2318–2321.
Franklin, T.J., Snow, G.A. (1989) *Biochemistry of Antimicrobial Action*, 4th edn, Chapman & Hall, London.
Freeman, R.S., Donoghue, D.J. (1991) *Biochemistry* **30**, 2293–2302.
Gille, G., Sigler, K., Hofer, M. (1993) *Journal of General Microbiology* **139**, 1627–1634.
Goodman, J.L., Winston, D.J., Greenfield, R.A., Chandraseka, P.H., Fox, B., Kaizer, H., Shadduck, R.K., Shea, T.C, Stiff, P. (1992) *New England Journal of Medicine* **326**, 845–851.
Greenspan, H.C., (1993) *Medical Hypothesis* **40**, 85–92.
Gross, E., Goldberg, D., Levitzki, A. (1992) *Nature* **360**, 762–764.
Guerin, B. (1991) In *The Yeasts* Vol. 4, 2nd edn (eds A.H. Rose and J.S. Harrison), Academic Press, London, pp. 541–600.
Gutteridge, J.M.C. (1993) *Free Radical Research Communications* **19**, 141–158.
Guzder S.M., Qiu, H., Sommers, C.H., Sung P., Prakash L., Prakash, S. (1994) *Nature* **367**, 91–94.
Halliwell, B. (1990) *Free Radical Research Communications* **9**, 1–32.
Halliwell, B., Gutteridge, J.M.C. (1989) *Free Radicals in Biology and Medicine,* 2nd edn, Oxford University Press, Oxford.
Halliwell, B., Gutteridge, J.M.C. (1990) *Archives of Biochemistry and Biophysics* **280**, 1–8.
Hardie, D.G. (1991) *Biochemical Messengers, Hormones Neurotransmitters, and Growth Factors*, Chapman & Hall, London.
Hartwell, L.H. (1992) *Cancer* **69**, 2615–2621.
Hawkins, J.D. (1991) *Gene Structure and Expression*, 2nd edn, Cambridge University Press, Cambridge.
Henschke, P.A., Rose, A.H. (1991) In *The Yeasts*, Vol. 4, 2nd edn (eds A.H. Rose and J.S. Harrison), Academic Press, London, pp. 297–345.
Herskowitz, I. (1992) *Nature* **357**, 190–191.
Jazwinski, S.M., Chen, J.B., Sun, J. (1993) *Advances in Experimental Medicine and Biology* **330**, 45–53.
Jones, A.L., Dowsett, M.J., Powles, T.J., Gallagher, C.J.,Coombes, R.C. (1991) *Eur. J. Cancer* **27**, 301.
Kashanchi, F., Piras, G., Radonovich, M.F., Duvall, J.F., Fattaey, A., Chiang, C.M., Roeder, R.G., Brady, J.N. (1994) *Nature* **367**, 295–298.
Kassavetic, G.A., Rigs, D.L., Negri, R., Nguyen, L.H., Geiduschek, E.P. (1989) *Molecular Cell Biology* **9**, 2551–2566.

Kelly, S.L., Rowe, J., Watson, P.F. (1991) *Biochemical Society Transactions* **19**, 796–798.
Kim, I.H., Kim, K., Rhee, S.G. (1989) *Proceedings of the National Academy of Sciences USA* **86**, 6018–6022.
King, D.J., Wiseman A. (1987) In *Enzyme Induction, Mutagen Activation and Carcinogen Testing in Yeast* (ed. A. Wiseman), Ellis Horwood, Chichester, pp. 115–157.
Kojima, S., Icho, T., Hayashi, M., Kajiwara, Y., Kitabatake, K., Kubota, K. (1993) *Journal of Pharmacology and Experimental Therapeutics* **266**, 1699–1704.
Korting, H.C., Blecher, P., Froschi, M., Braufalco, O. (1992) *Mycoses* **35**, 173–176.
Kupfer, D., Bulger, W.H. (1990) *Federation of European Biochemical Societies Letters* **261**, 59–62.
Kwoon S.J., Kim, K. Kim, I.H., Yoon, I.K., Park, J.W. (1993) *Biochemical and Biophysical Research Communications* **192**, 772–777.
Laughton, C.A., Niedle, S., Zuelebil, M.J.J.M., Sternberg, M.J.E. (1990) *Biochemical and Biophysical Research Communications* **171**, 1160–1167.
Laurence, J., Cook, H., Sikder, S.K. (1990) *Blood* **75**, 696–703.
Lee, J.C. (1991) In *The Yeasts*, Vol. 4, 2nd edn (eds A.H. Rose and J.S. Harrison), Academic Press, London, pp. 489–540.
Lewis, D.F.V., Rodrigues, A.D., Ioannides, C., Parke, D.V. (1989) *Journal of Biochemical Toxicology* **4**, 231–234.
Lim, Y.S., Kim, H.K., Uhm, T.B., Park, J.W., Kim, K., Kim, I.H. (1993) *Biochemical and Biophysical Research Communications* **192**, 273–280.
Lowndes, N.F., Johnson, A.L., Johnston, L.H. (1991) *Nature* **350**, 247–250.
Lowndes, N.F., Johnson, A.L., Breeden, L., Johnston, L.H. (1992) *Nature* **357**, 505–508.
Mager W.H., Ferreira, P.M. (1993) *Biochemical Journal* **290**, 1–13.
Mainwaring, W.I.P. (1991) In *Introdution to the Cellular and Molecular Biology of Cancer*, 2nd edn (eds L.M. Franks and N.M. Teich), Oxford University Press, Oxford, pp. 357–385.
Malloy, P.J., Zhao, X., Madani, N.D., Feldman, D. (1993) *Proceedings of the National Academy of Sciences USA* **90**, 1902–1906.
Malorni, W., Rivabene, R., Santini, M.T. and Donelli, G. (1993) *Federation of European Biochemical Societies Letters* **327**, 75–78.
Mani, C., Kupfer, D. (1991) *Cancer Research* **51**, 6052–6058.
Manser, E., Leung, T., Salihuddin, H., Zhao, Z.S., Lim, L. (1994) *Nature* **367**, 40–46.
McDonnell, D.P., Nawaz, Z., Densmore, C., Weigel, N.L., Pham, T.A., Clark, J.H., O'Malley, B.W. (1991) *Journal of Steroid Biochemistry and Molecular Biology* **39**, 291–298.
Metzger, D., White, J.H., Chambon, P. (1988) *Nature* **334**, 31–36.
Meunier, F. (1991) *Cancer Investigation* **9**, 151–158.
Mitchell, J.T., Allen, S.D., Jones, W.E. (1988) *Revista Iberica de Mycologia* **5**, 92.
Miyakawa, T., Oka, T., Tsuchiya, E., Fukui, S. (1989) *Journal of Bacteriology* **171**, 1417–1422.
Moll, T., Schwob, E., Koch, C., Moore, A., Auer, H., Nasmyth, K. (1993) *Philosophical Transactions of the Royal Society London—Series B; Biological Sciences* **340**, 351–360.
Moreno, S., Nurse, P. (1994) *Nature* **367**, 236–242.
Mori, K., Ma, W., Gething, M.J., Sambrook, J. (1993) *Cell* **74**, 743–756.
Motizuki, M., Tsurugi, K. (1992) *Biochemical and Biophysical Research Communications* **183**, 1191–1196.
Muhldorfer, S.M., Konig, H.J. (1990) *Mycoses* **33**, 291–296.

Muller, P.P., Trachsel, H. (1990) *European Journal of Biochemisty* **191**, 257–261.
Najid, A., Ratinaud, M.H. (1991) *Tumori* **77**, 385–390.
Nakajin, S., Takahashi, K., Shinoda, M. (1991) *Journal of Steroid Biochemistry and Molecular Biology* **38**, 95–99.
Nasmyth, K., Hunt, T. (1993) *Nature* **366**, 634–635.
Neer, E.J., Clapham, D.E. (1988) *Nature* **333**, 129–134.
Nes, W.D., Janssen, G.G., Crumley, F.G., Kalinowska, M., Akihisa, T. (1993) *Archives of Biochemistry and Biophysics* **300**, 724–746.
Newlon, C.S. (1989) In *The Yeasts*, Vol. 3, 2nd edn,, (eds A.H. Rose and J.S. Harrison), Academic Press, London, pp. 57–116.
Nightingale, S.D., Cal, S.Y., Peterson, D.M., Loss, S.D., Gamble, B.A., Watson, D.A., Manlone, C.P., Baker, J.E., Jockusch, J.D. (1992) *Acquired Immunodeficiency Syndrome* **6**, 191–194.
Odds, F.C. (1993) *Journal of Antimicrobial Chemotherapy* **31**, 463–472.
Ogita, K., Migamoto, S., Koide, H., Iwai, I., Oka, M., Ando, K., Kishimoto, H., Ikeda, K., Fukami, Y., Nishizuka, Y. (1990) *Proceedings of the National Academy of Sciences USA* **87**, 5011–5015.
O'Grady, J.F., Reade, P.C. (1992) *Carcinogenesis* **13**, 783–786.
Okorokov, L.A., Tanner, W., Lehle, L. (1993) *European Journal of Biochemistry* **216**, 573–577.
Oliver, S.G., Warmington, J.R. (1989) In *The Yeasts*, Vol. 3, 2nd edn (eds A.H. Rose and J.S. Harrison), Academic Press, London, pp. 117–160.
Pani, A., Marongiu, M.E., Lacolla, P. (1993) *Antiviral Research* **221**, 31–44.
Pardo, L.A., Lazo, P.S., Ramos, P.S. (1993) *Cellular Signalling* **5**, 435–441.
Park, H.O., Chant, J., Herskowitz, I. (1993) *Nature* **365**, 269–274.
Paule, M.R. (1990) *Nature* **344**, 819–820.
Pejin, D., Razmovski, R. (1993) *Folia Microbiologica* **38**, 141–146.
Pfaller, M., Wenzel, R. (1992) *European Journal of Clinical Microbiology and Infectious Diseases* **11**, 287–291.
Pietenpol, J.A., Vogelstein, B. (1993) *Nature* **365**, 17–18.
Polak, A. (1990) In *Chemotherapy of Fungal Diseases* (ed. J.F. Ryley), Springer-Verlag, Berlin, pp. 153–179.
Primig, M., Sockanathan, S., Auer, H., Nasmyth, K. (1992) *Nature* **358**, 593–597.
Quabeck, K., Muller, K.D., Beelen, D.W., Dermoumi, H., Kobel, M., Kraft, J., Ansorg, R., Schaefer, H.W. (1992) *Mycoses* **35**, 221–224.
Ratledge, C., Evans, C.T. (1989) In *The Yeasts*, Vol. 3, 2nd edn (eds A.H. Rose and J.S. Harrison), Academic Press, London, pp. 367–455.
Riedel, H., Hansen, H., Parissenti, A.M., Shieh, H.L., Zhu, J. (1993) *Journal of Cellular Biochemistry* **52**, 320–329.
Robinow, C.F., Johnson, B.F. (1991) In *The Yeasts*, Vol. 4, 2nd edn (eds A.H. Rose and J.S. Harrison), Academic Press, London, pp. 7–120.
Rose, A.H. (1989) In *Seventh International Symposium on Yeast*, John Wiley and Sons, Chichester, pp. 407–463.
Ruden, D.M., Junma, Y.L., Wood, K., Ptashne, M. (1991) *Nature* **350**, 250–252.
Saag, M.S., Cloud, G.A., Robinson, P., Meyer, R.D., Jacobson, J.M., Graybill, J.R., Sugar, A.M., Mcauliffe, V.J., Follansbee, S.E. (1992) *New England Journal of Medicine* **326**, 793–798.
Sakurai, H., Hiraoka, Y., Fukasawa, T. (1993) *Proceedings of the National Academy of Sciences USA* **90**, 8382–8386.
Scharer, E., Iggo, R. (1992) *Nucleic Acids Research* **20**, 1539–1547.
Siede, W., Friedberg, A.S., Friedberg, E.C. (1993) *Proceedings of the National Academy of Sciences USA* **90**, 7985–7989.

Sierkstra, L.N., Nouwen, N.P., Verbakel, J.M., Verrips, C.T. (1993) *Yeasts* **9**, 787–795.
Sharma, M.K., Buettner, G.R. (1993) *Free Radical Biology and Medicine* **14**, 649–653.
Staal, F.J., Roederer, M., Raju, P.A., Anderson, M.T., Ela, S.W., Herzenberg, L.A., Herzenberg, L.A. (1993) *AIDS Research and Human Retroviruses* **9**, 299–306.
Starovasnik, M.A., Davis, T.N., Klevit, R.E. (1993) *Biochemistry* **32**, 3261–3270.
Stewart, P.J., Stern, P.H. (1986) *Endocrinology* **118**, 125–131.
Strom, M., Vollmer, P., Tan, T.J., Gallwitz, D. (1993) *Nature* **361**, 736–739.
Sun, G.H., Ohya, Y., Anraku, Y. (1991) *Journal of Biological Chemistry* **266**, 7008–7015.
Swaffield, J.C., Bromberg, J.F., Johnston, S.A. (1992) *Nature* **357**, 698–700.
Tai, P.K., Chang, H., Albers, M.W., Schreiber, S.L., Toft, D.O., Faber, L.E. (1993) *Biochemistry* **32**, 8842–8847.
Tamai, K.T., Gralla, E.B., Ellerby, L.M., Valentine, J.S., Thiele, D.J. (1993) *Proceedings of the National Academy of Sciences USA* **90**, 8013–8017.
Tatsuka, M., Mitsui, H., Wada, M., Nagata, A., Nojima, H., Okayama, H. (1992) *Nature* **359**, 333–336.
Tuite, M.F. (1990) *The Biologist* **37**, 79–81.
Turner, M.J., Fields, C.E., Everman, D.B. (1991) *Biochemical Pharmacology* **41**, 1701–1705.
Uno, I., Fukam, K., Kato, H., Takenawa, T., Ishikawa, T. (1988) *Nature* **333**, 188–190.
Vanden Bossche, H. (1988) In *Sterol Biosynthesis Inhibitors* (eds D. Berg and M. Plempel), Ellis Horwood, Chichester, pp. 191–207.
Vanden Bossche, H., Willensens, G., Cools, W., Cornelissen, F., Lauwers, W.F., Cutsem, J.M. (1980) *Antimicrobial Agents and Chemotherapy* **17**, 922–928.
Vanden Bossche, H. Marichal, P., Gorrens, J., Geerts H., Janssen, P.A. (1988) *Annals of the New York Academy of Sciences* **544**, 191–207.
Vennin, P.H., Gougeon, E., Azab, M. (1992) *Lancet* **340**, 798.
Viviani, M.A. (1992) *Chemotherapy* **38**, 35–42.
Wilkie, D., Collier, D.C. (1987) In *Enzyme Induction, Mutagen Activation and Carcinogen Testing in Yeast*, (ed. A. Wiseman), Ellis Horwood, Chichester, pp. 12–40.
Williamson, D.H. (1991) In *The Yeasts* Vol. 4, 2nd edition (eds A.H. Rose and J.S. Harrison), Academic Press, London, pp. 433–488.
Wiseman, H. (1993) *Federation of European Biochemical Societies Letters* **326**, 285–288.
Wiseman, H. (1994a) *Trends in Pharmacological Sciences* **15**, 83–89.
Wiseman, H. (1994b) *Methods in Enzymology: Part D*, Volume 234, Chapter 61, 602–614.
Wiseman, H., Cannon, M., Arnstein, H.R.V. (1989) *Biochemical Society Transactions*, **17**, 1038–1039.
Wiseman, H., Cannon, M., Arnstein, H.R.V. (1990a) *Biochemical Society Transactions* **18** 557–558.
Wiseman, H., Cannon, M., Arnstein, H.R.V. (1990b) *Biochemical Society Transactions* **18**, 877–878.
Wiseman, H., Cannon, M., Arnstein, H.R.V. (1990c) *Biochemical Society Transactions* **18**, 1167–1168.
Wiseman, H., Cannon, M., Arnstein, H.R.V., Halliwell, B. (1990d) *Federation of European Biochemical Societies Letters* **274**, 107–110.
Wiseman, H., Smith, C., Arnstein, H.R.V., Halliwell, B., Cannon, M. (1991) *Chemico-Biological Interactions* **79**, 229–243.

Wiseman, H., Cannon, M., Arnstein, H.R.V., Barlow, D.J. (1992) *Biochimica et Biophysica Acta* **1138**, 197–202.
Wiseman, H., Cannon, M., Arnstein, H.R.V., Halliwell, B. (1993a) *Biochimica et Biophysica Acta* **1181**, 201–206.
Wiseman, H., Quinn, P., Halliwell, B. (1993b) *Federation of European Biochemical Societies Letters* **330**, 53–56.
Wiseman, H., Cannon, M., Arnstein H.R.V. (1994a) Submitted for publication.
Wiseman, H., Winkler, M., Wiseman A. (1994b) In *Handbook of Enzyme Biotechnology* (ed. A. Wiseman), Ellis Horwood, Chichester (in press).
Xiong, Y., Hannon, G.J., Zhang, H., Casso, D., Kobayashi, R., Beach, D. (1993) *Nature* **366**, 701–704.
Yeo, J.P., Alderuccio, F., Toh, B.H. (1994) *Nature* **367**, 288–291.

10

Tamoxifen: Brief Outline of Future Possibilities in Disease Control in Relation to Drug Design Strategies

PRESENT STATUS

Tamoxifen is used in the treatment of breast cancer and may be of use in the prevention of this disease. It is clear that tamoxifen is now recognised by most investigators to have beneficial effects on general health, such as protection against heart disease, bone wastage (oestrogenic effects) and osteoarthritis. It is of interest that a new derivative of tamoxifen has been designed for the treatment of prostatic cancer: future possibilities for improvement in specificity and efficacy are, therefore, now open to attempted prediction and assessment.

TAMOXIFEN: A SUMMARY OF ITS FUTURE?

Ongoing therapeutic use and the current prophylactic trials with tamoxifen should ensure further important basic research on this drug, and its designer derivatives. The molecular mechanisms of the development of clinically significant resistance of cancer to tamoxifen treatment are not clearly understood. This crucial problem is related to residual cancer cell growth, which may involve genetically controlled alterations in the cellular membrane, and changes therefore in associated transmembrane signalling events in the cell population during the course of prolonged treatment directed against the presenting tumour (Wiseman, 1994a).

The tamoxifen derivative droloxifene (3-hydroxytamoxifen) has several

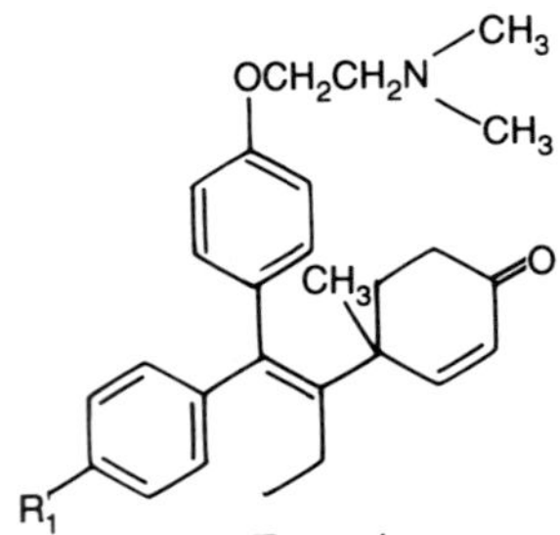

Tamandron

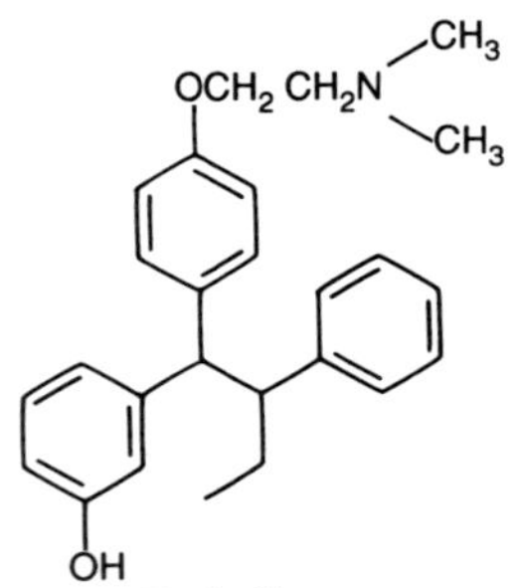

Droloxifene

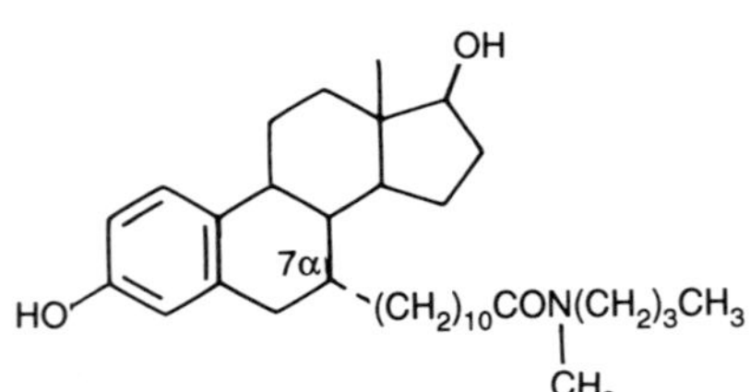

ICI 164, 384

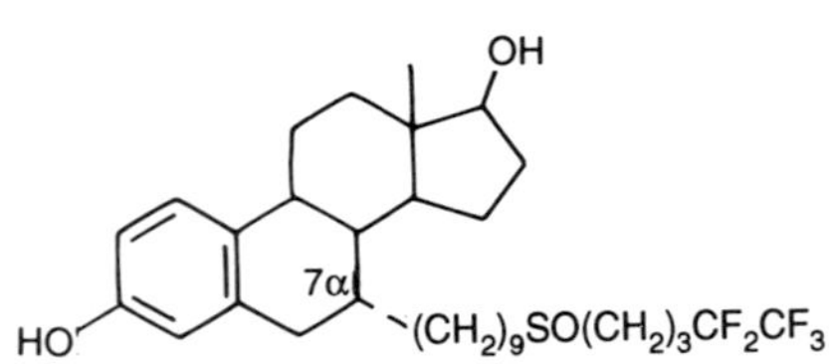

ICI 182,780

Figure 10.1. Structures of the tamoxifen derivatives tamandron and droloxifene, and the pure oestrogen antagonists ICI 164 384 and ICI 182 780

clinical advantages over tamoxifen: a shorter terminal elimination half-life, lower accumulation, improved drug tolerability and decreased risk of causing endometrial cancer. It is currently being used in a trial with women with advanced breast cancer. Another derivative of tamoxifen—tamandron (see Figure 10.1), for use in the treatment of cancer of the prostate—has now been synthesised (Potter and McCague, 1992) by altering one ring of tamoxifen so that it more closely mimics the steroid ring A of testosterone. In addition, a range of pure antioestrogens (tamoxifen is a partial oestrogen agonist), such as ICI 164 384 (see Figure 10.1)—a derivative of 17β-oestradiol—have been developed. ICI 164 384, a pure antagonist of oestrogen-simulated MCF-7 cell proliferation and invasiveness has been shown to inhibit the growth of an MCF-7 variant, dependent on tamoxifen for growth stimulation. It is of interest, therefore, that contrary to some suggestions that ICI 164 384 inhibits oestrogen receptor dimerisation and thus DNA binding, other studies have shown that this compound does not inhibit DNA binding of the oestrogen receptor *in vivo*, although it may reduce the affinity of the oestrogen receptor for its cognate response element. ICI 164 384 belongs to the same class of antihormones as tamoxifen (and 4-hydroxytamoxifen). Investigations are in progress with an oil depot formulation of ICI 182 780 (see Figure 10.1), a modified version of ICI 164 384 (these compounds display poor oral bioavailability) for use with breast cancer patients (De Friend *et al.*, 1994) including those who have suffered a relapse following the onset of resistance to therapy with tamoxifen (Wakeling, 1993).

It is important to appreciate that the cardioprotective plasma cholesterol-lowering action of tamoxifen arises from its partial oestrogen agonism action. Therefore, for pure antioestrogens used clinically antioxidant ability is likely to be crucial in achieving the full cardioprotection reported for tamoxifen, in which protection of low-density lipoproteins from oxidative damage may be the main contribution to the observed cardioprotection (Wiseman *et al.*, 1993; Wiseman 1994b). It is of interest, therefore, that ICI 164 384 was a good inhibitor of iron ion-dependent lipid peroxidation: in rat liver microsomes incubated with Fe(III)-ascorbate the overall order of effectiveness of the compounds tested as inhibitors of lipid peroxidation was 4-hydroxytamoxifen > 17β-oestradiol > tamoxifen > ICI 164 384; and in ox brain phospholipid liposomes incubated with Fe(III)-ascorbate the order was 4-hydroxytamoxifen > 17β-oestradiol > ICI 164 384 > tamoxifen (Wiseman, 1994c).

Cellular membranes should be viewed as important target sites for anticancer drugs, but this concept is remarkably under-developed. It is timely that this approach be extended through further studies on the antioxidant ability of tamoxifen (and redesigned derivatives) in cellular membranes arising from fluidity modulation (see Figure 10.2). This

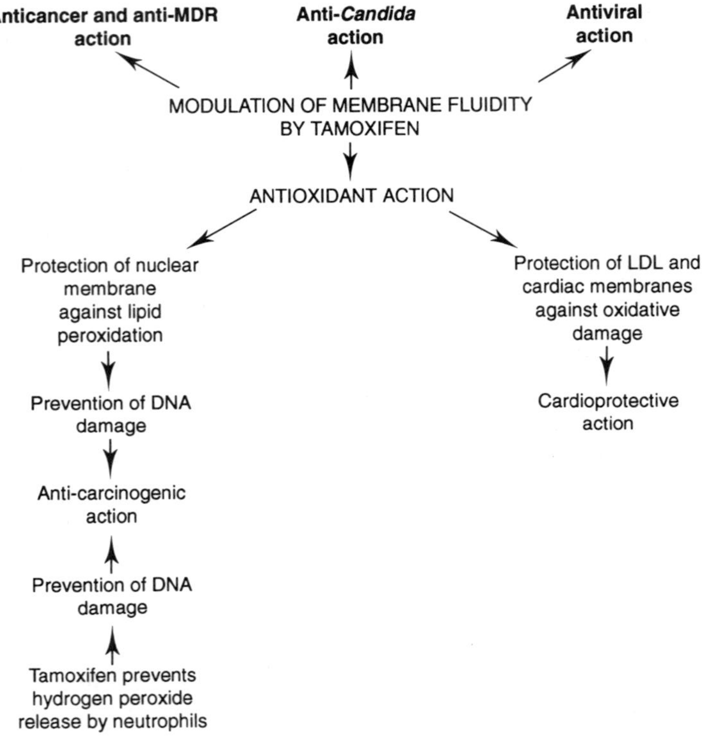

Figure 10.2. An overview of the membrane-mediated actions of tamoxifen

recognised mode of action of tamoxifen has important implications for its use in a variety of disease situations, because it provides an insight into the molecular basis of its clinical application. Such therapeutic application is already evident in the prevention and treatment of cancer and in the other beneficial health effects of tamoxifen, including its cardioprotectant action. Furthermore, potential for the use of tamoxifen in the prevention and treatment of some fungal and viral infections is now evident and this, along with indications of reversal of multidrug resistance (via inactivation of the P-170 glycoprotein), should ensure a continuing interest in tamoxifen and its derivatives. Considerable improvement of the therapeutic efficacy of tamoxifen and its derivatives, in particular to overcome the crucial problem of resistance due to a variety of molecular mechanisms, will no doubt emerge through molecular redesign strategies, using a combination of experimental approaches and computer-aided molecular modelling (Wiseman, 1994a).

REFERENCES

De Friend, D.J., Howell, A., Nicholson, R.I., Anderson, E., Dowsett, M., Mansel, R.E., Blamey, R.W., Bundred, N.J., Robertson, J.F., Saunders, C., Baum, M., Walton, P., Sutcliffe, F., Wakeling, A.E. (1994) *Cancer Research* **54**, 408–414.

Potter, G.A., McCague, R. (1992) *Journal of the Chemical Society of Chemical Communications* **8**, 635–637.

Wakeling, A.E. (1993) *Breast Cancer Research and Treatment* **25**, 1–10.

Wiseman, H. (1994a) *Trends in Pharmacological Sciences* **15**, 83–89.

Wiseman, H. (1994b) *Lancet* **343**, 598.

Wiseman, H. (1994c) *Biochemical Pharmacology* **47**, 493–498.

Wiseman, H., Paganga G., Rice-Evans, C., Halliwell, B. (1993) *Biochemical Journal* **292**, 635–638.

Index

Index compiled by Liza Weinkove